RENAL FAILURE – THE FACTS

Edited by **Momir Polenakovic**

Renal Failure – The Facts
Edited by Momir Polenakovic

Published by InTech
Janeza Trdine 9, 51000 Rijeka, Croatia

Publishing Process Manager Maja Bozicevic

Technical Editor Teodora Smiljanic

Cover Designer InTech Design Team

Additional hard copies can be obtained from orders@intechopen.com

Renal Failure – The Facts, Edited by Momir Polenakovic
p. cm.
ISBN 978-953-51-0630-2

For EU product safety concerns:
IN TECH d.o.o., Prolaz Marije Krucifikse Kozulić 3, 51000 Rijeka, Croatia,
info@intechopen.com or visit our website at intechopen.com.

Meet the editor

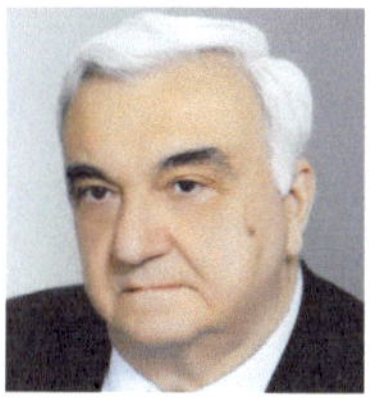

Professor Polenakovic is a Professor of Medicine – Nephrology. He is an outstanding researcher, educator and scientist, one of the founders of the nephrology in the Republic of Macedonia. He was a President - Macedonian Medical Association, President - Macedonian Society of Nephrology, Dialysis, Transplantation and Artificial Organs, Founder of the BANTAO Association (Balkan Cities Association of Nephrology, Dialysis, Transplantation and Artificial Organs). He has shown interest in the field of Glomerulonephritis, Tubulointerstitial Disease, ADPKD, Chronic Renal Failure, Artificial Organs (Kidney), Dialysis, Apheresis, Diabetic Nephropathy. He has published 480 papers on the subject of his work, out of which 157 are on Pub Med, as well as several chapters and books devoted to nephrology. He is an Editor in Chief of the journal "Prilozi" of the Macedonian Academy of Sciences and Arts (MASA). Head - Research Centre for Genetic Engineering and Biotechnology, MASA.

Contents

Preface

The book *Renal Failure – The Facts* consists of some facts about diagnosis, etiopathogenis and treatment of acute and chronic renal failure. Acute, as well as chronic renal failure is great medical problems and their treatment is a burden for the budget of each government.

Acute kidney injury (AKI), previously termed acute renal failure, is a frequent clinical condition in critically ill patients especially, in intensive care units (ICU). Its incidence varies from 1-7 % of all hospitalized patients to 30-50 % of patients in ICU. Irrespective of the progress being made in the understanding of the pathophysiology of AKI and its underlying processes and the advances in critical care medicine, mortality rate associated with AKI remains high especially in ICU patients at more than 50 %. In addition, a significant proportion of surviving patients (20 %) develops CKD and end-stage renal disease, requiring chronic renal replacement therapy. Long-term outcome is worse for patients after recovery from AKI, further impacting health care cost and quality of life. In developing countries, AKI is more common in young and pediatric patients, while in developed countries elderly patients are predominant. In critically ill patients the most common cause of AKI is sepsis, accounting for 50 % of all cases.

Chronic kidney disease (CKD) is a long-term condition which can arise from the damage to the kidneys from a variety of diseases. Patients with CKD are frequently asymptomatic until the disease is advanced. In 2002 the K/DOQI Clinical Practice Guidelines provided a definition of CKD which is now widely used around the world. Generally, cross-sectional population studies in a number of countries suggests an overall prevalence of CKD 1-5 of >10%. CKD appears to be an independent and significant risk factor for progressive cardio vascular disease (CVD). CVD accounts for ≈ 50% of the death in patients with CKD.

The purpose of the chapters is to present some important issues of diagnosis and causes of AKI, as well as caused by snakes and arthropods, after cardiac surgery, as well as some therapeutic achievements in AKI. Well presented are the psychological condition in patients on haemodialysis, as well as the treatment of diabetic uremics.

The book is aimed at clinicians with a special interest in nephrology (including consultants and specialist trainees in nephrology), but it should also prove to be a valuable resource for any generalists who encounter a nephrological problems in their day-to-day practice.

Momir H. Polenakovic
Macedonian Academy of Sciences and Arts
Republic of Macedonia

1

Risk Factors for Renal Failure: From Infancy to Adulthood

Silvio Maringhini*, Vitalba Azzolina, Rosa Cusumano and Ciro Corrado
Pediatric Nephrology Unit. U.O.C. Nefrologia Pediatrica, Ospedale dei Bambini "G. Di Cristina" A.R.N.A.S. "Civico, Di Cristina e Benfratelli", Palermo Italy

1. Introduction

Abnormal development of the kidneys and the urinary tract, genetic factors, acquired disease during infancy and childhood, wrong dietary habits and environmental factors may produce renal damage and cause renal insufficiency which may become clinically evident in adulthood. Prevention of renal insufficiency relies on early recognition of risk factors recognizable in childhood.

2. Risk factors for kidney disease

The incidence and progression of renal injury vary substantially among individuals who are at risk for kidney disease. Variability of risk for the occurrence and progression of Chronic Kidney Disease (CKD) suggests that biologically relevant characteristics may influence the occurrence or course of the renal disease. Prediction of increased risk of occurrence or progression of CKD may enable clinicians to identify individuals who may benefit from closer supervision of care or more intensive disease modifying interventions. Risk factors can be used to define at risk population that can be targeted for education and early intervention programs. These factors include familiarity of CKD, genetic factors, nephron number, low birth weight, perinatal programming, nutritional setting, hypertension and congenital abnormalities of the kidney and urinary tract (CAKUT) (Table 1).

Risk factors for Chronic Kidney Disease detectable in childhood
Family history of hypertension and kidney disease
Low birth weight
Perinatal kidney injury
Congenital injury
Hematuria and/or proteinuria
Urinary tract infection
High blood pressure
Overweight

Table 1.

*Corresponding Author

2.1 Familiarity of CKD

A family history of kidney disease (FAM) has been associated with an increased risk of end stage renal disease (ESRD). In a recent report FAM was identified as an independent risk factor for ESRD **[1]**. In 1998 Lei at al in large population case-control study found a correlation between FAM and ESRD, especially in patients with a strong FAM with an odds ratio of 7.4.**[2]**. In the same year Freedman et al. found a high prevalence (20%) of FAM in dialysis patients. The prevalence decreased with age, was higher among African-Americans than Caucasians **[3]**. Satko et al documented a three- to nine-fold greater risk of ESRD in individuals with a FAM of ESRD. He noted a marked racial variation in the familial aggregation of kidney disease, with high rates in African American **[4]**. Other authors documented a stronger association in blacks than whites, indicating specific ethnic differences **[5-6]**. Recently in USA it has been proposed the ESRD Networks Family History Project as a national CKD surveillance system for patients with stage 5 CKD to identify relatives of incident patients with ESRD who are 2 to 3 times as likely to have ESRD **[7]**.

2.2 Genetic factors

It is well known that genetic factors play a crucial role in CKD and ESRD [8] More recently, genome-wide association studies have yielded highly promising results suggesting a number of potential candidate genes and genomic regions that may contribute to the pathogenesis of CKD **[8]**. For example, common variants in the UMOD and PRKAG2 genes are associated with risk of chronic kidney disease **[9]**. Genome-wide association studies of CKD are beginning to define the genomic architecture of kidney disease and will impact our understanding of how genetic variation influences susceptibility to this condition.

The expression of genes is defined by their epigenetic state; prenatal factors may produce stable changes in expression of genes as documented in several studies. DNA methylation [10], oxidative stress in response to low protein diet in pregnancy [11], telomere length [12] which is regulated by telomerase enzymatic activity during fetal life have been implicated in fetal renal development and disesase, excess glucocorticoids in early life can permanently alter tissue glucocorticoid signalling. All these studies show that the mechanism involved in developmental programming are likely epigenetic rather than due to DNA sequence mutations. It is important to note that changes produced by epigenetic factors, differently from genetic changes, are potentially reversible.

2.3 Nephron number

The number of nephrons in humans ranges from 250.000 to 2.5 million with an average of about 1 million per kidney; this high variability is due to various causes. Nephrogenesis ends at 36 weeks of gestation, for this reason premature newborns may have a reduced nephron number; the same condition is observed in patients with kidney disease and in older patients due to age-related glomerulosclerosis. In the last 20 years many authors analyzed the association between nephron number and onset of renal disease later in life; most of these studies have been conducted in animals since it is difficult to determinate the number of glomeruli as measure of nephrons' number in humans. Nyengaard and Bendtsen performed in 1992 the first study that calculated the number of glomeruli in the kidneys of 37 Danes obtained at autopsy; they found a significant negative correlation between glomerular number and age **[13]**. Successively Keller et al. documented a significant reduced number of glomeruli in patients with hypertension compared to those who were normotensive **[14]**. More recently Zhang et al have documented a wide 4.5-fold variability in the number of glomeruli in children younger than 3 months ranging from 246,181 to 1,106,062 **[15]**.

2.4 Prematurity and low birth weight

Low birth weight (LBW) is defined by the World Health Organization as a birth weight of <2500 g. Intrauterine growth retardation (IUGR) is defined as weight below the tenth decile for birth weight.

Fetal growth is conditioned by multiple factors which include the composition of maternal body, alimentary habits during pregnancy, transport of nutrients through the placenta and others. The final consequence of the alteration of this factors determinate a fetal-growth reduction. The IUGR can be related to maternal undernutrition and/or placental insufficiency **[16]**. Placental insufficiency, usually associated with preeclampsia and maternal cardiovascular risk factors, is due to poor placentation. Maternal malnutrition is often related to wromg dietaty composition more than total calorie intake. In rats Langley-Evans et al have demonstrated that even short periods of maternal protein restriction during gestation in rats are associated with LBW and subsequent hypertension **[17]**. In humans, increased protein turnover at 18 weeks of gestation is associated with increased length of babies at birth [18**]**.

In humans, the causes of LBW are multifactorial: demographic factors, socio-economics status, poor maternal weight especially during pregnancy, shorter maternal height, maternal gestational weight gain below 7 kg, maternal hypertension, chronic infections, glucose intolerance or DM during pregnancy, maternal smoking or alcohol abuse, genetics, etc. Irving et al demonstrated that premature children, independently of birth weight, have an high risk of cardiovascular disease in adult age, thus making it very difficult to separate the effects of gestational age and birth weight **[19]**. However, the growth retardation for a given gestational age has greater relevance than the effect of prematurity on subsequent cardiovascular disease in adult age, as was demonstrated by Whincup et al **[20]**. The correlation between low birth weight and number of nephrons was reported by Ma˜ nalich et al.; they observed a mean reduction of 20% of the nephrons in children with LBW. **[21]**. The same observations was obtained by Hughson et al who documented that LBW is accompanied by fewer large-volume nephrons than in individuals with normal birth weights **[22]**.

Multiple animal models have demonstrated the association of LBW with later development of hypertension. The link between adult hypertension and LBW in these animal models appears to be mediated by a congenital nephron deficit showed by Vehaskari et al **[23]**. In humans many studies have reported higher blood pressures in those who had been of LBW. Barker et al first reported the association between hypertension in adult life and birth weight **[24]**. A study in Swedish children by Nilsson et al found a significant relation between birth weight and systolic arterial pressure **[25]**. Similar observations was done by Huxley et al **[26]**. In several studies, the relationship was more significant in girls than boys **[27]** and in woman than man **[28]**. The relationship between birth weight and blood pressure is also increased by accelerated postnatal growth **[29]** . Hoy et al in 1999 reported an association between low birth weight and CKD, observing increased rates of microalbuminuria in Australian Aborigines, a population with high rates of low birth weight **[30]**. In the last years many studies have documented that low birth weights contribute to high rates of early-onset chronic renal failure in United States patients, in ducth adolescents, and in young and adult Norwegians **[31-34]**. In a meta-analysis, White et al. found that the combined odds ratio (OR) for risk of albuminuria associated with low birth weight was 1.81 (1.19–2.77) and for ESRD 1.58 (1.33-1.88). They concluded that existing data indicate that low birth weight is associated with subsequent risk of CKD **[35]**. Recently, Hodgin et al. described an association between focal segmental glomerular sclerosis (FSGS) and prematurity and very low birth weight **[36]**.

2.5 Perinatal programming

The processes of development and maturation of organs occur continuously throughout the pre- and postnatal periods. Intrauterine growth is generally regulated by intrinsic growth potential, genetic endowment, and support of nutrients from the materno-uteroplacental unit. However, during the postnatal period growth may be affected by environmental conditions and genetic background. The environmental impact on a genetic program determine the renal perinatal programming of each individual. The term "fetal programming" describes the structural and functional adaptive phenomena in response to critical periods during fetal life and early postnatal growth. Perinatal programming may produce a reduced nephron number leading to the development of chronic kidney disease **[37]**. Several environmental stressors may act on specific genetic programming of low nephron number. The time at which an adverse factor is involved during gestation before completion of nephrogenesis may affect kidney growth **[38]**. A history of LBW and IUGR, vitamin A deficiency, urinary tract malformations, administration of nephrotoxic drugs may interact to increase potential nephron damage. Maternal nutrition may have an important influence on renal programming **[39]**. In rats, a restricted supply of nutrients to the mother during nephrogenesis contributed to a reduced number of glomeruli per kidney, activation of the renin-angiotensin system, glomerular enlargement, and hypertension in adult life **[40]**.

2.6 Hypertension

Maternal hypertension is a significant risk factor for LBW and is more prevalent among black than white women, making the population-attributable risk of LBW highest among babies of hypertensive black mothers **[41]**. Taittonen et al found that a history of mother's high blood pressure during pregnancy predicted future blood pressure more eminently than birth weight **[42]**.

Hypertension is one of the major causes of renal insufficiency in adults. It has been proven that children with higher blood pressure develop hypertension, cardiovascular diseases and renal failure as adults. The first study that found a correlation of adult blood pressure with childhood blood pressure was the Muscatine study in 1989 **[43]**. Successively the Bogalusa Heart study documented that childhood blood pressure predicts adult microalbuminuria in African Americans, but not in whites **[44]**. In the same group of patients it was found that diastolic blood pressure in children and increased blood pressure variability in children are significantly correlated with adult hypertension **[45-47]**.

2.7 Obesity

Obesity is a recognized risk factor for end-stage renal disease (ESRD) [48]. The increased blood pressure associated with obesity is accompanied by impaired pressure natriuresis.

The volume expansion is related to activation of the sympathetic nervous system and renin-angiotensin system. Obesity also causes renal vasodilation and glomerular hyperfiltration as compensatory mechanisms. In the long-term, these changes, along with the increased systemic arterial pressure, causes glomerular injury. Moreover obesity causes an increase of urinary protein excretion and gradual loss of nephron function that worsens with time and exacerbates hypertension. Overweight and obesity are associated with the metabolic syndrome and type II diabetes, a major cause of kidney disease; in obese patients renal failure progresses much more rapidly [49].

2.8 CAKUT

Congenital abnormalities of the kidney and urinary tract in most cases apparently are not associated with a reduced glomerular filtration rate (GFR) but the renal reserve may be reduced to the point that an increased demand by a growing body produces a drop in GFR. A recent review of Sanna-Cherchi et al evaluated the renal outcome in patients with CAKUT [50]. They found that patients with solitar kidney, usually considered to have good prognosis, have a higher risk for dialysis with an HR of 2.43 compared to patients with hypodysplasia or multicystic kidney. These data are in contrast to precedent studies that found a good prognosis of renal function in patients with unilateral agenesis [51]. In the last years many authors have looked for a correlation of CAKUT with genetic disorders [52].

2.9 Hematuria and proteinuria

Iseki et al in 1996 in a community mass screening found that proteinuria was the most useful predictor of ESRD (adjusted odds ratio 14.9, 95% confidence interval 10.9 to 20.2), and the next most potent predictor was hematuria (adjusted odds ratio 2.30, 95% confidence interval 1.62 to 3.28) [53]. In a recent paper Vivante A et Al found an increase of incidence of ESRD in patients (aged 16 to 25 year) with persistent asymptomatic isolated microscopic hematuria [54]. In 2011 a meta-analysis found that albuminuria is a risk factor for all-cause and cardiovascular mortality in high-risk populations [55].

2.10 Urinary tract infections and vesico-ureteral reflux

Vesicoureteral reflux (VUR) is a frequent condition in pediatric patients. Approximately 1/3 of patients who have had a urinary tract infection (UTI) have VUR and 9-20% of patients with prenatal hydronephrosis have VUR [56]. Children affected by VUR may develop reflux nephropathy (RN) and some of them chronic kidney disease (CKD). In a recent review Brakeman identifies the principal risk factors of progression of VUR to CKD: reduced glomerular filtration rate (GFR), bilateral VUR and/or renal scarring, grade V VUR, proteinuria, and hypertension. [57]. Ardissino et al found an estimated risk of end stage renal disease (ESRD) of 56% in italian children by age 20 years [58]

3. Evolution of renal damage

The pathogenesis of progressive renal functional deterioration is certainly multifactorial, and the decline in glomerular filtration rate varies in groups of patients with different nephropathies, but also in patients with the same disease. Some of these factors may be modifiable, particularly in children, and therapeutic interventions may result in a reduced rate of deterioration of renal function. The persistent deterioration of renal function may be a result of repeated and chronic insults to the renal parenchyma leading to permanent damage and/or to the adaptive hyperfiltration response of the kidney. The reduced glomerular filtration area due to congenital or acquired nephron deficit, according with the Brenner's hypothesis of "glomerular hyperfiltration", could expose to a higher risk of cardiovascular and renal disease in adulthood since the increased workload produces proteinuria with glomerulosclerosis, tubulointerstitial inflammation and fibrosis [59]. In addition to hyperfiltration and proteinuria, there is evidence that chronic renal hypoxia could be directly involved in the progression of CKD, particularly in progression of tubulointerstitial fibrosis. Chronic renal hypoxia could be elicited by several factors such as loss of peritubular capillaries (PTCs), decreased PTC flow, decreased nitric oxide production and/or bioavailability and activation of the renin-angiotensin system. With regard to this, Kang et al previously demonstrated that the inhibition of NOS accelerated renal damage in a remnant kidney model by eliciting PTC loss [60]. Recent evidence suggests that overweight and obesity play a role in renal-pressure natriuresis. Excessive weight gain increases renal tubular reabsorption and impairs pressure natriuresis, in part, through activation of the sympathetic and renin-angiotensin system as well as physical compression of the kidney. With prolonged obesity, there are also structural changes in the kidney (including enlargement of Bowman's space, increased glomerular cell proliferation, increased mesangial matrix, and thicker basement membranes, increased expression of glomerular transforming growth factor) that eventually cause loss of nephron function, further impairment of pressure natriuresis, and further increases in arterial pressure [61]. Finally, a number of genetic factors (eg, single nucleotide polymorphisms and modifier genes) may influence the immune response, inflammation, fibrosis, and atherosclerosis, possibly contributing to accelerated progression of CKD [62]. With respect to specific genes, apolipoprotein E (ApoE) polymorphisms may alter the risk of atherosclerotic disease, and therefore progression of CKD. The ApoE epsilon-2 allele is associated with elevated lipoprotein and triglyceride levels, whereas the ApoE epsilon-4 allele is associated with elevated levels of high density lipoprotein and lower triglycerides. In a secondary analysis of the Atherosclerosis Risk in Communities Study of 14,520 patients with a median follow-up of 14 years, individuals with an ApoE epsilon-4 allele (present in 30 percent) had a 15 percent reduction in risk of progression of CKD compared to individuals with ApoE epsilon-3 allele (present in 90 percent). The risk with the ApoE epsilon-2 allele was not significantly different compared with ApoE epsilon-3 [63]. Gene expression profiles within the kidney may help identify molecular prognostic factors in chronic renal disease. In the future, genetic testing and molecular analysis of renal biopsy specimens (and/or urine) may provide useful prognostic information.

The rate of progression to ESRD in childhood is inversely proportional to the baseline CrCl at presentation. In addition, genetic, familial, or ethnic predisposition may influence the rate of renal decline. As an example, African-Americans are more susceptible to CKD, and the rate of progression of CKD is higher among African-American males than other ethnic groups. The rate of progression of CKD is usually greatest during the two periods of rapid growth, infancy and puberty, when the sudden increase in body mass results in a rise in the filtration demands of the remaining nephrons [64]. Therefore children may have a normal glomerular filtration rate which sharply reduces in young adulthood. These events place increased demands upon the preexistent compromised kidney function. As a result, children with CKD should be closely monitored during these two periods for an accelerated progression of CKD. In addition to the increase in body mass, hormonal changes during puberty may also contribute to the rapid decline in renal function seen in adolescence.

4. Causes of renal injury and renal failure in children

Genetic and environmental factors are traditionally considered causes of human disease. Many genetic disorders may cause renal disease in childhood or in adults (Table 2) but also prenatal factors may produce stable changes in expression of genes. Studies from diverse populations suggest that fetal programming may be the origin of several intrauterine events that ultimately manifests as overt disease such as hypertension, type 2 diabetes, obesity, and chronic kidney disease (CKD) [65].

GENETIC KIDNEY DISEASE
Cystic disease
Polycistic Disease (ARPKD, ADPKD) Tuberous Sclerosis Von Hippel Lindau Syndrome Glomerulocystic Disease Medullary Cystic Disease (Nephronophthisis)
Glomerular Disease
Alport Syndrome Family Focal Glomerulosclerosis Congenital Nephrotic Syndrome Nail-Patella Syndrome Denys-Dash Syndrome
Tubular Disease
Dent Syndrome Distal tubular acidosis Lowe's syndrome Fanconi Syndrome Gitelman syndrome Bartter syndrome

Table 2.

In addition to prenatal conditions, adverse postnatal events must be taken in consideration: infections, drugs, trauma, systemic diseases etc. In fact, CKD in children, which has a much lower prevalence than in adults, is the result of a heterogeneous group of disorders (Figure 1). Congenital disease accounts for almost 60 percent of CKD cases and includes obstructive uropathy, renal hypoplasia, and renal dysplasia. Glomerular disorders are the second largest cause of childhood CKD and are present in 7 to 17 percent of children with CKD.

Glomerular disease is more common in children greater than 12 years of age. Focal segmental glomerulosclerosis (FSGS) is the most common glomerular disorder occurring in 9 percent of all CKD cases. Other causes account for approximately 25 percent of cases. In 18 percent of all cases of CKD, the underlying primary diagnosis is not identified (15 percent) or is unknown (3 percent). Other more uncommon causes of CKD in children include hemolytic-uremic syndrome, genetic disorders (eg, cystinosis, oxalosis, and hereditary nephritis), and interstitial nephritis.

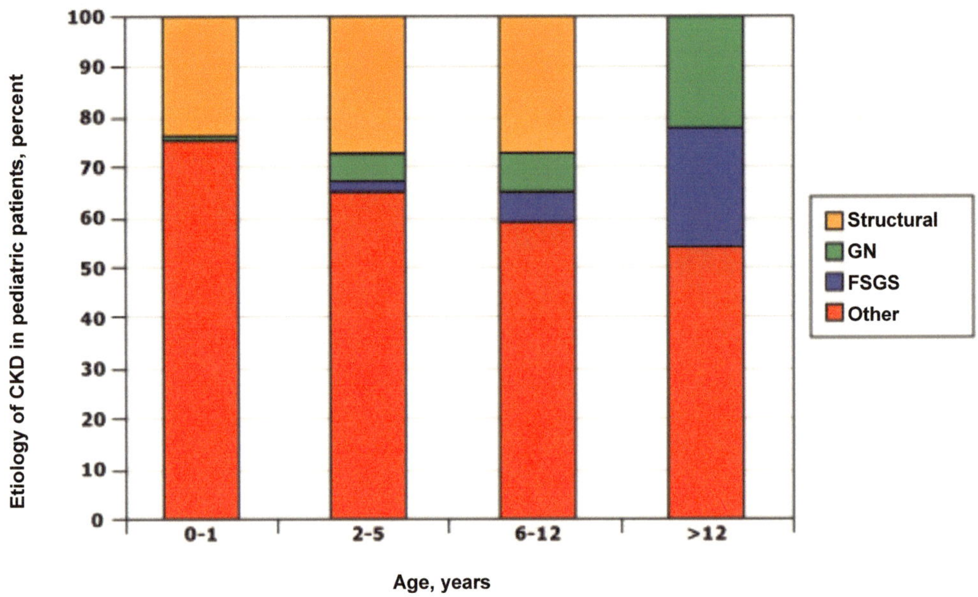

Fig. 1. FSGS: focal segmental glomerulosclerosis; GN: glomerulonephritis; Structural: structural anomalies of the kidney and urinary tract.
Adapted from: NAPRTCS: 2007 Annual Report, Rockville, MD, EMMES, 2007. Available at https://web.emmes.com/study/ped/announce.htm.

5. Prevention of renal diseases and kidney injury

Preventing renal impairment is an urgent challenge for medical practitioners. Several studies indicate that earlier stages of CKD can be detected through laboratory testing, and that early therapeutic interventions in the course of CKD are effective in slowing or preventing the progression toward ESRD and its associated complications [66]. Pediatricians and General Practioners should closely follow these infants, Health Care and Education providers should prioritize programs to stress the importance of preventive care and continuity of care especially for children of mothers with evidence of low propensity toward health promotion.

The NKF-K/DOQI guidelines for CKD, reviewed in Kidney Disease Improving Global Outcomes (KDIGO), recommend that all individuals should be assessed, as routine health examinations, to determine the increased risk for developing CKD. Patients who are at risk for developing CKD should be screened for hematuria with a urinalysis and with a urine test for proteinuria and a blood test for creatinine to estimate GFR. Depending upon the presence of particular risk factors, additional testing such as renal ultrasonography may be required, for example in patients with a family history of polycystic kidney disease. A formidable task for paediatricians is to prevent renal diseases that may develop in adult life. In order to achieve such goal, they should identify children at risk, counsel families to minimize any further renal risk factors such as smoking, obesity, and hypertension, and, in some cases together with a nephrologist, to institute pharmacologic therapy **[67].**

Strict blood pressure control has been shown to slow the progression of kidney disease and reduce the risk of cardiovascular disease. The National High Blood Pressure Education Program Working Group (NHBPEP) established guidelines for the definition of normal and elevated blood pressures (BP) in children by developing blood pressure percentiles based on gender, age, and height **[68].** Hypertension (HTN) is defined as either systolic and/or diastolic BP ≥95th percentile measured upon three or more occasions. Therapy includes both nonpharmacologic and pharmacologic interventions. Treatment should be initiated with conservative measures such as weight reduction, exercise, and dietary salt reduction. Pharmacologic therapy may be started in non responders; ACE inhibitors or angiotensin II receptor blockers (ARBs), that are the preferred antihypertensive agents as they reduce proteinuria and appear to be more beneficial in slowing the progression of CKD compared to other agents in patients with CKD [69-70].

Additional interventions that have been studied in adults with CKD include dietary protein restriction, lipid lowering therapy, and correction of anemia. However, results are inconclusive with respect to the impact of these interventions upon delaying the progression of CKD. In children, data have not shown a benefit of a low protein diet upon the progression of kidney disease CKD [71]. The current consensus by pediatric nephrology experts is to provide children with CKD the age appropriate recommended daily allowance for protein.

6. Treatment

The management of patients with CKD varies upon the severity of CKD. In the early stage it is important to treat reversible kidney dysfunction and prevent or slow the progression of kidney disease. In advanced stages (Stage 3 to 5) the management is focused on preventing and treating the complications of CKD, that include disorders of fluid and electrolytes, renal osteodystrophy, anemia, hypertension, dyslipidemia, growth impairment. The most common conditions with potentially recoverable kidney function are primarily due to decreased kidney perfusion or to the administration of nephrotoxic agents. Kidney hypoperfusion is produced by systemic hypotension, volume depletion from vomiting, diarrhea, diuretic use, or bleeding, and the administration of drugs that lower the kidney perfusion (such as nonsteroidal anti-inflammatory drugs, angiotensin converting enzyme [ACE] inhibitors, angiotensin II receptor blockers [ARBs]). Common nephrotoxic drugs include nonsteroidal anti-inflammatory agents, diagnostic agents (eg, radiographic contrast materials), and others (eg, aminoglycosides, amphotericin B, cyclosporine, and tacrolimus). The administration of such drugs, therefore, should be avoided or used with caution in patients with underlying CKD, with the assistance of therapeutic drug level monitoring. [72]

6.1 CKD complications

Major Problems in children with CKD
• Water and sodium retection • Hyperkalemia • Metabolic acidosis • Mineral metabolism and bone disease • Anemia • Nutrition • Growth

Table 3.

6.1.1 Water and sodium retention

It's present as GFR becomes severely decreased (ie, stages 4 and 5 disease), and it may result in volume overload. In general, a combination of dietary sodium restriction and diuretic therapy may correct the increased water balance. Dietary sodium intake should be decreased to 2 to 3 g/day and diuretic therapy includes loop diuretics such as furosemide given at a dose of 0.5 to 2 mg/kg per day [73].

6.1.2 Hyperkalemia

Hyperkalemia develops primarily because of inadequate potassium excretion due to a reduced GFR. Other factors that can contribute to elevated potassium levels include a high dietary potassium intake, metabolic acidosis, hypoaldosteronism (due in some cases to administration of an ACE inhibitor or an ARB), or an impaired cellular uptake of potassium. Management to prevent hyperkalemia in children with CKD consists in low potassium diet, administration of a loop diuretic (eg, furosemide) to increase urinary potassium loss, correction of acidosis with oral sodium bicarbonate [73].

6.1.3 Metabolic acidosis

Metabolic acidosis is characteristically present when the estimated GFR is less than 30 mL/min per 1.73 m2 (ie, stage 4 disease). Acidosis is associated with growth impairment because the body utilizes bone buffering to bind some of the excess hydrogen ions. Current guidelines by the K/DOQI working group are to maintain the serum bicarbonate level at or above 22 mEq/L . Sodium bicarbonate therapy is started at 1 to 2 mEq/kg per day in two to three divided doses, and the dose is titrated to the clinical target **[74].**

6.1.4 Mineral metabolism and bone disease

Alterations of mineral metabolism are an almost universal finding with progressive CKD due to abnormalities in the metabolism of calcium, phosphate, vitamin D, and parathyroid hormone (PTH) levels. If these abnormalities are not addressed, these changes result in kidney bone disease, referred to as renal osteodystrophy. The management and prevention of secondary hyperparathyroidism is complex and requires frequent monitoring and adjustment of therapy. The initial step is to correct phosphate retention by dietary restriction usually combined with either calcium-containing phosphate binders and/or sevelamer. The KDOQI guidelines recommend that treatment with calcitriol should be started when the serum 25-hydroxyvitamin D is <30 ng/mL (75 nmol/L), or when serum PTH is above the target range [75]. In adults, calcimimetics have been increasingly used to suppress PTH secretion and decrease the risk of hypercalcemia associated with calcitriol. These agents, which increase the sensitivity of the calcium-sensing receptor (CaSR) in the parathyroid gland to calcium, have not been adequately studied in the pediatric population.

6.1.5 Anemia

Anemia in CKD is due to reduced kidney erythropoietin production and generally develops when the GFR is below 30 mL/min per 1.73 m2. The treatment of anemia in children with CKD often includes iron supplementation and erythropoiesis stimulating agent (ESA). The K/DOQI guidelines recommend a target Hgb between 11 and 12 g/dL based upon consensus expert opinion. The initial ESA dose in older children not receiving dialysis is 80 to 120 u/kg per week, administered in two to three divided doses. Children younger than five years of age or children receiving dialysis frequently require higher doses (300 u/kg per week) [76-77].

6.1.6 Nutrition

Malnutrition is common in children with CKD because of poor appetite, decreased intestinal absorption of nutrients, and metabolic acidosis. Attention to nutrition is critical as it affects both the physical growth and neurocognitive development of children [78].

6.1.7 Growth

Growth failure has been long recognized in children with CKD. While the institution of recombinant human growth hormone (rHuGH) therapy can have a profound effect on the height velocity of children with CKD who are growing poorly, early recognition and management of malnutrition, renal osteodystrophy, acid-base abnormalities and electrolyte disturbances should take place prior to considering the institution of rHuGH. [79].

6.1.8 Renal replacement therapy

Once the estimated GFR declines to less than 30 mL/min per 1.73 m^2 (stage 4 CKD), it is time to start preparing the child and the family for renal replacement therapy. The family should be provided with information related to preemptive kidney transplantation, peritoneal dialysis, and hemodialysis. As in adults, some form of renal replacement therapy will generally be needed when the GFR falls below 15 mL/min per 1.73 m2 (stage 5 CKD). However, renal replacement therapy is often initiated before children reach these levels.

7. References

[1] Hsu C, Iribarren C, McCulloch C.E., Darbinian J, Go A. S.. Risk factors for end stage renal disease. Arch Intern Med 169 (4): 342-350, 2009

[2] Lei H.H, Perneger T.V., Klag M.J., Whelton P.K., Coresh J. Familial aggregation of renal disease in a population-based case-control study. JASN 9 1270-1276, 1998

[3] Freedman BI, Soucie M, McClellan W.M.: Family history of End-Stage Renal Disease among incident dialysis patients. J Am Soc Nephrol 8: 1942-1945, 1997.
[4] Satko SG, Freedman BI, Moossavi S. Genetic factors in end-stage renal disease. Kidney Int Suppl. Apr;(94):S46-9, 2005.
[5] Freedman BI, Spray BI, Tuttle AB, Buckalew VM Ir: The familial risk of end-stage renal disease in African Americans. Am J Kidney Dis 2 1: 387-393, 1993.
[6] Spray BI, Atassi NG, Tuttle AB, Freedman BI: Familial risk, age at onset, and cause of end-stage renal disease in white Americans.J Am Soc Nephrol 5: 1806-1 8 10, 1999.
[7] McClellan W.M., Satko SG, Gladstone E, Krisher JO, Narva AS, Freedman BI. Individuals with a family history of ESRD are a high-risk population for CKD: implications for targeted surveillance and interventions activities. Am J Kidney Dis 53 (Suppl 3) 100-106, 2009
[8] O'Seaghdha CM, Fox CS. Genetics of chronic kidney disease. Nephron Clin Pract.;118(1):55-63, 2011.
[9] Köttgen A. Genome-wide association studies in nephrology research. Am J Kidney Dis. 56(4):743-58), 2010.
[10] Dressler GR: Epigenetics, development, and the kidney. J Am Soc Nephrol; 19: 2060–2067, 2008
[11] Mohn A, Chiavaroli V, Cerruto M, et al. Increased oxidative stress in prepubertal children born small for gestational age. J Clin Endocrinol Metab; 92:1372–1378, 2007
[12] Nilsson PM, Lurbe E, Laurent S. The early life origins of vascular ageing and cardiovascular risk: the EVA syndrome. J Hypertens. 26(6):1049-57, 2008
[13] Nyengaard JR, Bendtsen TF Glomerular number and size in relation to age, kidney weight, and body surface in normal man. Anat Rec 232:194–201, 1992
[14] Keller G, Zimmer G, Mall G, Ritz E, Amann K. Nephron number in patients with primary hypertension. N Engl J Med 348:101–108, 2003.
[15] Zhang Z, Quinlan J, Hoy W, Hughson MD, Lemire M, Hudson T, Hueber PA, Benjamin A, Roy A, Pascuet E, Goodyer M, Raju C, Houghton F, Bertram J, Goodyer P. A common RET variant is associated with reduced newborn kidney size and function. J Am Soc Nephrol. 19(10):2027-34, 2008.
[16] Duggleby S, Jackson Aa: Relationship of maternal protein turnover and lean body mass during pregnancy and birth. Clin Sci 101:65–72, 2001
[17] Langley-Evans Sc, Phillips Gj, Benediktsson R, et al: Protein intake in pregnancy, placental glucocorticoid metabolism and the programming of hypertension in the rat. Placenta. 17:169–172, 1996.
[18] Henriksen T, Clausen T: The fetal origins hypothesis: Placental insufficiency and inheritance versus maternal malnutrition in well-nourished populations. Acta Obstet Gynecol Scand 81:112- 114, 2002.
[19] Irving J, Belton NR, Elton RA, et al: Adult cardiovascular risk factors in premature babies. Lancet 355:2135–2136, 2000.
[20] Whincup PH, Cook DG, Papacosta O: Do maternal and intrauterine risk factors influence blood pressure in childhood? Arch Dis Child 67:1423–1429, 1992.
[21] Ma˜ Nalich R, Reyes L, Herrera M, et al: Relationship between weight at birth and number and size of renal glomeruli in humans: A histomorphometric study. Kidney Int 58:770–773, 2000.

[22] Hughson M, Farris Ab Iii, Douglas-Denton R, et al: Glomerular number and size in autopsy kidneys: The relationship to birth weight. Kidney Int 63:2113-2122, 2003.
[23] Vehaskari Vm, Aviles Dh, Manning J: Prenatal programming of adult hypertension in the rat. Kidney Int 59:238-245, 2001
[24] Barker Dj, Osmond C: Low birth weight and hypertension. BMJ 297:134-135, 1988.
[25] Nilsson Pm, Ostergren Po, Nyberg P, et al: LBW is associated with elevated systolic blood pressure in adolescence: A prospective study of birth cohort of 149,378 Swedish boys. J Hypertens 15:1627-1631, 1997.
[26] Huxley Rr, Shiell Aw, Law Cm: The role of size at birth and postnatal catch-up growth in determining systolic blood pressure: A systematic review of the literature. J Hypertens 18:815-831, 2000.
[27] Whincup P, Cook D, Papacosta O, et al: Birth weight and blood pressure: Cross sectional and longitudinal relations in childhood. BMJ 311:773-776, 1995.
[28] Andersson Sw, Lapidus L, Niklasson A, et al: Blood pressure and hypertension in middle-aged women in relation to weight and length at birth: A follow-up study. J Hypertens 18:1753-1761, 2000.
[29] Huxley Rr, Shiell Aw, Law Cm: The role of size at birth and postnatal catch-up growth in determining systolic blood pressure: Asystematic review of the literature. J Hypertens 18:815-831, 2000.
[30] Hoy WE, Rees M, Kile E, Mathews JD, Wang Z. A new dimension to the Barker hypothesis: low birthweight and susceptibility to renal disease. Kidney Int 56:1072-1077. 1999.
[31] Lackland DT, Bendall HE, Osmond C, Egan BM, Barker DJ. Low birth weights contribute to high rates of early-onset chronic renal failure in the Southeastern United States. Arch Intern Med 160:1472-1476, 2000.
[32] Keijzer-Veen MG, Schrevel M, Finken MJ, Dekker FW, Nauta J, Hille ET, Frölich M, van der Heijden BJ, Dutch POPS-19 Collaborative Study Group. Microalbuminuria and lower glomerular filtration rate at young adult age in subjects born very premature and after intrauterine growth retardation. J Am Soc Nephrol 16:2762-2768, 2005.
[33] Hallan S, Euser AM, Irgens LM, Finken MJ, Holmen J, Dekker FW. Effect of intrauterine growth restriction on kidney function at young adult age: the Nord Trondelag Health (HUNT 2) Study. Am J Kidney Dis 51:10-20, 2008.
[34] Vikse BE, Irgens LM, Leivestad T, Hallan S, Iversen BM. Low birth weight increases risk for end-stage renal disease. J Am Soc Nephrol 19:151-157, 2008.
[35] White SL, Perkovic V, Cass A, Chang CL, Poulter NR, SpectorT, Haysom L, Craig JC, Salmi IA, Chadban SJ, Huxley RR. Is low birth weight an antecedent of CKD in later life? A systematic review of observational studies. Am J Kidney Dis 54:248-261, 2009.
[36] Hodgin JB, Rasoulpour M, Markowitz GS, D'Agati VD. Very low birth weight is a risk factor for secondary focal segmental glomerulosclerosis. Clin J Am Soc Nephrol 4:71-76, 2009.
[37] Ingelfinger JR: Disparities in renal endowment: causes and consequences. Adv Chronic Kidney Dis; 15: 107-114, 2008.
[38] Hotoura E, Argyropoulou M, Papadopoulou F, Giapros V, Drougia A, Nikolopoulos P, Andronikou S: Kidney development in the first year of life in small-for-gestational age preterm infants. Pediatr Radiol; 35:991-994, 2005.

[39] Barker DJ, Osmond C, Simmonds SJ, Wield GA: The relation of small head circumference and thinness at birth to death from cardiovascular disease in adult life. BMJ ; 306: 422–426. 1993.
[40] Woods LL, Ingelfinger JR, Nyengaard JR, Rasch R: Maternal protein restriction suppresses the newborn renin-angiotensin system and programs adult hypertension in rats. Pediatr Res; 49: 460–467, 2001.
[41] Fang J, Madhavan S, Alderman Mh: The influence of maternal hypertension on low birth weight: Differences among ethnic populations. Ethn Dis 9:369–376, 1999
[42] Taittonen L, Nuutinen M, Turtinen , Uhari M. Prenatal and postnatal factors in predicting later blood pressure among children: cardiovascular risk in young Finns. Pediatr. Res 40(4): 627-32, 1996
[43] Lauer RM, Clarke WR. Childhood risk factors for high adult blood pressure: the Muscatine Study. Pediatrics 84 (4): 633-41, 1989
[44] Hog S, Chen W, Srinivasan SR, Berenson GS. Childhood blood pressure predicts adult microalbuminuria in African Americans, but not in whites: the Bogalusa Heart Study. Am J. Hypertens 15 (12): 1036-41, 2002.
[45] Chen W, Srinivasan S. R., Ruan L, Mei H, Berenson G. Adult hypertension is associated with blood pressure variability in childhood in blacks and whites: the Bogalusa Heart Study. Am J. Hypertens 24(1): 77-82, 2011.
[46] Elkasabany AM, Urbina EM, Daniels SR, Berenson GS. Prediction of adult hypertension by K4 e K5 diastolic blood pressure in children: the Bogalusa Heart Study. J Pediatr 132 (4): 687-692, 1998.
[47] Bao W, Threefoot SA, Srinivasan SR, Berenson G.. Essential hypertension predicted by tracking of elevated blood pressure from childhood to adulthood: the Bogalusa Heart Study. Am J. Hypertens 8 (7): 657-65, 1995.
[48] Hall JE, Henegar JR, Dwyer TM, Liu J, Da Silva AA, Kuo JJ, Tallam L . Is obesity a major cause of chronic kidney disease? Adv Ren Replace Ther. Jan;11(1):41-54, 2004.
[49] Naumnik B, Myśliwiec M. Renal consequences of obesity. Med Sci Monit. 16 (8): 63-70, 2010.
[50] Sanna-Cherchi S, Ravani P, Corbani V, Parodi S, Haupt R, Piaggio G., Degli Innocenti M.L., Somenzi D, Trivelli A, Caridi G, Izzi C, Scolari F, Mattioli G, Allegri L, Ghiggeri G. M.. Renal outcome in patients with congenital anomalies of the kidney and urinary tract. Kidney Int (76): 528-533, 2009.
[51] Hedge S, Coulthard M. Renal agenesis and unilateral nephrectomy: what are the risks of living with a single kidney?. Pediatr Nephrol 24:439-446, 2009.
[52] Sanna-Cherchi S, Caridi G, Weng P. L., Scolari F, Perfumo F, Gharavi A. G., Ghiggeri G. M.. Genetic approaches to human renal agenesis/hypoplasia and dysplasia. Pediatr Nephrol 22: 1675-1684, 2007.
[53] Iseki K, Iseki C, Ikemiya Y, Fukiyama K. Risk of developing end-stage renal disease in a cohort of mass screening. Kidney Int. 49(3):800-5, 1996
[54] Vivante A. et Al. Persistent asymptomatic isolated microscopic hematuria in Israeli adolescents and young adults and risk for end-stage renal disease. JAMA. 17;306(7):729-36, 2011.
[55] Van Der Velde M et Al. Lower estimated glomerular filtration rate and higher albuminuria are associated with all-cause and cardiovascular mortality. A

collaborative meta-analysis of high-risk population cohorts. Kidney Int. 79(12):1341-52, 2011.
[56] Sargent M.A., "What is the normal prevalence of vesicoureteral reflux?" Pediatric Radiology, vol. 30, no. 9, pp. 587- 593, 2000.
[57] Brakeman P. Vesicoureteral Reflux, Reflux Nephropathy, and End-Stage Renal Disease. Advances in Urology, 50: 89. 5089-49, 2008.
[58] Ardissino G, Avolio L, Dacco V, Testa S, Marra G, Viganò S, Loi S, Caione P, De Castro R, De Pascale S, Marras E, Riccipetitoni G, Selvaggio G, Pedotti P, Claris-Appiani A, Ciofani A, Dello Strologo L, Lama G, Montini G, Verrina E; ItalKid Project. Long-term outcome of vesicoureteral reflux associated chronic renal failure in children. Data from the ItalKid Project. J Urol. 172(1):305-10, 2004
[59] Brenner BM, Garcia DL, Anderson S.. Glomeruli and blood pressure. Less of one, more the other?. Am J Hypertens 1:335-347, 1988
[60] Kriz W, LeHir M: Pathways to nephron loss starting from glomerular diseases - insights from animal models. Kidney Int 2005; 67: 404–419, 2005
[61] Hall J. E. The Kidney, Hypertension, and Obesity. Hypertension; 41;625-633, 2003.
[62] Nordfors L, Lindholm B, Stenvinkel P. End-stage renal disease--not an equal opportunity disease: the role of genetic polymorphisms. J Intern Med; 258:1-12, 2005
[63] Hsu CC, Kao WH, Coresh J, et al. Apolipoprotein E and progression of chronic kidney disease. JAMA; 293:2892-9, 2005
[64] Luyckx VA, Brenner BM: Low birth weight, nephron number, and kidney disease. Kidney Int Suppl: S68–S77, 2005
[65] Maringhini S, Corrado C, Maringhini G, Cusumano R, Azzolina V, Leone F. Early origin of adult renal disease. J Matern Fetal Neonatal Med Oct, 23 Suppl 3: 84-6. 2010.
[66] Pereira BJ. Optimization of pre-ESRD care: the key to improved dialysis outcomes Kidney Int. Jan;57(1):351-65. 2000
[67] Kidney Disease Outcomes Quality Initiative (K/DOQI). K/DOQI clinical practice guidelines on hypertension and antihypertensive agents in chronic kidney disease. Am J Kidney Dis ; 43:S1, 2004.
[68] The National High Blood Pressure Education Program Working Group (NHBPEP) guidelines. Pediatrics Oct;98. 649-58, 1996.
[69] Wühl E, Schaefer F. Therapeutic strategies to slow chronic kidney disease progression. Pediatr Nephrol; 23:705-16, 2008.
[70] ESCAPE Trial Group, Wühl E, Trivelli A, et al. Strict blood-pressure control and progression of renal failure in children. N Engl J Med 2009; 361:1639-50, 2009.
[71] Wingen AM, Fabian-Bach C, Schaefer F, Mehls O. Randomised multicentre study of a low-protein diet on the progression of chronic renal failure in children. European Study Group of Nutritional Treatment of Chronic Renal Failure in Childhood. Lancet; 349:1117. 1997).
[72] Andreev E, Koopman M, Arisz L SO. A rise in plasma creatinine that is not a sign of renal failure: which drugs can be responsible?J Intern Med (3) 246-247. 1999.
[73] Panel of Dietary Intakes for Electrolytes and Water, Standing Committee on the Scientific Evaluation of Dietary Reference Intakes, Food and Nutrition Board, Institute of Medicine. Dietary Reference Intakes for Water, Potassium, Sodium,

Chloride, and Sulfate. National Academic Press, Washington, DC 2004. Available at www.nap.edu/books/0309091691/html.

[74] National Kidney Foundation. K/DOQI clinical practice guidelines for nutrition in chronic renal failure: 2008 Update. Am J Kidney Dis; 53(Suppl 2):S1, 2009.

[75] National Kidney Foundation. K/DOQI clinical practice guidelines for bone metabolism and disease in children with chronic kidney disease. Am J Kidney Dis 2005; 46(Suppl1):S, 2005

[76] K/DOQI Clinical practice guidelines and clinical practice recommendations for anemia in chronic kidney disease. Am J Kidney Dis; 47(Suppl 3):S1, 2006.

[77] NKF-K/DOQI Clinical Practice Guidelines and Clinical practice recommendations for anemia in chronic kidney disease: 2007 update of hemoglobin target. Am J Kidney Dis; 50:474, 2007.

[78] National Kidney Foundation. K/DOQI clinical practice guidelines for nutrition in chronic renal failure: 2008 Update. Am J Kidney Dis; 53(Suppl 2):S1, 2009.

[79] Kidney Disease: Improving Global Outcomes (KDIGO) CKD-MBD Work Group. KDIGO clinical practice guideline for the diagnosis, evaluation, prevention, and treatment of Chronic Kidney Disease-Mineral and Bone Disorder (CKD-MBD). Kidney Int Suppl 2009.

2

The Pathogenesis of Acute Kidney Injury

Nicholas A. Barrett and Marlies Ostermann
Department of Critical Care,
Guy's and St Thomas' NHS Foundation Trust, London
UK

1. Introduction

Acute kidney injury (AKI) is common in critically ill patients affecting 20 - 60% of patients (Chertow, et al., 2005; de Mendonca, et al., 2000; Mehta, et al., 2005; Ostermann & Chang, 2008; Silvester, et al., 2001; Uchino, et al., 2005). The exact incidence varies depending on patient population, associated comorbid factors and criteria used to define AKI. Sepsis induced AKI accounts for approximately 50% of cases and AKI is commonly a manifestation of multiple organ dysfunction (Chertow, et al., 2005; de Mendonca, et al., 2000; Mehta, et al., 2005; Ostermann & Chang, 2008; Silvester, et al., 2001; Uchino, et al., 2005). Many patients with AKI have a mixed aetiology where the presence of sepsis, ischaemia and nephrotoxicity co-exist. Current management of AKI is supportive, ensuring adequate perfusion pressures, correction of fluid depletion, avoidance of nephrotoxins and when required institution of renal replacement therapy (RRT). Despite the widespread use of RRT in the intensive care unit (ICU), AKI is associated with an associated mortality risk of 40 – 90% depending on patient population (Chertow, et al., 2005; Ostermann & Chang, 2008; Silvester, et al., 2001). Furthermore, evidence has emerged that AKI survivors have an increased risk of chronic kidney disease, long-term dialysis, increased mortality and reduced quality of life (Johansen, et al., 2010; Lo, et al., 2009; Lopes, et al., 2010; Wald, et al., 2009). AKI is no longer viewed as a reversible bystander of critical illness but a significant contributor to short and long-term morbidity and mortality.

2. Renal physiology

2.1 Renal blood supply and oxygenation

The chief function of the kidneys (ie. filtration of plasma and formation of urine) dictates the renal flow to be much higher than necessary to meet the metabolic needs. The kidneys receive blood via the renal arteries which supply them with approximately 25% of cardiac output. The vascular supply of nephrons consists of glomerular afferent and efferent arterioles which branch into the peritubular arteries and vasa recta. Oxygen tensions in the kidney are low, decreasing from 70 mmHg in the cortex to 20 mmHg in the medulla. The unique microvasculature of the kidneys coupled with high oxygen demand from the tubular salt-water reabsorption make the kidneys, in particular the medulla highly sensitive to hypoxia (Brezis & Rosen, 1995; Evans, et al., 2008). As a result, the renal microcirculation is recognised as a key actor in the initiation and development of AKI.

Basal renal oxygen consumption is approximately 400mmol/min/100g. Due to the high renal blood flow, there is a low oxygen extraction (Valtin & Schafer, 1995). Energy dependent processes in the kidney are those related to basal cellular metabolism and those related to filtration and reabsorption of solutes. In conditions associated with decreased renal blood flow, there is a reduction in both glomerular filtration and tubular reabsorption followed by a reduction in oxygen consumption. This relationship holds until the threshold of approximately 150mL/min/100g blood flow at which point oxygen extraction increases. At a blood flow of approximately 75mL/min/100g tissue the capacity for increased oxygen extraction is exceeded and anaerobic metabolism and cellular ischaemia occur (Schlichtig, et al., 1991).

2.2 Renal energy utilisation

Aside from basal metabolic requirements the major energy dependent process in the kidney is the reabsorption of solute, especially sodium. From animal studies, it is well established that there is a linear relationship between the reabsorption of sodium and oxygen consumption within the kidney (Gullans & Mandel, 1992). The predominant method of ATP production within the kidney is oxidative metabolism. In the cortex, oxidative metabolism accounts for over 97% of ATP production whereas in the medulla, up to 33% of energy comes from glycolysis (Bernanke & Epstein, 1965). In the presence of renal cortical hypoxia, the predominant form of energy production changes to glycolysis, however, this can not sustain significant function of the renal cells above homeostasis (Gullans & Mandel, 1992).

3. Ischaemic Acute Kidney Injury

Ischaemic AKI can occur in several clinical settings ranging from hypotension due to fluid depletion, blood loss, sepsis or reduced cardiac output to the use of vasoactive drugs. Following a reduction in effective kidney perfusion, tubular cells are unable to maintain adequate intracellular ATP. This depletion of ATP leads to rapid disorganization of the cytoskeletal structure and disruption of tight intercellular junctions (Sharfuddin & Molitoris, 2011). in case of severe depletion, apoptosis or necrosis occur and cells die. All segments of the nephron can be affected during an ischaemic insult but the most commonly injured sites are the proximal and distal tubular cells. Sloughed tubular cells and cellular debris can obstruct the tubule lumen and ultimately cease glomerular filtration in that functional nephron.

A marked decrease in total kidney perfusion may cause global ischaemia, but more often, ischaemic injury occurs due to decreased regional perfusion without major change in global perfusion. Both ischaemia and sepsis can have profound effects on renal endothelial cells, resulting in microvascular dysregulation and continued ischaemia and further injury. Ischaemic injury results in endothelial cell activation, endothelial swelling, up-regulation of adhesion molecules and shedding of components of the glycocalyx. This, in combination with leucocyte activation, platelet aggregation, red cell trapping and activation of the coagulation pathway serve as the basis for vascular congestion of the microvasculature (Le Dorze, et al., 2009). In response, a range of inflammatory mediators are being released, including prostaglandins, endothelin and nitric oxide, that alter the balance of vasodilatation and constriction within the renal vasculature (Bonventre, 2004; Le Dorze, et al., 2009). Although the ultimate aim is to control intrarenal damage and to promote repair, these activated leucocytes and proinflammatory mediators are also thought to be responsible for distant effects in non-renal organs, in particular lungs, heart and brain (ie. principle of organ cross-talk).

4. Septic Acute Kidney Injury

Sepsis is a pathological state characterised by a systemic inflammatory response to infective agents. Septic shock is characterised by inadequate tissue perfusion and significant hypotension is usually present. There are a number of proposed mechanisms regarding the pathogenesis of septic AKI, including hypoperfusion at the systemic and/or microcirculatory level, apoptosis mediated by either the infective agents or cytokines released in response to infection as well as renal mitochondrial hibernation triggered by sepsis.

4.1 Histopathology

Our progress in understanding the pathogenesis of AKI in sepsis has been limited due to the paucity of histopathological studies performed in well-defined patient populations with sepsis. Results from studies have been inconsistent with varying reports of cellular necrosis, glomerular infiltration and microvascular thrombosis (Solez, et al., 1979).

Autopsy studies have similarly reported variable and inconsistent findings in sepsis-induced AKI including interstitial oedema, swelling of the tubular cells, tubular cell apoptosis and regeneration, as well as focal necrosis and micro-abscess formation (Lucas, 2007). Part of the difficulty with autopsy series is that autolysis of the kidney occurs rapidly after death which leads to difficulties in interpreting findings. In one study reporting on rapid autopsies (within 6 hours) of 20 patients who died from sepsis and multiple organ dysfunction, there was no evidence of cellular necrosis or apoptosis (Hotchkiss, et al., 1999). However, a more recent study of immediate (within 30 minutes) post-mortem renal histology in patients with septic shock demonstrated acute tubular lesions, glomerular leukocyte infiltration and tubular cell apoptosis which affected 2.9% of tubular cells (Lerolle, et al., 2010). In this study these patients had died in states of profound shock. Hypovolaemia and hyperlactataemia, suggestive of poor tissue perfusion correlated with the degree of histological change seen and it is not clear that the changes seen were due to shock and hypoperfusion or sepsis *per se*.

Animal models of sepsis-induced AKI exist and have also demonstrated inconsistent changes in renal histopathology (Heyman, et al., 2002; Rosen & Heyman, 2001). Furthermore, the microvasculature of the rat kidney is markedly different from that of humans (Rosen & Heyman, 2001) and none of the models adequately account for the resuscitation and supportive management seen in critically ill patients, making data difficult to extrapolate (Heyman, et al., 2002).

4.2 Haemodynamic changes

Experimental evidence for renal haemodynamic changes due to sepsis is inconsistent. Animal models variably demonstrate that with preserved systemic blood pressures there is either a reduction in renal blood flow causing decreased glomerular flow (Badr, et al., 1986; Kikeri, et al., 1986) or renovascular vasodilatation with a consequent increase in renal blood flow (Langenberg, et al., 2006; Ravikant & Lucas, 1977). In humans, techniques measuring renal blood flow using para-aminohippurate extraction and renal vein catheter thermodilution have demonstrated that renal blood flow is preserved in sepsis (Brenner, et al., 1990). A systematic review of human and animal trials found that the primary determinant of renal blood flow during sepsis was cardiac output and that even in the presence of preserved renal blood flow, there is a reduction in glomerular filtration and AKI continues to progress (Langenberg, et al., 2005). It remains unclear as to whether there is significant relative reduction in medullary blood flow in humans with sepsis but given that the renal medulla is normally exposed to relative hypoxia, it has been hypothesised that this may be exacerbated during sepsis leading to tubular cell dysfunction or death (Brezis & Rosen, 1995; Eckardt, et al., 2005). Sepsis also leads to damage of the endothelial glycocalyx which aggravates a breakdown of the vascular barrier and contributes to microcirculatory changes in septic AKI (Chappell, et al., 2009).

4.3 Apoptosis

Apoptosis has been demonstrated to occur in animal models of AKI (Bonegio & Lieberthal, 2002; Sharfuddin & Molitoris, 2011; Wan, et al., 2003). Apoptosis is thought to occur in response to a variety of insults including sepsis, ischaemia, inflammatory cytokines and bacterial lipo-polysaccharide. However, there is inconsistent evidence for the presence of significant apoptosis in kidneys from patients with sepsis at autopsy (Hotchkiss, et al., 1999; Lerolle, et al., 2010; Lucas, 2007). It remains uncertain that apoptosis, estimated at less than 3% in a recent study (Lerolle, et al., 2010), is occurring on a scale that would result in significant organ dysfunction and failure.

4.4 Bioenergetics

A recent hypothesis is that the organ dysfunction including AKI observed in sepsis is secondary to bioenergetic changes with mitochondrial down-regulation and hibernation (Singer, 2007a, 2007b; Singer, et al., 2004). There is some evidence that there is reversible mitochondrial dysfunction resulting in inadequate ATP generation and that this may underlie the organ dysfunction seen in sepsis (Singer, et al., 2004). Although not conclusively demonstrated in humans, there is evidence of decreased ATP and a reduction in activity of respiratory chain complexes associated with sepsis and septic shock (Brealey, et al., 2002).

4.5 Immune mechanisms

Another mechanism of renal failure associated with infection is that of immune-mediated glomerulonephritis (Naicker, et al., 2007). This occurs as a post-infectious condition and is usually related to streptococcal or viral diseases. The pathophysiological mechanism is immune-complex deposition leading to inflammation within the glomerulus and glomerulonephritis. Although well characterised following infection, there is no evidence that this mechanism is responsible for AKI associated with acute sepsis.

5. Repair of AKI

Renal tubular epithelial cells have high potential to regenerate after an ischaemic, septic or toxic insult. Minimally injured cells are repaired when blood flow is re-established. Viable cells proliferate and spread across denuded basement membrane and later regain their characteristics as tubular epithelial cells (Sharfuddin & Molitoris, 2011). There is evidence that progenitor cells, stem cells and mesenchymal stem cells have an important role in promoting tubular epithelial repair but also lead to chronic fibrosis. The benefit of infusions of mesenchymal cells to promote recovery of renal function in humans is currently under investigation (Humphreys & Bonventre, 2008). Endothelial cells have less regenerative capability. Decrease of peritubular capillary density has been observed several months after an episode of AKI (Basile, et al., 2001).

6. Conclusion

AKI is a common manifestation of multiple organ dysfunction observed in critically ill patients, especially in relation to sepsis and ischaemia. There is increasing evidence that independent of the exact aetiology, AKI should be regarded as an inflammatory condition with secondary effects on other organs. However, the exact underlying pathophysiology and pathology of human AKI remains incompletely understood.

7. References

Badr, K. F., Kelley, V. E., Rennke, H. G. & Brenner, B. M. (1986). Roles for thromboxane A2 and leukotrienes in endotoxin-induced acute renal failure. *Kidney International*, Vol. 30, No. pp. 474- 480.

Basile, D. P., Donohoe, D., Roethe, K. & Osborn, J. L. (2001). Renal ischemic injury results in permanent damage to peritubular capillaries and influences long-term function. *Am J Physiol Renal Physiol*, Vol. 281, No. 5, pp. F887-99.

Bernanke, D. & Epstein, F. A. (1965). Metabolism of the renal medulla. *Am J Physiol*, Vol. 208, No. pp. 541-545.

Bonegio, R. & Lieberthal, W. (2002). Role of apoptosis in the pathogenesis of acute renal failure. *Curr Opin Nephrol Hypertens*, Vol. 11, No. pp. 301–308.

Bonventre, J. V. (2004). Pathophysiology of ischemic acute renal failure. Inflammation, lung-kidney cross-talk, and biomarkers. *Contrib Nephrol*, Vol. 144, No. pp. 19-30.

Brealey, D., Brand, M. D. & Hargreaves, I. (2002). Association between mitochondrial dysfunction and severity and outcome of septic shock. *Lancet*, Vol. 360, No. pp. 219-223.

Brenner, M., Schaer, G. L., Mallory, D. L., Suffredini, A. F. & Parrillo, J. E. (1990). Detection of renal blood flow abnormalities in septic and critically ill patients using a newly designed indwelling thermodilution renal vein catheter. *Chest*, Vol. 98, No. 1, pp. 170-9.

Brezis, M. & Rosen, S. (1995). Hypoxia of the renal medulla: its implications for disease. *N Engl J Med*, Vol. 332, No. pp. 647–655.

Chappell, D., Westphal, M. & Jacob, M. (2009). The impact of the glycocalyx on microcirculatory oxygen distribution in critical illness. *Curr Opin Anaesthesiol*, Vol. 22, No. 2, pp. 155-162.

Chertow, G. M., Burdick, E., Honour, M., Bonventre, J. V. & Bates, D. W. (2005). Acute kidney injury, mortality, length of stand and costs in hospitalised patients. *J Am Soc Nephrol*, Vol. 16, No. pp. 3365-3370.

de Mendonca, A., Vincent, J. L., Suter, P. M., Moreno, R., Deardon, N. M., Antonelli, M., Takala, J., Sprung, C. & Cantraine, F. (2000). Acute renal failure in the ICU. Risk factors and outcome evaluated by the SOFA Score. *Intensive Care Medicine*, Vol. 26, No. 7, pp. 915–21.

Eckardt, K. U., Bernhardt, W. M., Weidemann, A., Warnecke, C., Rosenberger, C., Wiesener, M. S. & Willam, C. (2005). Role of hypoxia in the pathogenesis of renal disease. *Kidney Int*, Vol. 68, No. Suppl 99s, pp. S46-51.

Evans, R. G., Gardiner, B. S. & Smith, D. W. (2008). Intrarenal oxygenation: unique challenge and the biophysical basis of homeostasis. *Am J Physiol Renal Physiol*, Vol. 295, No. pp. F1259-F1270.

Gullans, S. R. & Mandel, L. J. (1992). Coupling of energy to transport in proximal and distal nephron. In: *The Kidney: Physiology and Pathophysiology*, Seldin, D. W. and Giebisch, G., pp, 1291-1337. Raven Press, New York.

Heyman, S. N., Lieberthal, W., Rogiers, P. & Bonventre, J. V. (2002). Animal models of acute tubular necrosis. *Current Opinion in Critical Care*, Vol. 8, No. pp. 526–534

Hotchkiss, R. S., Swanson, P. E., Freeman, B. D., Tinsley, K. W., Cobb, J. P., Matuschak, G. M., Buchman, T. G. & Karl, I. E. (1999). Apoptotic cell death in patients with sepsis, shock, and multiple organ dysfunction. *Crit Care Med*, Vol. 27, No. 7, pp. 1230-1251.

Humphreys, B. D. & Bonventre, J. V. (2008). Mesenchymal stem cells in acute kidney injury. *Annu Rev Med*, Vol. 59, No. pp. 311-325.

Johansen, K. L., Smith, M. W., Unruha, M. L., Siroka, A. M., O'Connor, T. Z. & Palevsky, P. M. (2010). Predictors of health utility among 60-day survivors of acute kidney injury in the Veterans Affairs/National Institutes of Health Acute Renal Failure Trial Network Study. *Clin J Am Soc Nephrol*, Vol. 5, No. 8, pp. 1366-1372.

Kikeri, D., Pennell, J. P., Hwang, K. H., Jacob, A. I., Richman, A. V. & Bourgoignie, J. J. (1986). Endotoxemic acute renal failure in awake rats. *Am J Physiol*, Vol. 250, No. 6 Pt 2, pp. F1098–F1106.

Langenberg, C., Bellomo, R., May, C., Wan, L., Egi, M. & Morgera, S. (2005). Renal blood flow in sepsis. *Crit Care*, Vol. 9, No. pp. R363-374.

Langenberg, C., Wan, L., Bagshaw, S. M., Egi, M., May, C. N. & Bellomo, R. (2006). Urinary biochemistry in experimental septic acute renal failure. *Nephrol Dial Transplant*, Vol. 21, No. pp. 3389-97.

Le Dorze, M., Legrand, M., Payen, D. & Ince, C. (2009). The role of the microcirculation in acute kidney injury. *Curr Opin Crit Care*, Vol. 15, No. 6, pp. 503-8.

Lerolle, N., Nochy, D., Guerot, E., Bruneval, P., Fagon, J., Diehl, J. & Hill, G. (2010). Histopathology of septic shock induced acute kidney injury: apoptosis and leukocytic infiltration. *Intensive Care Med*, Vol. 36, No. pp. 471-478.

Lo, L. J., Go, A. S. & Chertow, G. M. (2009). Dialysis requiring acute renal failure increases the risk of progressive chronic kidney disease. *Kidney Int*, Vol. 76, No. pp. 893-899.

Lopes, J., Fernandes, P., Jorge, S., Resina, C., Santos, C., Pereira, A., Neves, J., Antunes, F. & Gomes da Costa, A. (2010). Long-term risk of mortality after acute kidney injury in patients with sepsis: a contemporary analysis. . *BMC Nephrol*, Vol. 11, No. 9, pp.

Lucas, S. (2007). The autopsy pathology of sepsis-related death. *Current Diagnostic Pathology*, Vol. 13, No. pp. 375–388.

Mehta, R. L., Pascual, M. T. & Soroko, S. (2005). Spectrum of acute renal failure in the intensive care unit: The PICARD experience. *Kidney Int*, Vol. 66, No. 4, pp. 1613-1621.

Naicker, S., Fabian, J., Naidoo, S., Wadee, S., Paget, G. & Goetsch, S. (2007). Infection and glomerulonephritis. *Seminars in Immunopathology*, Vol. 29, No. 4, pp. 397-414.

Ostermann, M. & Chang, R. W. (2008). Correlation between the AKI classification and outcome. *Crit Care*, Vol. 12, No. 6, pp. R144.

Ravikant, T. & Lucas, T. E. (1977). Renal blood flow distribution in septic hyperdynamic pigs. *J Surg Res* Vol. 22, No. pp. 294–298.

Rosen, S. & Heyman, S. N. (2001). Difficulties in understanding human "acute tubular necrosis": Limited data and flawed animal models *Kidney International* Vol. 60, No. pp. 1220–1224.

Schlichtig, R., Kramer, D. J., Boston, J. R. & Pinsky, M. R. (1991). Renal O2 consumption during progressive haemorrhage. *J Appl Physiol*, Vol. 70, No. 5, pp. 1757-62.

Sharfuddin, A. A. & Molitoris, B. (2011). Pathophysiology of ischemic acute kidney injury. *Nat Rev Nephrol*, Vol. 7, No. 4, pp. 189-200.

Silvester, W., Bellomo, R. & Cole, L. (2001). Epidemiology, management, and outcome of severe acute renal failure of critical illness in Australia. *Crit Care Med*, Vol. 29, No. pp. 1910–1915.

Singer, M. (2007a). Mitochondrial function in sepsis: acute phase versus multiple organ failure. *Crit Care Med*, Vol. 35, No. pp. S441-8.

Singer, M. (2007b). Powering up failed organs. *Am J Respir Crit Care Med*, Vol. 176, No. pp. 733-4.

Singer, M., De Santis, V., Vitale, D. & Jeffcoate, W. (2004). Multiorgan failure is an adaptive, endocrine-mediated, metabolic response to overwhelming systemic inflammation. *Lancet*, Vol. 364, No. pp. 545-8.

Solez, K., Morel-Maroger, L. & Sraer, J.-D. (1979). The morphology of "acute tubular necrosis" in man: Analysis of 57 renal biopsies and a comparison with the glycerol model. *Medicine*, Vol. 58, No. pp. 362–376.

Uchino, S., Kellum, J. A., Bellomo, R., Doig, G. S., Morimatsu, H., Morgera, S., Schetz, M., Tan, I., Bouman, C., Macedo, E., Gibney, N., Tolwani, A. & Ronco, C. (2005). Acute renal failure in critically ill patients: a multinational, multicenter study. *Jama*, Vol. 294, No. 7, pp. 813-8.

Valtin, H. & Schafer, J. A. (1995). Renal hemodynamics and oxygen consumption. In: *Renal Function*, Valtin, H. and Schafer, J. A., pp, 95-114. Little, Brown and Company, New York.

Wald, R., Quinn, R. R., Luo, J., Li, P., Scales, D. C., Mamdani, M. M. & Ray, J. G. (2009). Chronic dialysis and death among survivors of acute kidney injury requiring dialysis. *JAMA*, Vol. 302, No. 11, pp. 1179-1185.

Wan, L., Bellomo, R., Di Giantomasso, D. & Ronco, C. (2003). The pathogenesis of septic acute renal failure. *Curr Opin Crit Care,* Vol. 9, No. 6, pp. 496-502.

3

Oxidative and Nitrosative Stress in the Ischemic Acute Renal Failure

Miguel G. Salom, B. Bonacasa, F. Rodríguez and F. J. Fenoy
Department of Physiology, University of Murcia
Spain

1. Introduction

Ischemic injury to the kidney is the most common cause of acute kidney injury. Despite intensive basic research and in critical care for decades it is still associated with high mortality rates of ~50% in the intensive care unit. It is observed in a variety of clinical situations such as cardiac arrest with recovery, organ transplantation, or heminephrectomy. Postischemic acute kidney injury is characterized by an abrupt decrease in glomerular filtration rate (GFR) (the hallmark feature of acute kidney injury), and increased renal vascular resistance that determines a persistent reduction in renal blood flow (RBF) and tubular injury. However, the pathophysiological mechanisms responsible for the postischemic renal injury and the profoundly depressed renal function remain incompletely understood. The accumulated data in the literature are compatible with the hypothesis that ischemic acute kidney injury is essentially a phenomenon of altered renal hemodynamics linked critically to endothelial cell dysfunction caused by the production of high levels of reactive oxygen species (ROS) and reactive nitrogen species (RNS), leading to decreased nitric oxide availability as a consequence of its destruction to form peroxynitrite, associated with an intracellular energy store depletion. The oxidative and nitrosative stress will produce lipid peroxidation, oxidative DNA damage and modification and inactivation of proteins that originates an inflammatory reaction characterized by endothelial activation and injury, enhanced endothelial cell-leukocyte adhesion, leukocyte entrapment, and a reduction in microvascular blood flow mainly affecting the renal outer medulla as indicated by the marked vascular congestion typically observed in this zone of the kidney. On the other hand, and depending on the severity of renal ischemia, tubular epithelial cells will undergo a varying degree of necrosis or apoptosis with tubular obstruction followed by both an anatomical and functional recovery. The way in which vascular and tubular epithelium recover determines the final status of the renal function, ranging from full recovery to chronic renal failure and ultimately to end-stage renal disease. Because of the importance of endothelial cells in this process, emphasis will be placed on the involvement of oxidative and nitrosative stress in causing endothelial dysfunction, the sources of oxygen and nitrogen reactive species, and the interactions between them, specially superoxide anion and nitric oxide because together they form peroxynitrite, a potent oxidant and nitrosant agent. Among other factors, the severity of acute kidney injury is mainly determined by the duration of the ischemia. Special attention will be paid to the vascular and hemodynamic changes produced in the outer medulla during renal ischemia/reperfusion, because this renal zone is physiologically nearly hypoxic. The role of heme oxygenase system and the gender differences in the susceptibility to ischemic acute renal failure will be also be revised

2. Morphologic and hemodynamic changes in ischemic acute kidney injury

In apparent disagreement with the severe impairment of renal function, histologic changes in acute kidney injury are relatively subtle, and necrosis (if present) is restricted to the outer medullary region of the kidney. Morphologic changes include effacement and loss of proximal tubule brush border, patchy loss of tubule cells with apoptosis limited to both proximal and distal tubules, focal areas of tubular dilation with distal tubular casts (consisting of Tamm-Horsfall protein and cellular debris) and areas of regeneration. Peritubular capillaries present endothelial injury with enhanced expression of adhesion molecules (e.g. intercellular adhesion molecule-1, E-selectin, P-selectin) and cell swelling that promote adhesion of platelets to endothelium, with subsequent leukocyte adhesion and adhesion of platelets to neutrophils which are then aggregated and trapped in narrow peritubular capillaries causing vascular congestion, with cessation and even reversal of blood flow (Brodsky et al, 2002; Yamamoto et al, 2002). Endothelial injury also iniciates an inflammatory response that can be enhanced by tubular cells through the generation of proinflammatory cytokines and chemotactic cytokines (Bonventre & Zuk, 2004; Friedewald & Rabb, 2004; Schrier et al, 2004; Devarajan, 2006).

Functionally, the ischemic insult is followed by an intense and persistent renal vasoconstriction that significantly reduces renal blood flow to ~50% of normal (Cristol et al, 1993; Lieberthal et al, 1989), and has dramatic consequences in the renal outer medulla due to the fact that it is physiologically on the verge of hypoxia. Through a poorly understood mechanism, this acute reduction in outer medullary blood flow is followed later by a situation of chronic hypoxia (Basile et al, 2001; López Conesa et al, 2001). The increased basal vascular tone is also accompanied by increased reactivity to vasoconstrictors and a decreased response of arterioles to vasodilators, with loss of autoregulation of renal blood flow and abnormal vascular reactivity characteristic of postischemic acute kidney injury (Bonventre & Weinberg, 2003). These changes have been attributed to altered prostaglandins synthesis, to the generation of reactive oxygen and nitrogen species, and/or to activation of inflammatory responses to ischemia and it seems to be critically linked to endothelial dysfunction and to the increased generation of reactive oxygen and nitrogen species (oxidative and nitrosative stress) with a decrease in nitric oxide availability.

3. Temporal course of ischemic acute renal failure

Clinically, ischemic acute renal failure has classically been divided into the "Initiation", "Maintenance" and "Recovery" phases (Sutton et al, 2002; Devarajan et al, 2006). Sutton et al (2002) proposed a fourth phase, the "Extension" phase.

The "Initiation" phase begins when cellular ATP content becomes depleted as a consequence of anoxia, with the resultant tubular epithelial, smooth muscle and endothelial cell injuries characterized by disruption of actin cytoskeleton that produces structural and functional tubular alterations, and renal vasculature abnormalities. The severity and extent of these injuries will be determined by the degree and duration of ischemia. From a functional point of view epithelial and endothelial cells become "activated" up-regulating a number of cytokines and chemokines such as interleukins -1, -6, and -8, monocyte chemoatractant protein-1, and tumor necrosis factor alpha, thus triggering the inflammatory cascade. A key event in the "activation" of endothelial cells is a decrease in nitric oxide production.

The "Extension" phase is determined by two major events, a state of continued hypoxia with decreased blood flow, stasis and red and white blood cells accumulation mainly affecting outer medulla, and an inflammatory response. Thus, endothelial dysfunction in this phase plays a key role in the continued ischemia of tubular cells as well as in the inflammatory response observed in ischemic acute renal failure. As a consequence of these changes, apoptosis and necrosis of tubular cells (mainly affecting outer medulla) is observed and glomerular filtration rate continues falling.

During the "Maintenance" phase cells undergo repair (with apoptosis, proliferation and migration of cells) to re-establish and maintain cell and structure integrity with a slow improving in cellular and tubular function. Glomerular filtration rate is maintained to a level determined by the severity and duration of ischemia. Renal blood flow recovers approaching preischemic levels. During the "Recovery" phase a slowly and progressive improvement towards normality is taking place.

During all these phases the initial endothelium dysfunction and its posterior recuperation are of key importance to overall recovery.

4. Importance of renal medulla in the renal response to ischemia

4.1 Susceptibility of renal medulla to hypoxia

Many studies indicate that the severity of post-ischemic renal injury depends on the state of persistent hypo-perfusion of the renal outer medulla. The susceptibility of renal medulla to hypoxia lies in the fact that: a) renal arteries and veins run strictly parallel and in close contact with each other over long distances, allowing oxygen to diffuse from the arterial to the venous system before it has entered the capillary bed; b) tubular segments of the outer medulla have a limited capacity for anaerobic energy generation and, thus, depend on its oxygen supply to maintain active transtubular sodium and the reabsorption and secretion of solutes. These facts are particularly relevant in the tubular segments of the outer medulla (S3 segment of proximal tubules and medullary thick ascending loop of Henle) where the combination of limited oxygen supply ($pO_2 < 25$ mmHg) and a high oxygen demand makes the outer medulla to be physiologically on the verge of hypoxia (Brezis & Rosen, 1995; Zhang & Edwards, 2002). A variety of physiologic mechanisms are involved in protecting the outer medulla against hypoxic injury, including nitric oxide, prostaglandins, heme oxygenase-1 and adenosine, all of which enhance medullary blood flow while down-regulate active tubular transport of sodium and solutes (Brezis et al, 1989; Brezis et al, 1991; Knight & Johns, 2005; Rosenberger et al, 2006). A number of studies have shown that nitric oxide is a main regulator of medullary blood flow. Inhibition of nitric oxide production is followed by a decrease in medullary pO_2 in control animals and medullary blood flow (Cowley et al, 2003; Fenoy et al, 1995; López-Conesa et al, 2001; Nakanishi et al, 1995; O´Connor et al, 2006; Rodríguez et al, 2010; Rosenberger et al, 2006). Therefore, the functional status of the renal medullary nitric oxide system after the ischemia-reperfusion injury is believed to be a major determinant in the development of renal failure.

4.2 Outer medulla and ischemia-reperfusion

The importance of outer medulla in the renal response to an ischemic event has been demonstrated by several studies. Basile et al (2001) observed that renal ischemia results in permanent damage to peritubular capillaries and influences long-term function. They measured a 30-50% reduction in peritubular capillary density in the outer medulla at 4, 8 and 40 weeks after ischemia and tubulointerstitial fibrosis with increased transforming growth factor-1 expression at 40 weeks. Moreover, they also demonstrated an increase in 2-pimonidazole staining (a hypoxia-sensitive marker) in outer medulla accompanied by proteinuria, interstitial fibrosis and renal functional loss. They also observed that chronic L-arginine administration in drinking water increased total renal blood flow, decreased 2-pimonidazole staining and attenuated or delayed the progression of chronic renal insufficiency after recovery from acute ischemic injury (Basile et al, 2003). On the other hand, López-Conesa et al (2001) reported that an antioxidant ameliorated the renal failure and prevented the outer medullary vasoconstriction observed after 45 min of renal ischemia, effects that seem to be dependent on the presence of nitric oxide and the scavenging of peroxynitrite. Taken together, data from these studies strongly suggest that the renal failure that follows an ischemic event is directly related to alterations in outer medullary blood flow and that these changes seems to be dependent on free radical production and nitric oxide bioavailability.

5. Free radicals in acute renal injury

Free radicals are small, diffusible molecules that have an unpaired electron and tend to be reactive and can participate in chain reactions in which a single free radical event can be propagated to damage multiple molecules. The generation of oxygen free radicals is mainly restricted to mitochondria. In a controlled process 4 electrons from the electron transport chain are added to molecular oxygen yielding two water molecules. These electrons additions generate sequentially superoxide anion, hydrogen peroxide and the hydroxyl radical before the addition of the final electron to produce water. Reactive oxygen species can be also endogenously generated from other enzymes such as NAD(P)H-oxidases, xanthine oxidases, cyclooxigenases, lipooxygenases, myeloperoxidases, or uncoupled nitric oxide synthases. Each of these free radicals is able of oxidizing surrounding biomolecules thus generating other potent oxidants such as hypochlorous acid (harnessed by phagocytes for bacterial killing) or peroxynitrite anion (formed by the reaction of equimolecular amounts of nitric oxide and superoxide). However, the idea that the effects of reactive oxygen species on cellular functions are always deleterious is no longer valid because a number of studies have demonstrated that under physiological conditions low concentrations of reactive oxygen species play an important role in the normal regulation of cell and organ function. In this regard Ignarro et al (1988) demonstrated that superoxide dismutase enhanced arterial relaxation induced by the infusion of acetylcholine, indicating that there is a physiological production of a small amount of superoxide that is normally counteracting the vasodilatory effect of nitric oxide. In the kidney, Zou & Cowley (2001) demonstrated a basal generation of superoxide anion in all renal zones with the highest production in the outer medulla. Nitric oxide is a known renal vasodilator and acts as a natriuretic agent; superoxide has been shown to decrease renal blood flow and sodium excretion (Majid & Nishiyama, 2002; Majid et al, 2004, 2005; López et al, 2003; Makino et al, 2002; Zou & Cowley, 2001). Thus, there is evidence suggesting that superoxide is an important physiologic modulator of endogenous NO activity, counteracting the effects of nitric oxide in the kidney, and that superoxide exerts a tonic regulatory action on renal medullary blood flow.

Under steady-state conditions free radicals are effectively eliminated by antioxidant defense mechanisms that include free radical scavenging enzymes (superoxide dismutase, catalase, or glutathione peroxidase) and abundant radical scavenging chemicals (reduced glutathione, cysteine, vitamins C and E) that prevent almost completely radical chain reactions. However, when present in excess, a condition known as oxidative stress, they exert deleterious effects including lipid peroxidation, oxidative DNA damage and protein oxidation and nitration that collectively lead to progressive endothelial and tubular cells damage described in the precedent section. Generation of high levels of reactive oxygen species during renal ischemia/reperfusion have been confirmed directly (Zweier et al, 1994; Salom et al, 2007) and indirectly by measuring the effects of oxidants on lipids, proteins and DNA and by determining the beneficial effects of free radicals scavenging with antioxidant enzymes like superoxide dismutase or catalase or with antioxidants allopurinol (a xanthine oxidase inhibitor), tempol (an superoxide dismutase mimetic), N-acetyl-L-cysteine (an antioxidant), or dimethylthiourea (a hydroxyl radical scavenger)(Chatterjee et al, 2000; López-Conesa et al, 2001; Nitescu et al, 2006; Noiri et al, 2001; Tsuji et al, 2009). However, these compounds also scavenge or inhibit the formation of peroxynitrite ($ONOO^-$) a highly reactive chemical specie derived from nitric oxide and superoxide. Peroxynitrite and other reactive nitrogen species act together with other reactive oxygen species to damage cells, causing what is known as nitrosative stress.

6. Renal vascular endothelium, nitric oxide and acute renal failure

6.1 Vascular endothelium and nitric oxide in renal function regulation

The endothelium is the thin layer of cells that lines the interior surface of blood vessels, forming an interface between circulating blood in the lumen and the rest of the vessel wall. The vascular endothelium regulates vascular permeability, and modulates vasomotor, inflammatory, and haemostatic responses and nitric oxide appears to play a key role in these regulatory functions (Bird, 2011; Michel, & Vanhoutte, 2010). Nitric oxide regulates vascular tone preventing abnormal constriction, inhibits platelet aggregation, the expression of adhesion molecules at the surface of endothelial cells thus inhibiting the adhesion and penetration of white blood cells, and the release and action of endothelin-1 (Michel & Vanhoutte, 2010).

6.1.1 Nitric Oxide System

Nitric oxide is a diatomic free-radical gas synthesized from L-arginine by a family of enzymes called nitric oxide synthases. There are three mammalian nitric oxide synthases isoforms: neuronal (nNOS), inducible (iNOS) and endothelial (eNOS). They share 50–60% homology at the amino acid level and have an N-terminal oxygenase domain with heme-, L-arginine-, tetrahydrobiopterin (BH4)-binding domains, a central calmodulin (CaM)-binding region, and a C-terminal reductase domain with NADPH, FAD, and FMN binding sites (Stuehr, 1997). Under physiological conditions, the dominant nitric oxide synthase isoform in the vasculature is endothelial nitric oxide synthase, which is dynamically regulated at the transcriptional, posttranscriptional, and posttranslational levels (see Rafikov R et al, 2011 for a comprehensible review of the posttranslational control of endothelial nitric oxide synthase). Nitric oxide synthesis requires binding of the Ca^{2+}/calmodulin complex, but also requires dimerization of endothelial nitric oxide synthase and cofactors binding for activity. In the inactive state, endothelial nitric oxide synthase is located in plasma membrane caveolae bound to inhibitory protein caveolin-1. When activated the increase in Ca^{2+}/CaM releases and dimerizes endothelial nitric oxide synthase and interacts with its associated proteins heat shock protein 90 and Akt, and cofactors in an active complex. This activation process requires phosphorylation/dephosphorylation of the enzyme at different sites of tyrosine (Tyr-81 and Tyr-657), serine (Ser-114, Ser-615, Ser-633, and Ser-1177), and threonine (Thr495). The enzymes cycles between the inactive state bound to caveolin-1 in caveolae to cytoplasma in the activated state. The production of nitric oxide in endothelium cells is induced by mechanical action (shear stress) and by agonists such as acetylcholine, bradykinin, or histamine. Nitric oxide freely diffuses through plasma membrane to the underlying smooth muscles and triggers their relaxation by stimulating soluble guanylate cyclase that increases cyclic guanosine monophosphate levels. Nitric oxide also diffuses to the endothelium surface where inhibits adhesion and aggregation of platelets, modulates the permeability of endothelium, and inhibits endothelium-leukocytes interaction by reducing the expression of adhesion molecules.

Nitric oxide also plays an important role in the regulation of the renal hemodynamic and excretory functions (Romero et al, 1992). Inhibition of nitric oxide synthesis has shown to worsen both cortical and medullary blood flow and oxygenation (Cowley et al, 2003; Brezis et al, 1991)., indicating that nitric oxide is important for the maintenance of renal blood flow after ischemia-reperfusion injury of the renal vascular bed.

6.2 Endothelial dysfunction and acute renal failure – Role of nitric oxide

Ischemia/reperfusion of the kidney is followed by endothelium dysfunction and injury that contribute to the impairment of renal perfusion and chronic hypoxia, with the subsequent epithelial cell injury and decrease in the glomerular filtration rate that are the hallmarks of acute renal failure. Endothelial dysfunction, defined as impaired vasorelaxation in response to endothelium-dependent vasodilators, has been observed during renal ischemia-reperfusion (Brezis & Rosen, 1995; Cristol et al, 1993; Erdely et al, 2003; Kher et al, 2005; Lieberthal et al, 1989; Salom et al, 1998). Cristol et al (1993) and Salom et al (1998) reported renal vasoconstriction and impairment of the vasodilator effect of acetylcholine after acute renal ischemia. They also found that the recovery of renal blood flow observed on reperfusion was prevented by the previous nitric oxide synthesis inhibition. Renal ischemia/reperfusion is accompanied by a persistent reduction in renal blood flow of greater magnitude in the outer medulla. Mechanisms involved in this persistent reduction in renal perfusion are incompletely understood, but it has been observed endothelial cell swelling and detachment with trapping of red blood cells and leukocytes that produce vascular congestion of renal microcirculation especially in outer medulla (Olof et al, 1991;

Hellberg et al, 1990a, 1990b; Mason et al, 1984; Solez et al, 1974). Endothelial dysfunction in the outer medulla could contribute to the tubular epithelial cell injury thus determining a progressive fall in glomerular filtration rate in the initial and extending phases of acute renal failure. The key role of endothelial dysfunction in acute renal ischemia was demonstrated by studies of Brodsky et al, (2002) who transplanted endothelial cells or surrogate cells expressing endothelial nitric oxide synthase into rats subjected to renal artery clamping. Implantation of endothelial cells or their surrogates in the renal microvasculature resulted in a dramatic functional protection of ischemic kidneys. These observations strongly suggest that endothelial cell dysfunction is the primary cause of the no-reflow phenomenon, which, when ameliorated, results in prevention of renal injury seen in acute renal failure.

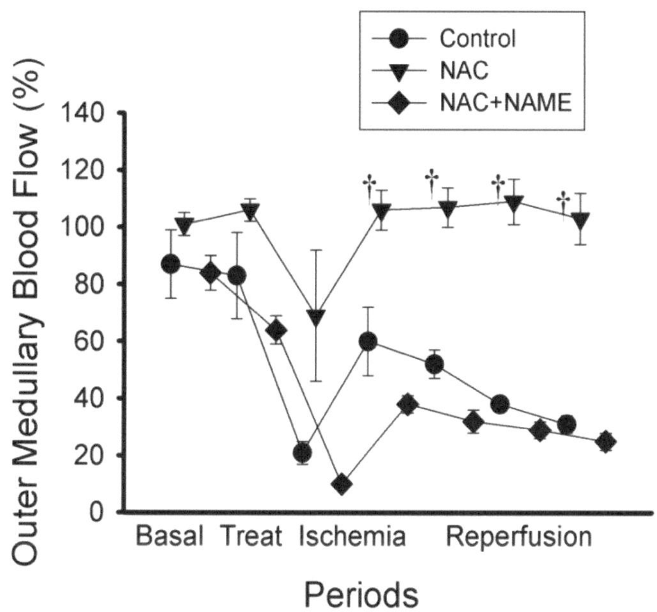

Fig. 1. Outer medullary blood flow during renal ischemia/reperfusion in SD rats.
% Change from the basal period in outer medullary blood flow during renal ischemia/reperfusion (45 min occlusion of renal artery) in Sprague-Dawley rats infused (Treat.) with saline (Control), N-acetyl-L-cysteine (150 mg/kg, as a bolus, plus 715 µg/kg/min) or L-Name (10 µg/kg/min), or L-Name + N-acetyl-L-cysteine).† Significant difference from the same experimental period of the control group (López-Conesa et al, 2001)

Endothelial dysfunction is an early event that is produced when oxygen free radicals are produced on reflow. Tsao et al (1990), Tsao & Lefer (1990) and Lefer & Ma (1991) in cardiac and splanchnic ischemia-reperfusion experiments demonstrated that endothelial dysfunction was related to reoxygenation and not to reflow and that this noxious effect can be prevented when free radical scavengers are infused before reperfusion. In the kidney, an increased free radical production has been demonstrated during reperfusion in *in vitro* (Kadkhodaee et al, 1995; Paller & Neumann, 1991) and *in vivo* experiments (Haraldsson et al, 1992; Nilsson et al, 1993). There is indirect evidence showing that endothelial dysfunction appears to be due to the generation of oxygen free radicals during reperfusion (Lieberthal, 1997; Salom et al, 1998). When infused before reperfusion, oxygen free radical scavengers exert a beneficial effect by preventing oxygen free radical production during reoxygenation (Baker et al, 1985; Hansson et al, 1990; Nilsson et al, 1993; Salom et al, 1998). In addition, the beneficial effect of some scavengers has been attributed to nitric oxide potentiation (Caramelo et al, 1996; López-Neblina et al, 1996; Salom et al, 1998), suggesting that the inactivation of nitric oxide by free radical is an important factor contributing to postischemic acute renal failure. This hypothesis was tested by López-Conesa et al, (2001) who found that N-acetyl-L-cysteine, a free radical scavenger, ameliorated the renal failure, and prevented the outer medullary vasoconstriction and the increase in plasma concentration of rhodamine 123 (index of peroxynitrite production) induced by renal ischemia. These results suggest that beneficial effects of N-acetyl-L-cysteine seem to be dependent on the presence of nitric oxide and the scavenging of peroxynitrite.

6.3 Ischemic preconditioning

Ischemic preconditioning is a phenomenon induced by brief ischemia and reperfusion periods that renders an organ more tolerant to subsequent sustained ischemia/reperfusion. In preconditioned kidneys, the sustained ischemia produces only small increases in plasma creatinine and in fractional sodium excretion, accompanied by markedly attenuated outer medullary congestion and leukocyte infiltration (Park et al, 2001, 2002). The mechanisms underlying this protective effect against injury are not well known. However, several candidates that could potentially serve as mediators of the preconditioning phenomenon have been identified. One of them, the nitric oxide synthase pathway, seems to be of importance. Park et al (2003) observed that prior ischemia results in prolonged increase in endothelial and inducible nitric oxide synthases (eNOS and iNOS). Torras et al (2002) observed that the protection afforded by ischemic preconditioning is abrogated by the inhibition of iNOS, and reproduced by a nitric oxide donor. Park et al (2003) showed that gene deletion of inducible (but not endothelial) nitric oxide synthase increases the kidney susceptibility to ischemia. In apparent contradiction, Yamasowa et al (2005) found that preconditioning in eNOS$^{+/+}$ mice markedly attenuated the renal dysfunction and improved the histological renal damage that follow ischemia/reperfusion (medullary congestion, intratubular casts or tubular necrosis). Preconditioning also prevented the marked decrease in endothelial nitric oxide synthase activity observed 6 hours after ischemia. (Yamasowa et al, 2005). The effects of preconditioning were abolished by a non-selective inhibitor of nitric oxide synthases, whereas aminoguanidine (a selective inhibitor of the inducible isoform) had no effect. A role for nitric oxide has also been reported by Jefayri et al (2000). Differences in the length of time between the first (preconditioning) and the second ischemic episode may explain differences observed between these studies. Park et al (2003) performed the second ischemia 1, 3, 4, 6, 10, or 12 weeks after the first (preconditioning) ischemia and at that time the expression of inducible but not endothelial nitric oxide synthase was significantly increased and nitric oxide levels before the second ischemia were high due to inducible isoform of the enzyme. In the study of Yamasowa et al (2005) the second ischemia was performed immediately after the preconditioning was finished (5 min). Yamasowa et al found that preconditioning prevents the decrease in endothelial nitric oxide synthase activity and prevented the increase in inducible nitric oxide synthase activity observed after 6 h of reperfusion. As Nakajima et al (2006) observed an increased production of superoxide in the first day after the ischemia, the inhibition of inducible nitric oxide synthase could theoretically prevent the formation of high levels of peroxynitrite. This could explain why inhibition of inducible nitric oxide synthase before the ischemia reduces renal ischemia/reperfusion injury (Chatterjee et al, 2002; Walker et al, 2000) and why inhibition of inducible nitric oxide synthase before the ischemia prevents renal microvascular hypoxia and inhibition of endothelial isoform aggravates renal function (Legrand et al, 2009). The data of these studies indicate that preconditioning protects the kidney partly by increasing nitric oxide levels due to the increase in endothelial (early protecting effect) or in the inducible nitric oxide synthase activity (long lasting protective effect). The studies of Nakajima et al (2006) who observed a significant attenuation of nitrotyrosine formation, neutrophil infiltration into renal tissues, and renal superoxide production, that were significantly attenuated by the preischemic treatment with a nitric oxide donor. Thus, a better understanding of ischemic preconditioning may help to unravel the underlying mechanisms of protection that mediate this tolerance against injury.

7. Oxidative and nitrosative stress and endothelial dysfunction in ischemic acute kidney injury

Endothelial dysfunction and oxidative stress are the main pathophysiological mechanisms of several diseases such as hypertension, atherosclerosis, dyslipidemia, diabetes mellitus, cardiovascular disease, renal failure and ischemia-reperfusion injury. Reactive oxygen species can modulate cellular function, receptor signals and immune responses in physiological conditions, but when present in excess, they mediate progressive endothelial damage through growth and migration of vascular smooth muscle and inflammatory cells, alteration of extracellular matrix, apoptosis of endothelial cells, activation of transcription factors (NFkB, AP-1), and over-expression of inflammatory cytokines and adhesion molecules (ICAM-1, VCAM-1 , E-selectin). Recent evidences suggest that the major source of reactive oxygen species is the NADPH-oxidase, especially activated by angiotensin II, shear stress and hyperglycemia. The unbalance between production of free radicals and the ability to neutralize them by antioxidant systems causes a condition of "oxidative stress". Reactive oxygen species alter vascular tone by increasing concentration of cytosolic calcium and especially causing a decreased availability of nitric oxide, the principal agent of endothelial function with vasodilating action (Urso & Caimi, 2011).

Ischemia/reperfusion is accompanied by an increase in radical oxygen species, a situation known as oxidative stress. The superoxide anion formed reacts with nitric oxide and inactivates nitric oxide (endothelial dysfunction) producing peroxynitrite, a highly reactive oxidant specie that exerts profound deleterious effects on renal function. The amount of peroxynitrite and, thus, the severity of postischemic acute kidney injury will depend on the relative concentration of both nitric oxide and superoxide (Miles et al, 1996) in such a way that the higher the nitric oxide concentration, the lower peroxynitrite will be formed and less renal damage will take place after ischemia. Renal nitric oxide levels increase dramatically during ischemia decreasing to near preischemic levels on reperfusion (Figure 1). The increase in nitric oxide concentration seems to be independent of nitric oxide synthases and appears to originate in tissue nitric oxide stores that release nitric oxide during ischemia (Salom et al, 2005). Combined with superoxide produced during ischemia, the nitric oxide increase appears to be responsible for an important part of the ensuing renal damage.

It has been reported that arterial ischemia produces an abrupt and significant increase in tissue nitric oxide concentration, which can last as long as ischemia is maintained and returns to preischemic levels during reperfusion. This phenomenon has been observed in kidney (Saito & Miyawaga, 2000) as well as in other organs (Lhuillier et al, 2003; Zweier et al, 1999). Although its physiological relevance is unclear, it may generate the high levels of peroxynitrite anion formed during reperfusion when a burst of superoxide anion reacts with the high levels of nitric oxide accumulated during ischemia (Miles et al, 1996), thus contributing to reperfusion damage. The mechanism responsible for these increased nitric oxide levels during renal ischemia is unknown, although it seems to be partially insensitive to nitric oxide synthesis inhibition, at least in liver and kidney (Lhuillier et al, 2003; Saito & Miyawaga, 2000). This is not surprising because nitric oxide synthase requires molecular oxygen. Therefore, during ischemia, nitric oxide must be released from other sources, such as tissue nitric oxide stores (Muller et al, 1996; Rodriguez et al, 2003; Sogo et al, 2000).

In the presence of oxygen, nitric oxide is synthesized from L-arginine through the action of nitric oxide synthase, and this gaseous hormone acts in the kidney by stimulating guanylyl cyclase and by inhibiting cytochrome *P*-450 (López et al, 2003). However, as soon as it is synthesized, nitric oxide avidly reacts with molecular oxygen, superoxide anion, and heme groups. The wide availability of these nitric oxide scavengers in all tissues argues against the simple diffusion-limited transport of free nitric oxide from synthase to cyclase or cytochrome. This implies that nitric oxide must be stabilized in vivo by reacting with carrier molecules that prolong its half-life and preserve its biological activity. This role may be subserved by biological molecules containing sulfhydryl groups that readily react with nitric oxide to form *S*-nitrosothiols (Stamler et al, 1992b), which are significantly more stable than nitric oxide itself and have been shown to be long-lasting and potent vasodilators. These compounds have been postulated to be biologically active intermediates in the mechanism of action of nitric oxide (Stamler 1992a). From this point of view, it has been shown that, at physiological concentrations, nitric oxide reacts with thiols in the presence of oxygen to form *S*-nitrosoglutathione (Kharitonov et al, 1995) and that nitric oxide circulates in mammalian plasma as nitrosothiols, mainly *S*-nitroso-serum albumin (Stamler et al, 1992a). The abundance of *S*-nitrosothiols in plasma compared with that of nitric oxide (3- to 4-fold) (Stamler et al, 1992a) suggests that plasma *S*-nitrosothiols may serve as a reservoir of nitric oxide, acting as an effective buffer (Lhuillier et al, 2003). This has also been shown in vascular tissue (Muller et al, 1996), where *S*-nitrosothiols are known to cause a prolonged nitric oxide-dependent relaxation (Sogo et al, 2000). These facts led us to hypothesize that renal ischemia induces an increase in tissue nitric oxide levels likely coming from tissue nitrosothiol stores and therefore that this phenomenon should be dependent on the presence of thiol groups in the tissue. In a study performed in our laboratories (Salom et al, 2005) we found that renal ischemia is followed by a rapid increase in intrarenal nitric oxide concentration that is maintained until reperfusion, when a fast drop in nitric oxide levels near preischemic values is observed. The increased nitric oxide concentration observed seems to be independent of nitric oxide synthase and appears to originate in tissue nitric oxide stores that release nitric oxide during ischemia.

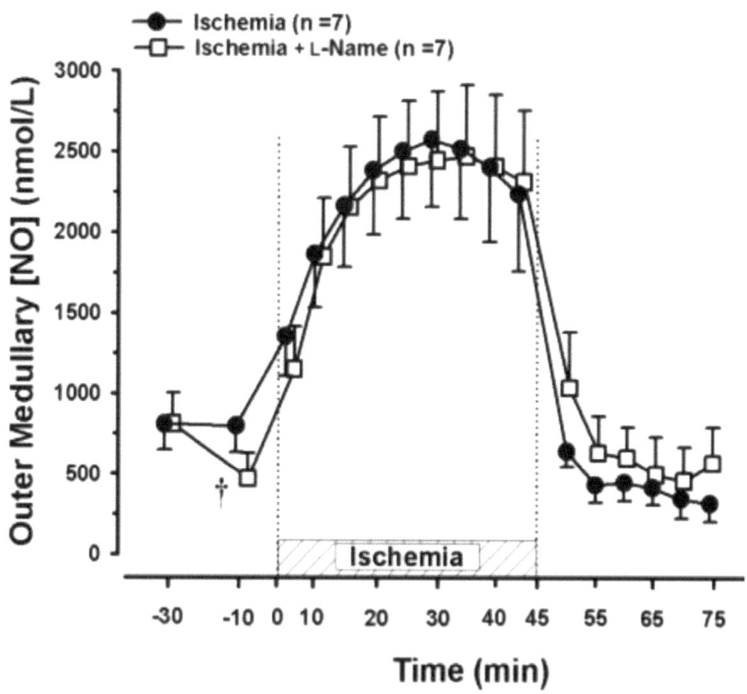

Fig. 2. Changes in nitric oxide levels in Outer Medulla during renal ischemia/reperfusion Changes in nitric oxide levels in outer medulla before, during and after a 45 min renal artery occlusion in SD rats infused with either saline (Ischemia) or L-Name (10 µg/kg/min, Ischemia + L-Name).).† Significant difference from the control period (-30 min) (Salom MG et al, 2005)

8. Sex differences in renal response to AKI

Females are known to suffer less severe renal I/R injury than males (Hutchens et al, 2008; Kang et al, 2004; Kher et al, 2005; Si et al, 2009; Wei et al, 2005; Xue et al, 2006) being the incidence of end stage renal disease approximately 50% higher in men than women. However, the mechanisms explaining this difference remain to be determined. It has been hypotethized that sex differences could be due to a higher renal constitutive nitric oxide synthase activity and/or increased nitric oxide bioavailability in females that protects the kidney against I/R injury (Chambliss & Shaul, 2002). However, lower, higher, or similar levels of endothelial and neuronal nitric oxide synthase expression in renal homogenates, cortex, and medulla of males and females have been reported (Erdely et al, 2003; Ji et al, 2005; Reckelhoff et al, 1998; Rodriguez et al, 2010; Wang et al, 2006; Wangensteen et al, 2004). However, the physiological meaning of nitric oxide synthase expression alone is uncertain, because dissociation between nitric oxide synthase expression and activity has been reported (Reckelhoff et al, 1998). The fact that nitric oxide availability depends not only on nitric oxide synthase expression and activity but also on the production of reactive oxygen species (because they inactivate nitric oxide in a concentration-dependent manner) also implies that sex differences could be due to a lower oxidative stress in females leading to increased nitric oxide levels (Arnal et al, 1996; Barbacanne et al, 1999) compared with males (Brandes & Mügge, 1997). Thus, the reduced susceptibility of females to I/R injury may be due to a greater nitric oxide synthase activation, nitric oxide bioavailability, and/or lower free radicals formation during ischemia and early reperfusion, resulting in a less severe acute renal failure. In a recent study performed in our laboratory (Rodríguez et al 2010) we evaluated sex differences in outer medullary changes of nitric oxide and peroxynitrite levels during 45 min of ischemia and 60 min of reperfusion in SD rats. No sex differences were observed in endothelial and neuronal nitric oxide synthases nor in nitric oxide and peroxynitrite levels. We also found that a 45-min ischemia was followed after 24 h of reperfusion by a postischemic renal failure in males but not in females. This sex difference was associated with lower nitric oxide and greater peroxynitrite and 3-nitrotyrosine levels in males during ischemia, indicating increased oxidative and nitrosative stress. Pretreatment with the antioxidants N-acetyl-L-cysteine or ebselen abolished sex differences in peroxynitrite, nitrotyrosine, and glomerular filtration rate, suggesting that a greater oxidative and nitrosative stress worsens renal damage in males. Taken together, the data in the present study strongly suggest that the resistance of females to renal failure may be related to a greater renal tissular antioxidant capacity that could blunt the conversion of nitric oxide to peroxynitrite during ischemia.

9. Role of heme oxygenase system in renal I/R

Heme is a ubiquitous molecule with an active iron center with high affinity for oxygen which allows for transport of oxygen in hemoglobin and myoglobin. Heme also serves as the catalytic site in a variety of proteins involved in cell metabolism including respiratory chain cytochromes and numerous cytochrome P450 isoenzymes (Maines, 1997). Oxidative stress destabilizes heme proteins, leading to free heme release, which has prooxidant and toxic effects through free radical formation, and lipid peroxidation in renal tissues, (Akagi et al, 2002).

Intracellular free levels are tightly controlled in most cells and tissues by heme oxigenases (HO) which catalyze the initial and rate limiting step in heme catabolism (Tenhunen et al, 1968). Oxidative cleavage of heme molecules by HO yields equimolar quantities of biliverdin (BV), carbon monoxide (CO), and Fe^{+2}. Biliverdin undergoes further degradation to bilirubin (BR) by the cytosolic biliverdin reductase. All HO-derived products are biologically active substances: biliverdin and iron are believe to subserve antioxidant and prooxidant mechanisms, respectively (Abraham et al, 1997), whereas HO-derived CO exerts exerts vasorelaxant (Zhang et al, 2001), antiapoptotic, and anti-inflammatory effects.

Oxidative stress promotes the upregulation of the inducible isoform of heme oxygenase (HO-1) (Motterlini et al, 2002), which is expressed, along with the constitutive HO-2 isoform, in renal vascular and tubular structures in renal cortex and medulla (Abraham et al, 2009). HO-1 and HO-2 catalyze the same reaction and have similar cofactors requirements, but they differ with respect to the regulation and expression pattern. HO-2 accounts for the bulk of renal HO activity in normal conditions, whereas HO-1 operates as an inducible enzyme with low renal levels in the healthy kidney (Da Silva, 2001), but markedly increased in pathological conditions associated to hypoxia and inflammation (Otterbein et al, 2003).

Ischemia compromises organ function, which is further aggravated upon reperfusion, as a consequence of endothelial dysfunction, high levels of oxidative stress, altered renal hemodynamic, and activation of the immune response. HO-1 prior to the induction of I/R results in functional protection in ischemic renal failure (Maines, 1999), which is partially mediated by reduction of oxidative and nitrosative stress during ischemia (Salom et al, 2007). Moreover, in the same way that HO metabolites maintain renal medullary perfusion (Zou et al, 2000), glomerular filtration rate and renal blood flow (Arregui B, 2004) in physiological conditions, HO-1 induction preserved postischemic medullary blood flow and GFR, in ischemic renal failure, (Salom et al, 2007). Overall, HO-1 induction might have multiple beneficial functions in I/R injury a) by reducing oxidative stress insults b) by preserving alteration of renal hemodynamic which contributes greatly to the subsequent renal failure and c) via suppression of the immune response through its anti-inflammatory actions, (Kotsch et al, 2007).

The molecular mechanisms underlying the protective role of HO induction in I/R injury are complex and likely multifactorial. Increased HO-1 activity in acute renal ischemia would result in the removal of the potent cell stressor heme (Akagi et al, 2005), but protection is also a consequence of the production of biologically active metabolites, i.e, CO, and BV. In this regard, the preadministration of exogenous CO donors in vivo have demonstrated functional protection comparable to HO-1 induction, pointing out to CO as a key component of the protection associated with HO-1 induction (Vera et al, 2005). Moreover, studies combining inhaled CO and infused bilirubin in rat renal transplantation demonstrated synergistic effects on glomerular filtration rate and renal blood flow (Nakao et al, 2005) suggesting also a role of bilirubin production in cytoprotection against ischemia/reperfusion injury. Finally, HO induction, through a variety of mechanisms, can reduce NO synthesis and, consequently, diminish augmented peroxynitrite formation during ischemia (Salom MG, 2007).

10. Concluding remarks, perspectives and significance

Ischemic injury to the renal vasculature may play an important role in the pathogenesis of both early and chronic ischemic acute kidney injury (AKI). Established and new data support the suggestion that vascular injury, in particular endothelial cell injury, participates in the extent and maintenance of AKI. Early alterations in peritubular capillary blood flow during reperfusion has been documented and associated with loss of normal endothelial cell function, which can be replaced pharmacologically or with cell replacement interventions. Distorted peritubular capillary morphology is associated with loss of barrier function that may contribute to early alterations in vascular stasis. In addition, ischemia induces alterations in endothelial cells that may promote inflammation and procoagulant activity, thus contributing to vascular congestion. Reductions in microvasculature density may play a critical part in the progression of chronic kidney disease following initial recovery from ischemia/reperfusion-induced AKI. The exact nature of how capillary loss alters renal function and predisposes renal disease is thought to be due at least in part to oxidative and nitrosative stress causing an endothelial balance between nitric oxide and peroxynitrite. Restoring the imbalance between nitric oxide and peroxynitrite will ameliorate endothelial dysfunction thus improving renal function. Finally, the loss of endothelial cell function may represent an important therapeutic target in which nitric oxide, vascular trophic support, and/or endothelial progenitor cells may show potential importance in ameliorating the acute and/or chronic effects of ischemic AKI. The use of drugs like statins that increase hemo oxygenase-1 expression, and restores the normal imbalance beween nitric oxide and peroxynitrite (Heeba et al, 2009) and reduce postischemic renal failure (Gueler et al, 2002) seem to be promissory.

11. Grants

This work was supported by grants BFV 2006-06998 (Ministerio de Educación y Ciencia) and 05812/PI/07 (Fundación Séneca).

12. References

Abraham NG, Cao J, Sacerdoti D, Li X, Drummond G (2009). Heme oxygenase: the key to renal function regulation. *American Journal of Physiology*, 297(5):F1137-F1152

Abraham NG, Drummond GS, Lutton JD, Kappas A (1997). The biological significance and physiological role of heme oxygenase. *Cell Physiology and Biochemistry*, 247: 725,732

Akagi R, Takahashi T, & Sassa S. (2002). Fundamental role of heme oxygenase in the protection against ischemic acute renal failure. *Japanese Journal of Pharmacology*, 88: 127-132.

Akagi R, Takahashi T, Sassa S (2005). Cytoprotective effects of heme oxygenase in acute renal failure. *Contributions in Nephrology*, 148:70-85

Arnal JF, Clamens S, Pechel C, Negre-Salvayre A, Allera C, Girolami JP, Salvayre R, & Bayard F. (1996). Ethinylestradiol does not enhance the expression of nitric oxide synthase in bovine endothelial cells but increases the release of bioactive nitric oxide by inhibiting superoxide anion production. *Proceedings of the National Academy of Sciences USA* 93: 4108–4113.

Arregui B, López B, García Salom M, Valero F, Navarro C, Fenoy FJ (2004). Acute renal hemodynamic effects of dimanganese decacarbonyl and cobalt protoporphyrin. *Kidney International*, 65(2): 564-574

Baker GL, Corry RJ, & Autor AP. (1985). Oxygen free radical induced damage in kidneys subjected to warm ischemia and reperfusion. *Annals of Surgery*, 202:628-641

Barbacanne MA, Rami J, Michel JB, Souchard JP, Philippe M, Besombes JP, Bayard F, & Arnal JF. (1999). Estradiol increases rat aorta endothelium-derived relaxing factor (EDRF) activity without changes in endothelial NO synthase gene expression: possible role of decreased endothelium-derived superoxide anion production. *Cardiovascular Research* 41: 672–681

Basile DP, Donohoe DL, Roethe K, & Mattson DL. (2003). Chronic renal hypoxia after acute ischemic injury: effects of L-arginine on hypoxia and secondary damage. *American Journal of Physiology*, 284: F338-F348

Basile DP, Donohoe DL, Roethe K, & Osborn JL. (2001). Renal ischemia injury results in permanent damage to peritubular capillaries and influences long-term function. *American Journal of Physiology*, 281:F887-F899

Bird IM. (2011). Endothelial nitric oxide synthase activation and nitric oxide function: new light through old windows. Journal of Endocrinology, 210(3):239-241

Bonventre JV, & Weinberg J. (2003). Recent advances in the pathophysiology of ischemic acute renal failure. *Journal of American Society of Nephrology*, 14:2199-2210

Bonventre JV, & Zuk A. (2004). Ischemic acute renal failure: An inflammatory disease?. *Kidney International*, 66(2):480-485

Brandes RP, & Mügge A. (1997). Gender differences in the generation of superoxide anions in the rat aorta. *Life Science* 60: 391-396

Brezis M, & Rosen S. (1995). Hypoxia of the renal medulla: Its implications for disease. *New England Journal of Medicine*, 332:647-655

Brezis M, Heyman SN, Dinour D, Epstein FH, & Rosen S. (1991). Role of nitric oxide in renal medullary oxygenation. Studies in isolated and intact rat kidneys. *Journal of Clinical Investigation*, 88: 390-395

Brezis M, Rosen S, & Epstein FH. (1989). The pathophysiological implications of medullary hypoxia. *American Journal of Kidney Disease*, 13(3):253-258

Brodsky SV, Yamamoto T, Tada T, Kim B, Chen J, Kajiya F, & Goligorsky MS. (2002). Endothelial dysfunction in ischemic acute renal failure: Rescue by transplanted endothelial cells. *American Journal of Physiology*, 282: F1140–F1149

Caramelo C, Espinosa G, Manzarbeitia F, Cernadas MR, Pérez Tejerizo G, Tan D, Mosquera JR, Digiuni E, Montón M, Millás I, Hernando L, Casado S, & López-Farré A. (1996). Role of endothelium-related mechanisms in the pathophysiology of renal ischemia/reperfusión in normal rabbits. *Circulation Research*, 79:1031-1038

Chambliss KL, Shaul PW. (2002). Estrogen modulation of endothelial nitric oxide. *Endocrinology Reviews* 23: 665–686

Chatterjee PK, Cuzzocrea S, Brown PAJ, Zacharowski K, Stewart KN, Mota-Filipe H, & Thiemermann C. (2000). Tempol, a membrane-permeable radical scavenger, reduces oxidant stress-mediated renal dysfunction and injury in the rat. *Kidney International*, 58:658-673

Chatterjee PK, Nimesh SA, Patel SA, Kvale EO, Cuzzocrea S, Brown PAJ, Stewart KN, Mota-Filipe H, & Thiemermann C. (2002). Inhibition of inducible nitric oxide synthase reduces renal ischemia/reperfusion injury. *Kidney International*, 61: 862-871

Cowley AW Jr, Mori T, Mattson D, & Zou A-P. (2003). Role of renal NO production in the regulation of medullary blood flow. *American Journal of Physiology*, 284:R1355–R1369.

Cowley AW Jr. (2008). Renal medullary oxidative stress, pressure-natriuresis, and hypertension. *Hypertension*, 52:777-786

Cristol JP, Thiemermann C, Mitchell JA, Walder C, & Vane JR. (1993). Support of renal blood flow after ischemic-reperfusion injury by endogenous formation of nitric oxide and cyclo-oxygenase vasodilator metabolites. *British Journal of Pharmacology*, 109: 188-194

Da Silva, JL, Zand BA, Yang LM, Sabaawy HE, Lianos E, Abraham NG (2001). Heme oxygenase isoform-specific expression and distribution in the rat kidney. *Kidney International*, 59: 1448-1457

Devarajan P. (2006). Update on mechanism of ischemic acute kidney injury. *The Journal of the American Society of Nephrology*, 17:1503-1520

Erdely A, Greenfeld Z, Wagner L, & Baylis C. (2003). Sexual dimorphism in the aging kidney: Effects of injury and nitric oxide system. *Kidney International*, 63:1021–1026

Fenoy FJ, Ferrer P, Carbonell LF, & Salom MG. (1995).Role of nitric oxide on papillary blood flow and pressure-natriuresis. *Hypertension*, 25:408-414.

Friedewald JJ, & Rabb H. (2004). Inflammatory cells in ischemic acute renal failure. *Kidney International*, 66(2):486-491

Goligorsky MS, Brodsky SV, & Noiri E. (2004). NO bioavailability, endothelial dysfunction, and acute renal failure: new insights into pathophysiology. *Seminars in Nephrology,* 24:316-323

Gueler F, Rong S, Park JK, Fiebeler A, Menne J, Elger M, Mueller DN, Hampich F, Dechend R, Kunter U, Luft FC, & Haller H. (2002). Postischemic acute renal failure is reduced by short-term statin treatment in a rat model. *Journal of American Society of Nephrology,* 13: 2288–2298

Hansson R, Bratell S, Burian P, Bylund-Fellenius AC, Jonsson O, Lundgren O, Lunstam S, Pettersson S, & Schersten T. (1990). Renal function during reperfusion after warm ischemia in rabbits: an experimental study on the possible protective effects of pretreatment with oxygen free radical scavengers or lidoflazine. *Acta Physiologica Scandinavica,* 139;39-46

Haraldsson G, Nilsson U, Bratell S, Pettersson S, Scherstçen T, Akerlund S, & Johnsson O. (1992). ESR-measurement of production of oxygen radicals in vivo before and after renal ischaemia in the rabbit. *Acta Physiological Scandinavica,* 146(1):99-105

Heeba G, Moselhy ME, Hassan M, Khalifa M, Gryglewski R, & Malinski T. (2009). Anti-atherogenic effect of statins: role of nitric oxide, peroxynitrite and hem oxygenase-1. *British Journal of Pharmacology,* 156:1256-66

Hellberg POA, Källskog Ö, & Wolgast M. (1990b) Nephron function in the early phase of ischemic renal failure. Significance of erythrocyte trapping. *Kidney International,* 38: 432–439

Hellberg POA, Källskog Ö, Öjteg G, & Wolgast M. (1990a). Peritubular capillary permeability and intravascular RBC aggregation after ischemia: effects of neutrophils. *American Journal of Physiology,* 258: F1018–F1025

Hutchens MP, Dunlap J, Hurn PD, & Jarnberg PO. (2008). Renal ischemia: does sex matter? *Anesthesia and Analgesia,* 107: 239–249

Ignarro LJ, Byrns RE, Buga GM, Wood KS, & Chaudhuri G. (1988). Pharmacological evidence that endothelium-derived relaxing factor is nitric oxide: use of pyrogallol and superoxide dismutase to study endothelium-dependent and nitric oxide-elicited vascular smooth muscle relaxation. *The Journal of Pharmacology and Experimental Therapeutics,* 244(1):181-189

Jaimes EA, Sweeney C, & Raij L. (2001). Effects of the reactive oxygen species hydrogen peroxide and hypochlorite on endothelial nitric oxide production. *Hypertension,* 38:877-883

Jefayri MK, Grace PA, & Mathie RT. (2000). Attenuation of reperfusion-injury by renal ischaemic preconditioning: the role of nitric oxide. *British Journal of Urology International,* 85:1007-1013

Ji X, Pesce C, Zheng W, Kim J, Zhang Y, Menini S, Haywood JR, & Sandberg K. (2005). Sex differences in renal injury and nitric oxide production in renal wrap hypertension. *American Journal of Physiology* 288: H43–H47

Kadkhodaee M, Endre ZH, Towner RA, & Cross M. (1995). Hydroxyl radical generation following ischemia-reperfusion in cell-free perfused rat kidney. *Biochimica et Biophysica Acta,* 1243(2): 169-174

Kakoki M, Hirata Y, Hayakawa H, Suzuki E, Nagata D, Tojo A, Nishimatsu H, Nakanishi N, Hattori Y, Kikuchi K, Nagano T, & Omata M.. (2000). Effects of tetrahydrobiopterin on endotelial dysfunction in rats with ischemic acute renal failure. *The Journal of the American Society of Nephrology*, 11:301-309

Kang DH, Yu ES, Yoon KI, & Johnson R. (2004). The impact of gender on progression of renal disease. Potential role of estrogen-mediated vascular endothelial growth factor regulation and vascular protection. *American Journal of Pathology*, 164: 679–688

Kharitonov VG, Sundquist AR, & Sharma VS. (1995). Kinetics of nitrosation of thiols by nitric oxide in the presence of oxygen. *Journal of Biological Chemistry*, 270: 28158–28164.

Kher A, Meldrum KK, Wang M, Tsaia BM, Pitchera JM, & Meldruma DR. (2005). Cellular and molecular mechanisms of sex differences in renal ischemia-reperfusion injury. *Cardiovascular Research*, 67: 594–603

Knight S, & Johns EJ. (2005). Effect of COX inhibitors and NO on renal hemodynamics following ischemia-reperfusion injury in normotensive and hypertensive rats. *American Journal of Physiology*, 289:F1072-F1077

Kotsch K, Martins PN, Klemz R, Janssen U, Gerstmayer B, Dernier A, Reutzel-Selke A, Kuckelkorn U, Tullius SG, Volk HD(2007). Heme oxygenase-1 ameliorates ischemia/reperfusion injury by targeting dendritic cell maturation and migration. *Antioxidant Redox Signaling*, 9(12):2049-2063

Lefer AM, & Ma X-L. (1991). Endothelial dysfunction in splanchnic circulation following ischemia and reperfusion. *Journal of Cardiovascular Pharmacology*, 17(Suppl 3):S186-S190

Legrand M, Almac E, Milk eg, Johannes T, Kandil A, Bezemer R, Payen D, & Ince C. (2009). L-NIL prevents renal microvascular hypoxia and increase of renal oxygen consumption after ischemia-reperfusion in rats. *American Journal of Physiology*, 296:F1109-F1117

Lhuillier F, Parmentier P, Goudable J, Crova P, Delafosse B, Annat G, Cespuglio R, & Viale JP. (2003). Hepatic ischemia is associated with an increase in liver parenchyma nitric oxide that is in part enzyme-independent. *Anaesthesiology* 98: 373–378

Lieberthal W, Wolf EF, Rennke HG, Valeri CR, & Levinsky NG. (1989). Renal ischemia and reperfusion impair endothelium-dependent vascular relaxation. *American Journal of Physiology*, 256:F894-F900

Lopez B, Salom MG, Arregui B, Valero F, & Fenoy FJ. (2003). Role of superoxide in modulating the renal effects of angiotensin II. *Hypertension*, 42: 1150–6.

López Conesa E, Valero F, Nadal JC, Fenoy F, López B, Arregui B, & Salom MG. (2001). N-acetyl-L-cysteine improves renal medullary hypoperfusion in acute renal failure. *American Journal of Physiology*, 281:R730-R737

Lopez-Neblina F, Toledo-Pereyra LH, Mirmiran R, & Paez-Rollys AJ. (1996). Time dependence of Na-nitroprusside administration in the prevention of neutrophil infiltration in the rat ischemic kidney. *Transplantation*, 61(2):179-183

Maines MD (1997). The heme oxygenase system: a regulator of second messenger gases. *Annual Review of Pharmacology and Toxicology*, 37: 517-554

Maines MD, Raju VS, & Panahian N. (1999). Spin trap (*N-t*-butyl-_-phenylnitrone)-mediated suprainduction of heme oxygenase-1 in kidney ischemia/reperfusion model: role of the oxygenase in protection against oxidative injury. *Journal of Pharmacology and Experimental Therapeutics*, 291: 911–919

Majid DSA, & Nishiyama A. (2002). Nitric oxide blockade enhances renal reponses to superoxide dismutase inhibition in dogs. *Hypertension,* 39:293–297.

Majid DSA, Nishiyama A, Jackson KE, & Castillo A. (2004). Inhibition of nitric oxide synthase enhances superoxide activity in canine kidney. *American Journal of Physiology,* 287: R27–R32

Majid DSA, Nishiyama A, Jackson KE, & Castillo A. (2005). Superoxide scavenging attenuates renal responses to ANG II during nitric oxide synthase inhibition in anesthetized dogs. *American Journal of Physiology,* 288: F412–F419

Makino A, Skelton MM, Zou AP, Roman RJ, & Cowley Jr AW. (2002). Increased renal medullary oxidative stress produces hypertension. *Hypertension* 39: 667–672.

Mason J, Thorhorst J, & Welsch J. (1984). Role of medullary perfusion defect in the pathogenesis of ischemic renal failure. *Kidney International,* 24: 27–36

Michel T, & Vanhoutte PM. (2010). Cell signaling and NO production. *European Journal of Physiology,* 459:

Miles AM, Scott Bolhle D, Glassbrenner PA, Hansert B, Wink DA & Grisham MB. (1996). Modulation of superoxide-dependent oxidation and hydroxylation reactions by nitric oxide. *Journal of Biological Chemistry,* 271: 40-47

Motterlini R, Green CJ, Foresti R (2002). Regulation of heme oxygenase-1 by redox signals involving nitric oxide. *Antioxidant and Redox Signaling,* 4(4):615-624

Muller B, Kleschyov AL, & Stoclet JC. (1996). Evidence for *N*-acetylcysteinesensitive nitric oxide storage as dinitrosyl-iron complexes in lipopolysaccharide-treated rat aorta. *British Journal of Pharmacology,* 119: 1281–1285

Nakajima A, Ueda K, Takaoka M, Yoshimi Y, & Matsumura Y. (2006). Opposite effects of pre- and postischemic treatments with nitric oxide dono ron ischemia/reperfusión-induced renal injury. *The Journal of Pharmacology and Experimental Therapeutics,* 316: 1038-1046

Nakanishi K, Mattson DL, & Cowley AW Jr. (1995). Role of renal medullary blood flow in the development of L-Name hypertension in rats. *American Journal of Physiology,* 268:R317-R323

Nakao A, Neto JS, Kanno S, Stolz DB, Kimizuka K, Liu F, Bach FH, Billiar TR, Choi AM, Otterbein LE, Murase N (2005). Protection against ischemia/reperfusion injury in cardiac and renal transplantation with carbon monoxide, biliverdin and both. *American Journal of Transplant,* 5(2):282-291

Nilsson UA, Haraldsson G, Bratell S, Sorensen V, Akerlund A, Pettersonn S, Schersten T, & Jonsson O. (1993). ESR-measurement of oxygen radicals in vivo after renal ischemia of the rabbit. Effect of pretreatment with superoxide dismutase and heparin. *Acta Physiologica Scandinavica,* 147:263-279

Nitescu N, Grimberg E, Ricksten S-E, & Guron G. (2006). Effects of N-acetyl-Lcysteine on renal haemodynamics and function in early ischaemi-reperfusion injury in rats. *Clinical and Experimental Pharmacology and Physiology,* 33:53-57

Nitescu N, Ricksten SE, Marcussen N, Haraldsson B, Nilsson U, Basu S, Guron G. (2006). N-acetylcysteine attenuates kidney injury in rats subjected to renal ischaemia-reperfusion. *Nephrology and Dialysis Transplantation,* 21(5):1240-7

Noiri E, Nakao A, Uchida K, Tsukahara H, Ohno M, Fujita T, Brodsky S, & Goligorsky MS. (2001). Oxidative and nitrosative stress in acute renal ischemia. *American Journal of Physiology,* 281:F948-F957

Noiri E, Peresleni T, Miller F, & Goligorsky MS. (1996). In vivo targeting of inducible NO synthase with oligodeoxynucleotides protects rat kidney against ischemia. *Journal of Clinical Investigation*, 97(10): 2377-2383

O'Connor PM, Kett MM, Anderson WP, & Evans RG, (2006). Renal medullary tissue oxygenation is dependent on both cortical and medullary blood flow. *American Journal of Physiology*, 290: F688-F694

Olof P, Hellberg A, Källskog O, & Wolgast M.(1991). Red cell trapping and postischemic renal blood flow. Differences between the cortex, outer and inner medulla. *Kidney Intrnational*, 40(4):625-631.

Otterbein LE, Soares MP, Yamashita K, Bach FH (2003). *Heme oxygenase-1: unleashing the protective properties of heme. Trends in Immunology*, 24(8):449-455

Paller MS, & Neumann TV. (1991). Reactive oxygen species and rat renal epithelial cells during hypoxia and reoxygenation. *Kidney International*, 40(6):1041-1049

Park KM, Byun J-Y, Kramers C, Kim JI, Huang PL, & Bonventre JV. (2003). Inducible nitric oxide synthase is an important contributor to prolonged protective effects of ischemic preconditioning in the mouse kidney. *The Journal of the Biological Chemistry*, 278(29):27256-27266

Park KM, Chen A, & Bonventre JV. (2001). Prevention of kidney ischemia/reperfusion-induced functional injury and JNK, p38, and MAPK kinase activation by remote ischemic pretreatment. *Journal of Biology and Chemistry*,276(15):11870-11876

Park KM, Kramers C, Vayssier-Taussat M, Chen A, & Bonventre JV. (2002). Prevention of kidney ischemia/reperfusion-induced functional injury, MAPK and MAPK kinase activation, and inflammation by remote transient ureteral obstruction. *Journal of Biology and Chemistry*,277(3):2040-2049

Pfeilschifter J, Eberhardt W, & Huwiler A. (2003). Nitric oxide and mechanisms of redox signaling. *Journal of the American Society of Nephrology*, 14:S237-S240

Polytarchou C, & Papadimitriou E. (2005).Antioxidants inhibit human endothelial cell functions through down-regulation of endothelial nitric oxide synthase activity. *European Journal of Pharmacology*, 510(1-2):31-38

Rabelink TJ, & van Zonneveld AJ. (2006) Coupling eNOS uncoupling to the innate immune response. *Arteriosclerosis, Thrombosis, and Vascular Biolology*, 26:2585–2587

Rafikov R, Fonseca FV, Kumar S, Pardo D, Darragh C, Elms S, Fulton D, & Black SM. (2011). eNOS activation and NO function: Structural motifs responsible for the posttranslational control of endothelial nitric oxide synthase activity. *Journal of Endocrinology*, 210:271-284

Reckelhoff JF, Hennington BS, Moore AG, Blanchard EJ, & Cameron J. (1998). Gender differences in the renal nitric oxide (NO) system: dissociation between expression of endothelial NO synthase and renal hemodynamic response to nitric oxide inhibition. *American Journal of Hypertension*, 11: 97–104

Rodríguez F, Nieto-Cerón S, Fenoy FJ, López B, Hernández I, Rodado Martinez R, González Soriano MJ, & Salom MG. (2010). Sex differences in nitrosative stress during renal ischemia. *American Journal of Physiology*, 299: R1387–R1395

Rodriguez J, Maloney RE, Rassaf T, Bryan NS, & Feelisch M. (2003) Chemical nature of nitric oxide storage forms in rat vascular tissue. *Proceedings of the National Academy of Sciences, USA* 100: 336–341

Romero JC, Lahera V, Salom MG, & Biondi LM. (1992). Role of the endothelium-dependent relaxing factor Nitric Oxide on renal function. *Journal of the American Society of Nephrology*, 2: 1371-1387

Rosenberger C, Mandriota S, Jürgensen JS, Wiesener MS, Hörstrup JH, Frei U, Ratcliffe PJ, Maxwell PH, Bachmann S, & Eckardt K-U. (2002). Expression of Hypoxia-Inducible Factor-1α and -2α in Hypoxic and Ischemic Rat Kidneys. *Journal of the American Society of Nephrology*, 13: 1721–1732

Rosenberger C, Rosen S, & Heyman SN. (2006). Renal parenchymal oxygenation and hypoxia adaptation in acute kidney injury. *Clinical and Experimental Pharmacology and Physiology*, 33(10):980-988

Saito M, & Miyagawa I. (2000). Real-time monitoring of nitric oxide in ischemia-reperfusion rat kidney. *Urology Research*, 28: 141–146

Salom MG, Arregui B, Carbonell LF, Ruiz F, González-Mora JL, & Fenoy FJ. (2005). Renal ischemia induces an increase in nitric oxide levels from tissue stores. *American Journal of Physiology*, 289: R1459–R1466

Salom MG, Nieto-Cerón S, Rodríguez F, López B, Hernández I, Gil J, Martínez-Losa A, & Fenoy FJ. (2007). Heme-oxygenase-1 induction improves ischemic renal failure. Role of nitric oxide and peroxynitrite. *American Journal of Physiology*, 293: H3542–H3549

Salom MG, Ramírez P, Carbonell LF, López Conesa E, Cartagena J, Quesada T, Parrilla P, & Fenoy FJ. (1998). Protective effect of N-acetyl-L-cysteine on the renal failure induced by inferior vena cava occlusion. *Transplantation*, 65:1315-1321

Schrier RW, Wang W, Poole B, & Mitra A. (2004). Acute renal failure: definitions, diagnosis, pathogenesis, and therapy. *The Journal of Clinical Investigations*, 114(1):5-14

Si H, Banga RS, Kapitsinou P, Ramaiah M, Lawrence J, Kambhampati G, Gruenwald A, Bottinger E, Glicklich D, Tellis V, Greenstein S, Thomas DB, Pullman J, Fazzari M, & Susztak K. (2009). Human and murine kidneys show gender- and species-specific gene expression differences in response to injury. *PLoS One*, 4(3):e4802. Epub 2009

Sogo N, Campanella C, Webb DJ, & Megson IL. (2000). *S*-nitrosothiols cause prolonged, nitric oxide-mediated relaxation in human saphenous vein and internal mammary artery: therapeutic potential in bypass surgery. *British Journal of Pharmacology*, 131: 1236–1244

Solez K, Kramer EC, Fox JA, Heptinstall RH. (1974). Medullary plasma flow and intravascular leukocyte accumulation in acute renal failure. *Kidney International*, 6(1):24-37

Stamler JS, Jaraki O, Osborne J, Simon DI, Keaney J, Vita J, Singel D, Valeri CR, & Loscalzo J. (1992a). Nitric oxide circulates in mammalian plasma primarily as an S-nitroso adduct of serum albumin. *Proceedings of the Nationall Academy of Sciences, USA*, 89: 7674–7677

Stamler JS, Simon DI, Osborne JA, Mullins ME, Jaraki O, Michel T, Singel DJ, & Loscalzo J. (1992b) *S*-nitrosylation of proteins with nitric oxide: synthesis and characterization of biologically active compounds. *Proceedings of the Nationall Academy of Sciences USA* 89: 444–448

Stuehr DJ. (1997). Structure–function aspects in the nitric oxide synthases. *Annual Review of Pharmacology and Toxicology*, 37: 339–359

Summers W, & Jamison RL. (1971). The non-reflow phenomenon in renal ischemia. *Laboratory Investigation*, 25:635-643

Sutton TA, Fisher CJ, & Molitoris BA.(2002). Microvascular endothelial injury and dysfunction during ischemic acute renal failure. *Kidney International*, 62(5):1539-1549

Tenhunen R, Marver HS, Schmid R (1968). The enzymatic conversion of heme to bilirubin by microsomal heme oxygenase. *Proceedings of the National Academy of Sciences, U S A.*, 61(2):748-755

Torras J, Herrero-Fresneda I, Lloberas N, Riera M, Cruzado JM[a], & Grinyó JM[a]. (2002). Promising effects of ischemic preconditioning in renal transplantation. *Kidney International*, 61:2218-2227

Tsao PS, & Lefer AM. (1990). Time course and mechanism of endothelial dysfunction in isolated ischemic and hypoxic perfused rat hearts. *American Journal of Physiology*, 259:H1660-H1666

Tsao PS, Aoki N, Lefer DJ, Johnson G III, & Lefer AM. (1990). Time course of endothelial dysfunction and myocardial injury during myocardial ischemia and reperfusion in the cat. *Circulation*, 82:1402-1412

Tsuji T, Kato A, Yasuda H, Miyaji T, Luo J, Sakao Y, Ito H, Fujigaki Y, & Hishida A. (2009). The dimethylthiourea-induced attenuation of cisplatin nephrotoxicity is associated with the augmented induction of heat shock proteins. *Toxicology and Applied Pharmacology*, 234(2):202-208

Urso C, & Caimi G. (2011). Oxidative stress and endothelial dysfunction. *Minerva Medical*, 102(1):59-77

Vera T, Henegar JR, Drummond HA, Rimoldi JM, & Stec DE. (2005). Protective effect of carbon monoxide-releasing compounds in ischemia-induced acute renal failure. *Journal of the American Society of Nephrology*, 16(4):950-958

Walker LM, Walker PD, Imam SZ, Ali SF, & Mayeux PR. (2000). Evidence for peroxynitrite formation in renal ischemia-reperfusion injury: Studies with the inducible Nitric Oxide Synthase inhibitor L-N^6-(1-iminoethyl)lysine. *Journal of Pharmacology and Experimental Therapeutics*, 295:4177-22

Walker LM, York JL, Imam SZ, Ali SF, Muldrew KL, & Mayeux PR. (2001). Oxidative stress and reactive nitrogen species generation during renal ischemia. *Toxicological Sciences*, 63: 143-148

Wang X, Desai K, Juurlink BHJ, de Champlain J, & Wu L. (2006). Gender-related differences in advanced glycation endproducts, oxidative stress markers and nitric oxide synthases in rats. *Kidney International*, 69: 281–287

Wangensteen R, Moreno JM, Sainz J, Rodríguez-Gómez I, ChamorroV, Luna de D J, Osuna A, & Vargas F. (2004). Gender difference in the role of endothelium-derived relaxing factors modulating renal vascular reactivity. *European Journal of Pharmacology*, 486: 281–288

Wei Q, Wang MH, & Dong Z. (2005). Differential gender differences in ischemic and nephrotoxic acute renal failure. *American Journal of Nephrology*, 25: 491–499

Wu F, Park F, Cowley AW Jr, & Mattson DL. (1999). Quantification of nitric oxide synthase activity in microdissected segments of the rat kidney. *American Journal of Physiology*, 276: F874–F881

Yamamoto T, Tada T, Brodsky SV, Tanaka H, Noiri E, Kajiya F, & Goligorsky MS. (2002). Intravital videomicroscopy of peritubular capillaries in renal ischemia. *American Journal of Physiology,* 282: F1150–F1155

Yamasowa H, Shimizu S, Inoue T, Takaoka M & Matsumura Y. (2005). Endothelial nitric oxide contributes to the renal protective effects of ischemic preconditioning. *The Journal of Pharmacology and Experimental Therapeutics,* 312: 153-159

Zhang F, Kaide JI, Rodriguez-Mulero F, Abraham NG, Nasjletti A (2001). Vasoregulatory function of the heme-heme oxygenase-carbon monoxide system. *American Journal of Hypertension:* 14(6 Pt 2):62S-67S

Zhang W, & Edwards A. (2002). Oxygen transport across vasa recta in the renal medulla. *American Journal of Physiology,* 283:H1042-H1055

Zhang W, Pibulsonggram, & Edwards A. (2004). Determinants of basal nitric oxide concentration in the renal medullary microcirculation. *American Journal of Physiology,* 287:F1189-F1203

Zhang ZG, Chopp M, Bailey F, and Malinski T. Nitric oxide changes in the rat brain after transient middle cerebral artery occlusion. *Journal of Neurology Sciences,* 128: 22–27, 1995.

Zou A-P, & Cowley AW Jr. (1997). Nitric oxide in renal cortex and medulla: an in vivo microdialysis study. *Hypertension,* 29:194-198

Zou AP, & Cowley Jr AW. (2001). Production and actions of superoxide in the renal medulla. *Hypertension,* 37: 547–553.

Zou, AP, Billington H, Su N, & Cowley AW, Jr. (2000). Expression and actions of heme oxygenase in the renal medulla of rats. *Hypertension,* 35:342-347

4

Immunological and Molecular Mechanisms Leading to Fibrosis: Origin of Renal Myofibroblasts

Leonóra Himer[1], Erna Sziksz[1], Tivadar Tulassay[1,2] and Ádám Vannay[1]
[1]*Research Group for Paediatrics and Nephrology, Semmelweis University and Hungarian Academy of Sciences, Budapest,*
[2]*First Department of Paediatrics, Semmelweis University, Budapest*
Hungary

1. Introduction

There are about quarter of million patients on chronic renal replacement therapy in Europe, and the estimated number of patients with chronic kidney disease, stages 1-4 is about tenfold higher. Interestingly, regardless of the initiating cause (infection, autoimmune response, chemical insult, radiation or tissue injury etc.), the mechanism of fibrosis is similar in the different chronic kidney diseases and characterized by inflammation. In general, the damaged glomerular or tubular cells release danger signals (Anders, 2010; McDonald et al., 2010) and produce chemotactic stimuli, which trigger the rapid recruitment of leukocytes. The infiltrating immune and the damaged renal cells then produce high levels of proinflammatory cytokines, growth factors, chemokines and adhesion molecules which contribute to glomerular/tubular injury, accumulation of further leukocytes and myofibroblasts, which are the effector cells of renal fibrosis. However the origin of the myofibroblasts is still controversial recent hypotheses suggest that myofibroblasts can originate from different renal cells, such as epithelial and endothelial cells, pericytes or the bone marrow derived fibrocytes. The thus generated myofibroblasts then serves as the key cellular mediator of renal fibrosis. Myofibroblasts have migratory capacity, are resistant to apoptosis, produce several growth factors and cytokines and according to our present knowledge these cells are the main source of the collagen-I and collagen-III rich extracellular matrix in the fibrous tissue. Organ fibrosis is characterized by excessive deposit of extracellular matrix (ECM) leading to glomerular sclerosis and renal tubule-interstitium fibrosis. The excessive deposition of fibrous tissue replaces healthy kidney tissue; the nephrons disappear and the kidney function gradually declines. In this chapter we will summarize our knowledge about the role of immune cells and molecular changes leading to generation of renal myofibroblasts.

2. Role of immune system

Progressive renal diseases always have an inflammatory component, characterized by the infiltration of different leukocytes, overexpression of inflammatory genes and release of proinflammatory cytokines. In the following paragraphs we will summarise the role of the different immune cells in the pathomechanism of renal fibrosis.

2.1 Neutrophil granulocytes

Neutrophil granulocytes are polymorphonuclear cells, which constitute the majority of circulating leukocytes and respond quickly to chemotactic stimuli. They are the first immune cells, which migrate to the inflamed tissue and eliminate the pathogens and tissue debris by enzymatic degradation or by reactive oxygen species; moreover, they attract and activate further immune cells by producing different chemokines and cytokines. These cells are generally regarded as short-lived and terminally differentiated leukocytes. Kidney injury leads to the rapid influx of neutrophils and subsequent monocyte and other leukocyte recruitment (Machida et al., 2010). Damaged renal cells produce different cytokines and chemokines (e.g.: interleukin (IL)-8 (Hang et al., 2000; Topley et al., 2005), IL-17 (Kitching et al., 2011) macrophage inflammatory protein (MIP)-1, monocyte chemoattractant protein (MCP)-1 (Li et al., 2005)) which - among other leukocytes – efficiently attract neutrophils. Neutrophils become activated by immune complexes became trapped in the glomerulus or through pattern recognition receptors by damage associated or pathogen-associated molecular patterns (DAMP/PAMP) signals (like macrophages, see in details later). In response to specific stimuli, neutrophils have the capacity to synthesize several factors such as extracellular matrix and antimicrobial proteins (defensins), reactive oxygen species, cytokines (IL-1-β, tumor necrosis factor (TNF)-α) and chemokines (IL-8, MIPs) that can contribute in regulating the inflammatory response (Cassatella, 1999; Sawyer et al., 1989; Fantone & Ward, 1985). Neutrophils are able to generate arachidonic acid-derived lipid mediators, such as leukotriene B4, which is also a potent chemoattractant for leukocytes (Busse, 1998). Neutrophils have been shown to generate prostaglandin E2 and tromboxane via the inducible cyclooxigenase 2 pathway (Maloney et al, 1998). Prostaglandine E2 has both pro-and anti-inflammatory properties, for example it regulates vascular permeability, so contribute the accumulation of immune cells to the target tissue. Many of these cytokine-, lipid- and oxygen-derived mediators are regulated by nuclear factor (NF)-κB activation, which supports neutrophils in direct pathogen killing (Blackwell et al., 1997). Although these important host defense functions, neutrophils also have an destructive capacity and can elicit significant tissue damage. For example, in antineutrophil cytoplasmic antibody - associated diseases immune complexes became trapped on the endothelial surface in the vasculature of glomerulus, and the local activation of neutrophils and monocytes may disrupt the integrity of tissue architecture (Weidner et al., 2004). Human polymorphonuclear cells may be activated by particulate uromodulin (also known as: Tamm-Horsfall glycoprotein), which is the most abundant protein excreted in the urine under physiological conditions, but its biological function is still not fully understood (Rampoldi et al., 2011). Neutrophil-uromodulin interaction in the renal interstitium is characterized by the activation of the respiratory burst, as well as by comprehensive polymorphonuclear cell degranulations, which lead to marked tissue damage and eventually result in interstitial fibrosis (Horton et al., 1990). Ichino et al has been detected a marked upregulation of neutrophil-gelatinase associated lipocalin at the mRNA and protein levels in a rat model of renal scarring. This molecule has been proposed over the past years as emergent biomarkers for the early and accurate diagnosis and monitoring of acute kidney injury (Ichino et al., 2010). After they completed their role in the damaged kidney, neutrophils undergo apoptotic cell death. The phagocytic uptake of apoptotic neutrophils (and other cells) and other anti-inflammatory signals favor macrophage polarization toward anti-inflammatory (M2c) or profibrotic (M2a) M2 phenotypes (Swaminathan & Griffin, 2008). Furthermore, tumor-conditioned granulocytes may play a role in priming macrophages toward either an M1 or M2 phenotype (Tsuda et al., 2004).

2.2 Monocytes and macrophages

Cells of monocyte/macrophage lineage are always present and are the predominant infiltrating cell type both in experimental models and in human chronic kidney diseases (CKDs). Macrophages produce a wide variety of different cytokines, chemokines and growth factors, reactive oxygen and nitrogen species, matrix metalloproteinases and component of the extracellular matrix. Thus, the presence of macrophages often correlates with the degree of fibrosis, so infiltrated macrophages has been considered to be key effector cells by modulating inflammatory response and subsequent proliferation of myofibroblasts, extracellular matrix deposition and other fibrotic processes (Eddy, 1995). However, a significant number of reports noted an inverse correlation between the number of interstitial macrophages and the degree of fibrosis, especially at the later stage of the CKD. Therefore macrophages are also assumed to have a role in the repair processes of the injured kidney (Kushiyama et al., 2010; Cochrane et al., 2005). How is it possible that macrophages have functions, which are so different from each other? Recent works indicates that recruited monocytes may differentiate into at least two different types of tissue macrophages (Anders & Riu, 2011). Renal infection (bacterial or fungal cell wall components, viruses), degraded ECM or cell necrosis induces the differentiation of proinflammatory, "classically activated" M1 macrophages that may exacerbate renal cell damage. In contrast, uptake of apoptotic cells induces "alternatively activated" M2 macrophages, which have anti-inflammatory (M2c/suppressor), profibrotic (M2a/wound healing) or fibrolytic (M2b) properties (Gordon & Taylor, 2005; Mosser & Edwards, 2008; Mantovani et al., 2004). In renal fibrosis, classically and alternatively activated macrophage functions are not always sharply separated from each other, since some factors are required in the development and functions of both types.

2.2.1 Classically activated 'M1' macrophages

Tissue injury triggers a rapid influx of neutrophils that is followed by an increased adhesion of circulating monocytes to the activated endothelial surfaces and their subsequent extravasation into the renal interstitium (Muller, 2009). In obstructive nephropathy, flow cytometric analysis revealed a marked increase in cell counts of macrophages in the obstructed kidney. The depletion of Mac-1/CD11b+ monocyte lineages including macrophages and dendritic cells attenuated renal fibrosis, thus suggesting the importance of monocyte lineage in the development of the early phase of renal fibrotic diseases (Machida et al., 2010). Duffield et al. also showed that macrophage depletion reduced the number of interstitial myofibroblasts and CD4+ T lymhocytes, and attenuated the degree of fibrosis in the diseased kidney (Duffield et al., 2005). Renal epithelial, capillary endothelial cells and infiltrated leukocytes produce various chemokines, which are responsible for the early recruitment of macrophages into the injured tissue (Crisman et al., 2001). For example the levels of CC chemokines (MCP-1/CCL-2, macrophage inhibitory protein (MIP)-1α/CCL-3, "regulated on activation normal T cell expressed and secreted" (RANTES/CCL-5)) are quickly increased after unilateral ureteral obstruction (UUO) (Vielhauer et al., 2001). Targeted deletion or blockade of these chemokines (Wada et al., 2004; Li et al., 2005) or chemokine receptors (Kitagawa et al., 2004; Eis et al., 2004) primarily interrupted the initial phase of macrophage infiltration and resulted in reduced inflammation and subsequent renal fibrosis. Also at the early stage of inflammation, DAMP (such as ATP, uric acid, hypomethylated DNA) or PAMP (such as bacterial lipopolysaccharide), lipoteichoic acid, peptidoglycan, double-stranded RNA, unmethylated CpG motifs) activate Toll-like (TLR) and other pattern recognition receptors of leukocytes and inherent renal cells. TLR activation on the monocytes and the presence of interferon (IFN)-γ are essential for the expression of interferon-related factor 5. It is required for the complete activation of NF-κB signaling and thus for the maturation of the proinflammatory M1 macrophage phenotype (Krausgruber et al., 2011). However, after the early inflammation response, in the progressive fibrotic stage macrophage activation may occur in TLR-independent pathways as well (Chowdhury et al., 2010). In addition, in the most types of glomerulonephritis, immune complexes can deposit in the glomerulus and bind leukocyte receptors including activating immunoglobulin Fc receptors and complement receptors to activate macrophages with similar activation and cytokine release pattern that described for DAMP/PAMP signals (Ravetch et al., 2001). The mature proinflammatory M1 macrophages then release matrix-metalloproteases (MMPs), which may induce the destruction of vascular and tubular basement membranes and further migration of inflammatory and fibrotic cells into the interstitial space (Song et al., 2000; Gibbs et al., 1999). MMPs also promote the degradation of ECM that results small ECM fragments, which can serve as immunstimulatory DAMP signals to maintain M1 macrophage phenotype (Sorokin, 2004). Stimulation of the production of MMPs by M1 macrophages during the later stages of fibrosis may shift the equilibrium towards ECM degradation and play an important anti-fibrotic role (see below). In M1 macrophages NF-κB is activated early after renal damage and controls the expression of multiple proinflammatory factors, such as chemokines (to recruit additional immune cells), adhesion molecules (to help the leukocyte adhesion and extravasation into the tissue), proinflammatory cytokines (to activate tissue or accumulated immune cells), lipid mediators and reactive oxygen species that support neutrophils in direct pathogen killing (Blackwell & Christman 1997). Furthermore, in M1 macrophages the synthesis of inducible nitric oxide synthase is also triggered by NF-κB proinflammatory pathway (Musial & Eissa, 2001). Nitric oxide (NO) produced by inducible nitric oxide synthase has a well known protective function against renal fibrosis (Hochberg et al., 2000; Morrissey et al., 1996). M1 macrophages express Major Histocompatibility Complex (MHC) class II molecules on their cell surface, so have antigen-presenting capacity to activate naive T cells by antigen-specific manner. In this process macrophage IL-12 and IL-18 as a cofactor play an important role, because they promote the generation of T helper (Th)1 cell phenotype and potentially maintenance of proinflammatory Th1 responses (Kitching et al., 2005). M1 macrophages produce one of the most important proinflammatory cytokine IL-6, which have a significant role in releasing acute phase proteins from the liver, which is an early sign of inflammation. Elevated levels of the acute phase C-reactive protein may promote early renal inflammation and fibrosis by the activation of both proinflammatory NF-κB and profibrotic transforming growth factor (TGF)-β/Smad signaling pathways (Li et al., 2011). Following renal damage, renal epithelial cells, denditic cells and M1 macrophages release large amount of TNF-α, which has a paracrine/autocrine effect on macrophage activation. TNF-α mediates proapoptotic effects to limit the survival of activated immune cells (Wajant et al., 2003), but also induces activation and apoptosis of renal mesangial cells (Misseri et al., 2005; Duffield et al., 2000). NF-κB regulates the expression of TNF-α, which in turn may activate NF-κB (Ozes et al., 1999). Like TNF-α, after renal injury IL-1 cytokine levels are also upregulated. IL-1 may contribute to the development of renal interstitial injury and fibrosis, because IL-1 receptor blockade decreases the number of infiltrated macrophages and alpha smooth muscle actin (α-SMA)+ myofibroblasts (Yamagishi et al., 2001).

2.2.2 Alternatively activated 'M2' macrophages

Apoptotic cells of the injured kidney are rapidly recognized and phagocytosed by macrophages. This process effectively promotes their differentiation into alternatively activated M2 macrophages (Ricardo et al., 2008; Fadok et al., 1998). M2 macrophages express typically high-level of scavenger and mannose receptors, which may promote macrophage activation and phagocytosis by a TLR-independent manner. Besides the phagocytosis of apoptotic cells, the induction of M2 macrophages requires other anti-inflammatory signals favor macrophage polarization, like Th2 or regulatory T (Treg) cytokines and other anti-inflammatory agents such as corticosteroids (Goerdt & Orfanos, 1999). Like M1 macrophages, M2 macrophages are also characterized by expression of MHC class II molecules, and have antigen-presenting capacity to activate naive T cells towards Th2 or Treg phenotype (Gordon, 2003). The phagocytosis of the apoptotic cells that generated during the early immune response especially promotes the differentiation of anti-inflammatory M2c/supressor phenotype (Swaminathan & Griffin, 2008). Regulatory T cells via release of IL-10 and TGF-β are also required to the polarization of macrophages towards type M2c. M2c macrophages attenuate organ injury by downregulating inflammation, predominantly the Th1 response (Herbert et al., 2004). They secrete anti-inflammatory mediators, such as IL-10, TGF-β and other immune suppressive factors (Mosser & Edwards, 2008). Furthermore, M2c macrophages play a positive role in epithelial (tubular reepithelization) and vascular (angiogenesis) repair and tissue remodeling. Insufficient tissue repair lead to increased secretion of different profibrotic cytokines and growth factors such as TGF-β (Kaneto et al., 1993) or platelet derived growth factor receptor (PDGF) (Fellström et al., 1989), which promote the differentiation of macrophages into M2a/wound healing macrophages that accelerate fibrogenesis (Gurtner et al., 2008). This process is supported by Th2 cells that release IL-4 and IL-13 cytokines, which further promote the polarization of M2a macrophage phenotype (Mantovani et al., 2004). M2a macrophages preferentially express the macrophage scavenger receptor (CD204), the mannose receptor (CD206) and fibronectin-1 which provide signals for tissue repair and proliferation. M2a macrophages are characterized by the generation of arginase-1, which may enhance collagen biosynthesis by supressing proinflammatory NO production (Bronte & Zanovello, 2005). Interestingly organ fibrosis may be reversible. Recently the role of fibrolytic M2b macrophages was demonstrated in this process. Actually M2b macrophages have the potential to limit or reverse fibrogenesis by the secretion of different matrix metalloproteinases (Ronco & Chatziantoniou, 2008). MMPs have a digestive capacity against ECM proteins (especially against collagen IV and denatured collagen I) without concomitant secretion of proinflammatory cytokines. Indeed MMPs have dual role in renal inflammation and fibrosis (Zeisberg et al., 2006). During UUO the expression of tissue inhibitor of metalloproteinases-1 (TIMP-1) and -2 (TIMP-2), which are the main regulators of MMP synthesis can vary. Increased TIMP activity during the early phase of renal fibrosis lead to the decreased expression of MMP-2 and MMP-9 in the obstructed kidneys, which inhibits the degradation of ECM components. However, TIMP expression is attenuated in the chronic stage of UUO, which allows MMP synthesis by fibrolytic macrophages and ECM degradation, so collagen levels may return to control values (Sharma et al., 1995; Kim et al., 2001). Recent studies demonstrated that the early inhibition of MMP-2 activity ameliorates renal fibrosis, but MMP-2 inhibition during the late phase of fibrosis may results in more severe disease progression (Nishida et al., 2007; Lutz et al., 2005).

2.3 Dendritic cells

Dendritic cells (DCs) are antigen-presenting innate immune cells, which belong to the mononuclear phagocyte system and fulfill a sentinel function. In the obstructed kidney, flow cytometric analysis showed– beside other leukocytes - increased number of F4/80+ macrophages and dendritic cells (Machida et al., 2010). Kitamoto et al. demonstrated in the early stage of UUO, that either F4/80+ monocytes/macrophages, F4/80+ dendritic cells, or both cell types contribute to the development of renal fibrosis and tubular apoptosis (Kitamoto et al., 2009). Other studies found that DC accumulation in the interstitium is associated with the loss of renal function and the progression of tubulointerstitial fibrosis (Wu et al., 2006; Zhou et al., 2009). According to their typical antigen and chemokine expression and the tendency to migrate toward inflamed tissue DCs are differentiated either myeloid (mDC) or plasmacytoid phenotype (pDC). Myeloid DCs are characterized by the expression of CD11c/blood dendritic cell antigen 1, while the specific marker of plasmacytoid DCs is the CD11c/ blood dendritic cell antigen 2. Verkade et al. showed an impaired terminal differentiation of mDCs in patients with severe chronic kidney disease (Verkade et al., 2007). Tucci et al found that the number of peripheral pDCs is correlated with the degree of lupus nephritis, whereas mDCs were almost absent in the glomeruli. In this disease only IL-18R+ pDCs were susceptible to increased expression of IL-18 and relocate within the glomeruli, where they triggers the resident T cells, thus promoting renal damage (Tucci et al., 2008, 2009). Infiltrated DCs become activated through pattern recognition receptors by DAMP/PAMP signals or by immune complexes via Fc receptors or complement receptors. These dendritic cells are the early source of the proinflammatory mediators after acute kidney injury and play a specific role in recruitment and activation of effector/memory T cells. The capacity of macrophages and dendritic cells to present antigens on MHC molecules and additionally produce IL-12/IL-23 or IL-10 strongly influences the outcome of the Th1/Th17 or Th2 T cell response (Langenkamp et al., 2000; Dong et al., 2008; Liu et al, 1998). Dendritic cell-specific intercellular adhesion molecule 3-grabbing nonintegrin (DC-SIGN) is a marker of dendritic cells, which is important for DC in migrating, recognizing, antigen presenting and in initiating T cell responses. In a nephritis model, the expression of DC-SIGN, which was mainly expressed on tubular epithelial cells and DCs correlated with the degree of fibrosis, and was elevated by TNF-α treatment. These results suggest that DC-SIGN plays an important role in renal fibrosis by DC-mediated immuno-inflammatory responses (Zhou et al., 2009). Angiotensin II (Ang II) mediates proinflammatory effect also in the relationship of DCs, because AngII blockade with the Ang II receptor antagonist valsartan inhibited the local accumulation of dendritic cells and attenuated renal tubulointerstitial damage in rat fibrotic renal tissue (Wu et al, 2006). Muller et al demonstrated by using human renin and angiotensinogen double-transgenic rats, that Ang II induces DC migration directly, whereas *in vivo* TNF-α is involved in DC infiltration and maturation (Muller et al., 2002).

2.4 Mast cells

Mast cells (MCs) are known to participate in the pathogenesis of tubulointerstitial fibrosis in the different kidney diseases (Colvin et al., 1974; Pavone-Macaluso, 1960). MCs are present in every vascularized tissue, including the kidney (Kitamura, 1989). The localization of MCs is mainly interstitial, or in smaller extent periglomerular, but they have were never found in the glomeruli (Ehara & Shigematsu, 1998; Hiromura et al., 1998). MCs can be identified by their specific granular proteoglycans content by staining with metachromatic dyes or by using immunohistochemical staining with anti-tryptase and anti-chymase antibodies. In general, three MC subtypes are present in the kidney: the tryptase-positive mucosal type, the double-positive tryptase–chymase connective tissue type, and the third chymase-positive type MCs. The ratio of the different subtypes of MCs (in the renal interstitium can differ in the various renal diseases (Beil et al., 1998). There are certain factors, which can promote the recruitment of MCs into the damaged kidney. Perhaps the most well known is the stem cell factor, which is known as the prototypic growth factor for MCs. Stem cell factor is produced mainly by tubular epithelial cells and by infiltrating interstitial leukocytes (El-Koraie et al., 2001). TGF-β also has been described as a powerful chemoattractant for MCs (Gruber et al., 1994). In addition to these factors, IL-9, a Th2 cytokine, may enhance survival and proliferation of MCs (Godfraind et al., 1998). The activation of mast cells takes place by different ways: while the classical pathway of mast cell activation is through Immunglobulin (Ig)E-Fcε receptor crosslinking (Beaven & Metzger, 1993), the alternative way includes the activation of pattern recognition (such as TLRs) (McCurdy et al., 2001; Supajatura et al., 2002) or complement receptors (Prodeus et al., 1997). Activated MCs have a capacity to secrete a large variety of inflammatory mediators such as a range of bioactive amines and proteoglycans; histamine, which is a potent vasodilator and enhance vascular permeability; lipid mediators such as prostaglandins and leukotrienes, which are potent chemoattractants for CD8+ T cells and a large set of chemokines and cytokines, which are able to recruiting and activating leukocytes (Galli et al., 2005). Furthermore, they promote the vascular endothelial expression of selectins and adhesion molecules, which indirectly support leukocyte recruitment (Meng et al., 1995). MCs also have a direct immunoregulatory role by interacting with T cells, B cells, and dendritic cells (Galli et al., 2005). They are able to present antigens to naive T cells in an MHC-restricted manner (Dimitriadou et al., 1998) and influence T cell differentiation towards Th2 (by IL-4, IL-10 and histamin) (Jutel et al., 2002) or Th17 phenotype (Nakae et al., 2007). Furthermore, MCs seem to be essential to induce the development of Tregs that limit the infiltration of autoreactive T cells, and mediate peripheral tolerance (Lu et al., 2006). Experimental studies suggest that degranulation of MCs leads to the release of TGF-β, TNF-α, MCP-1, fibroblast growth factor (FGF), vascular endothelial growth factor (VEGF), IL-4 and MMP-9 and a variety of unique proteases, principally tryptase and chymase (Holdsworth & Summers, 2008), which contribute to progressive fibrogenesis (Cairns & Walls, 1997). Tryptase is prestored in cytoplasmic granules of MCs and has potent proteolytic activity against ECM proteins (Payne & Kam, 2004) and it supports the proliferation of fibroblasts and the synthesis of type I collagen (Cairns & Walls, 1997). Chymase can activate MMP-2 and MMP-9, disrupt of tight junction proteins (Scudamore et al., 1998) and involved in the activation of renin-angiotensin system (Huang et al., 2003). On the other hand MCs can also participate in tissue remodeling and restoration of the normal kidney homeostasis (Bradding et al., 2006; Bankl & Valent, 2002). For example heparin produced by MCs is a potent anti-thrombotic, anti-inflammatory, anti-coagulant and anti-fibrotic agent, which is able to modulate renal fibroblast proliferation by arachidonic acid-derived lipid mediators such as leukotriene and prostaglandin (Clarkson et al., 1998) or by inhibition of TGF-β (Miyazawa et al., 2004).

2.5 T lymphocytes

T lymphocytes are main effector cells of adaptive immune system and activated by specific antigen stimuli. Although macrophages constitute the predominant infiltrating cell population of the injured kidneys, increased number of T lymphocytes were also observed in chronic renal diseases. It is also well known that the degree of tubulointerstitial fibrosis is related to the number of infiltrating T cell, implying their role in the fibrotic process (Tapmeier et al., 2010). In accordance with this observation Niedermayer et al. have shown that lymphocyte deficiency cause a substantial reduction in collagen I deposition in the obstructed kidney (Niedermayer et al., 2009). In the early phase of renal injury chemoattractants released by damaged and infiltrating immune cells directing the migration of activated T lymphocytes into the injured tissue. In this process CC (RANTES/CCL5), CXC (IP-10/CXCL10) chemokines, MIPs, lipid mediators (leukotriene) and anaphylatoxic complement fragments play a pivotal role (Kuroiwa et al., 2000). The activation of T cells occurs by antigenspecific manner. Antigens are presented by MHC molecules expressed on the cell surface of antigen-presenting cells (dendritic cells, macrophages, B cells) and recognized by T cell receptor/CD3 complex, which are the specific antigen-recognizing receptors of T lymphocytes. There are two different populations of the effector T lymphocytes: while CD8+ cytotoxic T cells have a direct cell-killing activity, Th cells are characterized by the expression of CD4 costimulator molecule and release a wide range of cytokines to mediate immune functions. Endogen antigens are presented on MHC type I molecules to CD8+ T cells, while exogen antigens are presented on MHC type II molecules to CD4+ T cells. After antigen recognition T cells become activated effector T cells or long-lived memory T cells. Cytokines released by the antigen presenting cells, such as macrophages and dendritic cells play a pivotal role in polarization of CD4+ T cells to different Th subtypes: IL-12 and IL-18 as a cofactor promote the generation of Th1 phenotype and the proinflammatory Th1-type cellular immune response. In Goldblatt hypertensive rats antihypertensive therapy induces a significant proinflammatory Th1 immune response with increased Th1-type chemokine (IP-10) and cytokine (IFN-γ) expression (Steinmetz et al., 2007). Similarly, the absence of Ang II type 1 receptor (AT1) in AT1R KO mice is associated with Th1-type immune response (Ouyang et al., 2005). IFN-γ, which is secreted by Th1 cells (and also other immune cells) is required to the classical activation of M1-type macrophages, which have proinflammatory but not fibrotic properties. These data suggest that Th1 cells mediate proinflammatory, rather than fibrotic effects. Th2 lymphocytes may mediate the activation of alternatively activated M2 type macrophages by producing IL-4, IL-5, IL-10, IL-13 and TGF-β. The activated M2 macrophages may promote fibrotic diseases and mediate collagen synthesis, suggesting the role of Th2-mediated immune response in fibrotic process (Wynn, 2004). Beside Th1-Th2 polarization, the Treg-Th17 axis is the other important player of immune response observed in chronic kidney diseases. Foxp3+ Treg have immunoregulatory and anti-inflammatory role via release of TGF-β and IL-10 (Mu et al., 2005). IL-10-secreting Treg cells suppress the activation of Th1, Th2 and Th17 cells, thus ameliorate the severity of inflammatory process, for example in mice with lupus nephritis (Zhang et al., 2010). Treg cells may promote the polarization of monocytes towards M2 macrophages, which may mediate profibrotic effects. Th17 cells produce IL-17 (IL-17A), IL-17F, IL-21, IL-22 which may promote inflammation by directly causing tissue injury and enhancing secretion of proinflammatory cytokines and chemokines by resident cells. This results in augmented infiltration of leukocytes, mainly neutrophils to the injured tissue where they induce inflammation (Turner et al., 2010). Dudas et al. described that IL-17A also mediate proinflammatory/profibrotic activity on proximal tubule epithelial cells that may contribute to allograft rejection (Dudas et al., 2011). In general both CD8 and CD4 positive cells may directly stimulate the migration, proliferation and differentiation of renal cells resulting in the accumulation of α-SMA positive myofibroblasts. T cells may also act indirectly on the infiltrating macrophage population by inducing a profibrotic phenotype, which, in turn, secrete pro-proliferative and profibrotic cytokines and growth factors (for example PDGF, TGF-β). Moreover, T cells may directly interact with epithelial cells to induce secretion of cytokines and growth factors that, in turn, act on fibroblasts (Strutz & Neilson, 1994).

2.6 B lymphocytes

B lymphocytes are effector cells of the adaptive immune system. B cells are activated through their specific antigen-recognizing B cell receptor complex on T cell dependent or independent manner. Activated B cells mature to plasma cells and mediate humoral immune response by producing specific antibodies or differentiate into long-lived memory B cells. B cells themselves may also act as antigen presenting cells and influence T cell response in the lymphoid folliculi. B cells may contribute to renal fibrosis in different ways, but their exact role in the process is less known. On the one hand autoantibodies produced by B cells are largely present in immune complexes, which may accumulate in the glomeruli in severe autoimmune and kidney diseases and activate innate immune cells by their immunoglobulin Fc receptors. Autoantibody synthesis could also occur after bacterial or viral infection, oxidant synthesis, or T cell mediated immunity.

On the other hand infiltrated B cells have an important role in renal interstitial inflammation: indeed, Heller et al. found that mature B cells formed a prominent part of the renal interstitial infiltrating cells in renal biopsies from patients with acute or chronic interstitial nephritis and IgA nephropathy. The expression of CXCL13, which is a chemoattractant for B cells, was elevated in these inflamed kidneys. CXCL13 level was correlated with the infiltrated B cell number and contributed to the formation of intrarenal lymphoid follicle-like structures, which might represent an intrarenal immune system (Heller et al., 2007). B cell activating factor - which belongs to TNF superfamily - has an important role in the development and survival of B lymphocytes. Xu et al. demonstrated in kidney allograft biopsies, that B cell activating factor expression may be associated with the development of antibody-mediated allograft rejection and renal interstitial fibrosis in kidney transplants (Xu et al., 2009). Moreover, IgG4-associated tubulointerstitial nephritis is characterized by high levels of serum IgG4 and IgE and a significant number of IgG4-producing plasma cells in the renal fibrotic lesions (Saeki et al., 2007; Raissian et al., 2011).

2.7 Complement activation

Complement system is an essential, and conserved part of the immune system, defends the host against invading pathogens, prevents immune complex disease and aids the acquired immune response. It consists of a number of small proteins, which are generally synthesized by the liver and normally circulating in the blood as inactive precursors. In response to several triggers, proteases (convertases) cleave the specific proteins of the complement system and initiate a cascade of further cleavages. Finally the activated complement proteins as multimeric membrane attack complexes bind to the surface of target cells and and lyse them (Lesher & Song, 2010). Immune complexes contain a large amount of complement fragments, which may accumulate in the glomeruli in different autoimmune diseases and activate the innate immune cells by their complement receptors. Detection of complement deposition in the glomerulus using immunochemistry has become an important element of the histological analysis of renal biopsies, and is key to the diagnosis of many types of glomerulonephritis. In recent years it has become evident that complement activation is involved in the pathogenesis of other types of renal disease including progressive tubulointerstitial fibrosis (Brown et al., 2007). For example, deficiency in the expression of C5 (Boor et al., 2007), C4d (Xu et al., 2009) or C6 (He et al., 2005) complement fragments caused reduced renal damage and interstitial fibrosis in different kidney diseases. Blocking the receptors of the potent anaphylatoxins C5a and C3a lead to significantly reduced renal leukocyte infiltration, tubulointerstitial inflammation and fibrosis (Boor et al., 2007; Bao et al., 2011).

3. Important molecular pathways

In addition to the above mentioned activation of the immune cells the increased amount of different cytokines and growth factors are also participate in the accumulation of the ECM in renal the interstitium along the tubules. To date more than a dozen different cytokines (IFNγ, IL-1), growth factors (TGF, connective tissue growth factor, bone morphogenic protein, Insulin-like growth factor-1, TNFα) and other molecules (Ang II, NO) have been demonstrated to induce interstitial inflammation, maturation of myofibroblasts and degradation or production of ECM. Here we are going to summarize our knowledge about TGFβ, Ang II and PDGF and their downstream signaling pathways.

3.1 Transforming Growth Factor β (TGF β)

TGFβ is a member of the TGFβ superfamily that include activins, inhibins and bone morfogenic proteins (Peng, 2003). In the healthy kidney TGFβ participate in the maintaining of the homeostasis. However, when the kidney is exposed to an injury then TGFβ is excessively produced by the resident renal cells and also by the infiltrating leukocytes (Border & Noble, 1993; Coimbra et al., 1996; Eddy, 2000). Fukuda et al. (Fukuda et al., 2001) using in situ hybridization and immunohistochemistry demonstrated that TGFβ1 is mainly expressed by mesangial and epithelial cells of the glomeruli and the distal tubules in the healthy kidneys. Following UUO they observed increased TGFβ1 expression in the renal tubular epithelial cells of the renal cortex and outer medulla and also in the infiltrating macrophages. Indeed similar upregulation of TGFβ is present in every animal model of chronic renal disease and also in humans (Ketteler et al., 1994).

TGFβ1 and its isoforms (TGFβ2 and 3) are secreted as precursos in a complex with latent TGFβ binding proteins. TGFβ become active when it is cleaved by plasmin, thrombospondin-1 or reactive oxygen species and thus dissociated from latent TGFβ binding proteins. The activated TGFβ then form dimers and bind to their type I and II cell-surface serin/threonine kinase receptors (TBR I and TBR II, respectively). So far two TBR I (activin like receptor kinase 1 and 5) and one TBR II (TGFBR2) have been have been shown to bind TGFβ. TGFβ first binds to the constitutively active TBR II followed by the phosphorylation of the glycine/serin rich domain of the TBR I to create activated receptor heterodimer. Subsequently the activated receptor complex phosphorilates the downstream signaling mediators such as SMAD2/3, ERK1/2, Jun N-terminal Kinase 1/2 (Matsuzaki & Okazaki, 2006). In the injured tissue TGFβ through its activated signaling pathways can trigger the increased production and decreased degradation of ECM (Pohlers et al., 2009) and thus the renal fibrosis. Koesters et al. showed marked peritubular fibrosis in the double transgenic mice overexpressing TGFβ1 in their tubular epithelial cells (Koesters et al., 2010). They observed the proliferation of the peritubular cells and the deposition of collagen type I rich ECM. Moreover, they observed the TGFβ1 dependent autophagy of the tubular cells which may represent a novel mechanism of tubular decomposition. On the other hand Isaka et al. demonstrated that introduction of antisense oligodeoxynucleotides against TGFβ1 into interstitial fibroblasts block the interstitial fibrosis in rats with unilateral ureteral obstruction (Isaka et al., 2000). Similarly, Miyajima et al. observed that administration of neutralizing anti-TGFβ1 antibody attenuate the tubular apoptosis in a rat model of UUO (Miyajima et al., 2000). Also Decorin, which is an ECM protein that bind TGFβ, or soluble TGFβ receptor have been also shown to inhibit renal fibrosis (Peters et al., 1997; De Heer et al., 2000).

3.2 Renin-Angiotensin System

The RAS is the most important regulator of blood pressure, fluid and electrolyte homeostasis. The different components of the Renin-Angiotensin System, such as angiotensinogen, renin, AngI, angiotensin converting enzyme (ACE) Ang II, aldosterone and Ang II type I and II (AT1, AT2, respectively) receptors are all present in the kidney. Renin acts on angiotensinogen to form AngI, which is then converted by ACE to Ang II. The effects of Ang II are mediated by two high affinity receptors, AT1 and AT2. Since the overall abundance of AT1 receptors significantly exceeds that of AT2 type receptors in the adult kidney the most effects of Ang II are mediated through the AT1 receptor (Siragy, 2004). AT1 receptors are distributed on the luminal surface of the renal tubules, including proximal tubule, thick ascending limb of loop of Henle, distal tubule, macula densa and collecting duct (Allen et al., 2000). Recently the urinary angiotensinogen (Kim et al., 2011) and the intrarenal Ang II level (Del Prete et al., 2003) have been demonstrated to correlate with the severity of the chronic renal disease. As Ang II plays a key role in regulation of vascular tone (Cockcroft et al., 1995) and may induce proteinuria (Ren et al., 2011), oxidative stress, inflammation and renal fibrosis (Benigni et al., 2010) it is not surprising that ACE inhibitors or AT1 receptor antagonists have a renoprotective effect, which is independent from their antihypertensive effect (Mallamaci et al., 2011). Actually, the captopril trial on patients with type I diabetic nephropathy patients has shown a 50 % reduction in the end point of death by captopril administration (Lewis et al, 2003). Although the clinical relevance of Ang II in chronic renal disease is obvious, its precise role is still unclear. It is well known that Ang II may induce EMT on the epithelial cells in vitro. However, since the significance of in vivo

EMT is strongly questioned the in vivo relevance of Ang II on EMT is also questionable. Recently Kang et al. revealed that Ang II may decrease the NF-E2-related factor 2 (Nrf2) mediated signaling in murine renal epithelial TCMK-1 cells (Kang et al., 2011). Nrf2 is a transcriptional factor which by binding to the antioxidant response element on the promoter of different antioxidant genes can induce their expression. Kang et al. suggested that Ang II by inducing activating transcription factor 3 expression could inhibit the Nrf2 mediated upregulation of the antioxidant genes. Ang II increases vascular permeability via the release of prostaglandins and VEGF; contribute to the recruitment of inflammatory cells into the tissue through the regulation of adhesion molecules, chemokines (MCP-1, RANTES) and other molecules (osteopontin, see above) by resident cells; could directly activate infiltrating immunocompetent cells by cytokines (such as IL-6). AT1R or AT2R blockade (Esteban et al., 2003; Kellner et al., 2006) or treatment with ACE inhibitors (Ishidoya et al., 1995) greatly reduced monocyte/macrophage infiltration in short-term UUO, and AT1R-deficient macrophages have impaired phagocytic function (Nishida et al., 2002). Finally Ang II also may increase the expression of other molecules that play a pivotal role in organ fibrosis inducing TGFβ, TNFα or PDGF or bFGF (Rüster & Wolf, 2011). Moreover Ang II can potentiate the effect of TGFβ on the expression of SMA in TCMK-1 cells. Furthermore, AngII participates in tissue repair and remodeling, through the regulation of cell growth and matrix synthesis (Suzuki et al., 2003).

3.3 Platelet Derived Growth Factor (PDGF)

PDGF is a growth factor that regulates multiple cell function, such as cell growth (Bonner, 2004) or division and in particular in formation of blood vessels (Hellberg et al., 2010). Recently, its role in organ fibrosis has been also suggested (Trojanowska, 2008). PDGF family consist of five homo- or heterodimeric growth factors (PDGF-AA, -AB, -BB, -CC and -DD). PDGF-A has two splice variant, a longer (≈16 kD) which is retained to the cell surface and a shorter, which is released into the extracellular space. PDGF-AA and -BB can bind to different ECM proteins. PDGF-CC and -DD were identified just recently. PDGF-CC and -DD are secreted in a latent form and cleavage of the N terminal CUB (complement subcomponent C1r/C1s, Uegf and Bmp1) domain is required for their activation. While PDGF-CC is activated by tissue type plasminogen activator and plasmin PDGF-DD is activated by urokinase type plasminogen activator. Many inherent renal cell express one or more PDGF isoforms, such as pericytes (Winkler et al., 2010), podocytes (Changsirikulchai et al., 2002), endothelial (Eitner et al., 2003), tubular epithelial (Eitner et al., 2002) and smooth muscle cells (Seifert et al., 1998). The different isoforms of PDGF bind to the homo- or heterodimeric tyrosine kinase receptors (PDGFR-αα, -ββ and -αβ). The specifity and affinity of the different PDGF monomers to the α or β chain of the receptor PDGFRs are different. While PDGF-A can bind to the α, PDGF-B to the α and β chains. The receptor affinity of PDGF-C and –D is less characterized, but it is likely that similarly to PDGF-B they can bind to the α and β chain as well. Upon receptor binding the α and β chains dimerize and possesses tyrosine kinase activity. After autophosphorylation the PDGFRs provide docking site for downstream signaling molecules containing SH2 (Floege J, 2008), SH3, PTB, PH (Andrae et al., 2008) and other domains thus activating several signaling pathways such as MAPK, PLCγ or PI3K (Ostendorf et al., 2011). Increased expression of the different PDGF isoforms was observed in most if not all animal models of kidney injury. PDGFR-α chain, which is the receptor for PDGF-A and -C is widely expressed in the different renal cell types, such as myofibroblasts, mesangial and smooth muscle cells (Alpers et al., 1993). Interestingly, while infusion of high doses of PDGF-A (5mg/kg) did not induced renal lesion (Tang et al., 1996) inhibition of PDGF-C with a neutralizing antibody exhibited a significant reduction of renal fibrosis, myofibroblast accumulation and decreased leukocyte infiltration in a mice model of UUO (Eitner et al., 2008). PDGF-BB has a central proliferative effect on the mesangial cells. Actually infusion of PDGF-BB into of healthy rats led to increased mesangial cell proliferation and accumulation of the mesangial matrix (Tang et al., 1996). More recently, the role of PDGF has been suggested in the transformation of pericytes, the main source of myofibroblasts, into myofibroblasts following kidney injury (Chen et al., 2011). Inhibition of PDGFR-α or PDGFR-β signaling with a neutralizing antibody or with Imatinib, a PDGF tyrosine kinase inhibitor, treatment the UUO induced differentiation and proliferation of the pericytes decreased. The treatment of the animals with a neutralizing antibody against PDGFR-α or PDGFR-β reduced the UUO induced macrophage infiltration, renal TGFβ, PDGF and CCL2 expression and renal fibrosis. Hence PDGFR-α and PDGFR-β are potential candidates for antifibrotic therapy in the future.

4. Origin of myofibroblasts

Understanding the origin of myofibroblasts in the kidney is great interest because these cells are responsible for scar formation in fibrotic kidney diseases. Myofibroblasts have migratory capacity, are resistant to apoptosis, and can produce different components of the extracellular matrix, growth factors, cytokines and therefore contribute to organ fibrosis and to the maintenance of inflammation (Zeisberg et al., 2008). Actually, in the healthy kidney there are no known endogenous myofibroblasts. In the fibrotic kidney (as in other organs) the origin of the renal myofibroblast is still controversial, however there are some hypotheses. Recently the derivation of myofibroblasts from epithelial or endothelial cells, fibrocytes and pericytes has been suggested (Fig. 1.).

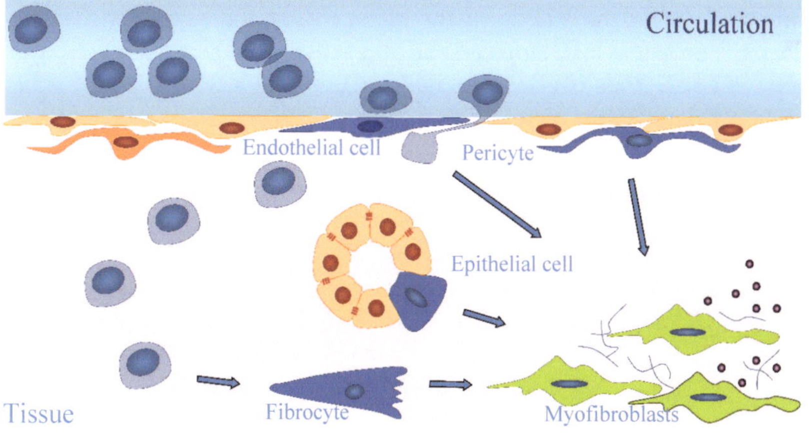

Fig. 1. Different possible origins of the myofibroblasts. There are different hypothesis about the possible origin of the myofibroblasts, which are effector cells of the organ fibrosis. The derivation of the myofibroblasts from endothelial and epithelial cells, from fibrocytes and pericytes (also known as perivascular cells, resident fibroblast or Rouget cells) has been suggested.

4.1 Epithelial-mesenchymal transition (EMT)

A hypothesis that recently has become popular is the mesenchymal transition of the renal tubular epithelial cells. The process when the epithelial cells lose their polarity and epithelial adhesion properties and starts the de novo synthesis of mesenchymal markers, such as αSMA is the so called EMT. This process is already well known in different physiological and pathological processes, notably in embryogenesis, carcinogenesis (Kalluri & Weinberg, 2009). The first remarkable evidence of EMT in the fibrotic kidney was demonstrated by Ng et al (Ng et al., 1998). They investigated the localization of αSMA after 1-21 weeks of 5/6 nephrectomy of Sprague-Dawley rats. In normal kidneys in situ hybridization and immunohistochemical staining revealed the mRNA or protein expression of αSMA only in the vascular smooth muscle cells. Later on the 3rd week after the 5/6 nephrectomy, mRNA and protein expression of αSMA was present in the proximal tubular epithelial cells (TEC) as well. Indeed they observed a gradually increasing number of αSMA+ TEC peaking at week 9. Moreover, about 70% of the αSMA+ TEC were proliferating based on their proliferating cell nuclear antigen positivity. Finally these cells became elongated separated from their neighboring cells and appeared to migrate into the renal interstitium through the damaged basement membrane. These original observations were confirmed at the ultrasructural level of the renal tubules by electron microscopy. They found that in the early transformed TECs contain large round or oval shaped nucleus, several mitochondria indicating the activation of these cells. Characteristic microfilaments and dense bodies (stress fibers) were present in the transformed TECs, lying next to the damaged TBM. Later in advanced state of EMT TECs exhibit elongated morphology and abundant microfilaments and dense bodies. At this stage microfilaments are diffusely fill the entire cytoplasm of TECs. Later Iwano et al. strengthened the hypothesis of in vivo EMT using genetic fate mapping method (Iwano et al., 2002). Briefly, they developed transgen mice that express Cre recombinase under the promoter of γGT. As γGT is a brush border protein, its promoter is active only in the proximal TECs (PTEC). These γGT-Cre mice were then bred with a R26R reporter mice (Fig. 2). In the PTECs of the bigenic mice the expressed Cre recombinase mediates the excision of the loxP stop cassette and activate the expression of β galactosidase from the gene of LacZ. Thus irreversibly marking the PTECs with β galactosidase, despite the subsequent phenotypic changes.

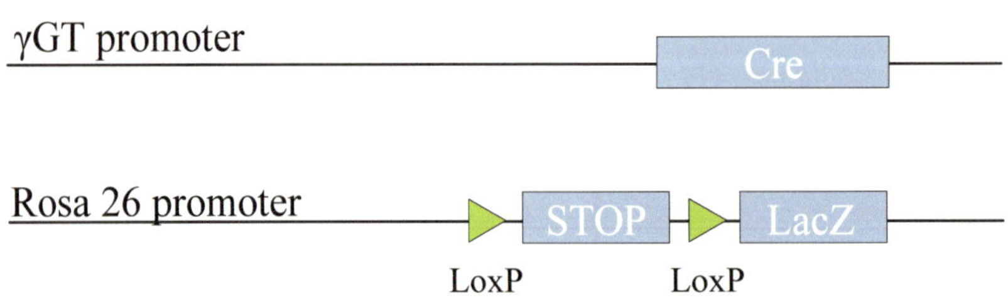

Fig. 2. Model of transgen mice that express Cre recombinase under the promoter of γGT. These γGT-Cre mice were then bred with a R26R reporter mice.

Later, ten days after UUO the PTECs of the double transgenic, γGT-Cre; R26R mice started to express (beside β galactosidase) fibroblast specific protein-1 (FSP-1), suggesting the EMT of TECs (Fig. 3/b; LacZ-red and FSP1-green, merge-yellow). Some of these FSP-1 and β galactosidase double positive PTECs also began to take an elongated shape of myofibroblasts (Fig. 3/b; arrows). Moreover, these double positive cells appeared in the fibrotic tissues surrounding the tubules (Fig. 3/c and d). Finally by counting the FSP1 and LacZ immunopositive cells in the renal interstitium, they suggested that after 10 days of UUO about 36% of the myofibroblasts originate from the renal tubular epithelial cells.

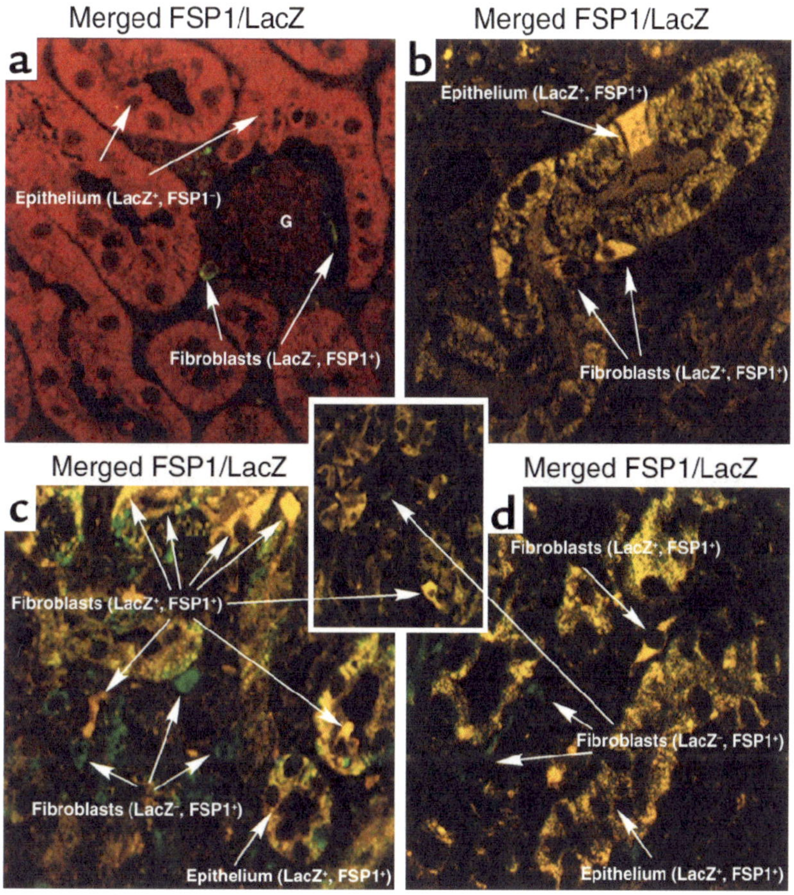

Fig. 3. Confocal microscopy images of contralateral (a) and injured (b, c and d) kidneys 10 days after the UUO (Iwano et al., 2002). Proximal tubular epithelial cells are stained with an anti-β galactosidase antibody (red) and the fibroblasts with an anti-FSP1 antibody (green). (b, c, d) Ten days after the onset of UUO the β galactosidase positive PTECs also expressed FSP-1 (β galactosidase+/FSP-1+ PTECs cells staining yellow), suggesting the mesenchymal transition of cells. (b, c, d) Some of these FSP-1+ PTECs (arrow) had the elongated shape of myofibroblasts, and appeared in the fibrotic tissues surrounding the tubules. (After Iwano et al., 2002)

Subsequently numerous in vitro studies confirmed the original observation of Ng (Ng et al., 1998) and Iwano et al. (Iwano et al., 2002). These studies on different cell lines (HK-2, HEK298, NRK) and on primer renal tubular epithelial cells have clearly shown that epithelial cells when exposed to hypoxia, reactive oxygen species, advanced glycation end products, pro-fibrotic cytokines, TGF-β1, angiotensin II (ANGII), platelet-derived growth factor, epidermal growth factor and fibroblast growth factor-2 (Liu, 2010) growth factors or metalloproteinases (Yang & Liu, 2001) may undergo EMT. During EMT these molecules activate different signaling pathways on a coordinated manner. As a result the Ras/Rho GTPase, Rho-activated kinase, c-Src tyrozin kinase, Integrin-linked kinase, Wnt-1, Smad 2 and 3, p38 mitogen-activated protein kinase, extracellular signal-regulated kinase (ERK) and phosphatidil-inositol-3 kinase (PI3K) signaling pathways can be activated (Thiery & Sleeman, 2006). Activation of these signaling pathways leads to the phenotypical conversion of the TECs. During EMT TECs lose their cellular polarity, downregulate epithelial markers and acquire mesenchymal features, such as the de novo synthesis of α-SMA. Finally the epithelial cells are transformed to myofibroblasts as a determinative step in renal fibrosis (Iwano et al., 2002). In the 2008 EMT congress in Cold Spring Harbor according to the in vivo and in vitro findings this process that led to tissue scaring was defined as type II EMT. Based on these studies EMT has been widely accepted as one of the main mechanism by which myofibroblast formed during renal fibrosis. However the presence of this phenomenon, even on primer epithelial cells is evident in vitro, recently it has been questioned in vivo. Unfortunately, the results of Iwano et al. have not been confirmed by other groups. In contrast others using genetic fate mapping techniques were not able to demonstrate any evidence of EMT in vivo. Humphreys et al. developed two transgenic Cre driver mice that express bacterial Cre recombinase under the regulation of Six2 or HoxB7 promoters (Humphreys et al., 2010) (Fig. 4/A). Both Six2 and HoxB7 are transcriptional factors that transiently expressed during development. Six2 is expressed only in those cells of metanephric mesenchyme that are fated to be epithelial cell of the proximal or distal tubules. HoxB7 is expressed in the cells of ureteric bund that are fated to be the cells of the collecting duct. These transgenic mice were bred with R26R reporter mice expressing β galactosidase. In the kidney samples of the healthy Six2-Cre; R262 bigenic mice strong epithelial β galactosidase activity was present in the podocytes and in the whole tubulus until the collecting duct. In case of HoxB7-Cre; R262 double transgenic mice this positivity was restricted to the epithelia of the collecting duct (Figure 4/B). Fourteen days after the UUO there was no change in the localization of β galactosidase activity. β galactosidase activity was present in the epithelial cell of the bigenic mice (Six2-Cre; R262 or HoxB7-Cre; R262), but none of the αSMA positive interstitial cells were positive for β galactosidase activity. These results strongly suggest that epithelial cells do not leave their original place, behind the basement membrane and they do not migrate into the interstitium of the ureteral obstructed kidney.

Based on these conflicting data it is not evident whether in vivo EMT is an existing process in the fibrotic kidney or not. While in vitro data strongly suggest the existence of EMT in vivo studies of Humphreys et al. and others suggest that TECs do not invade the basement membrane and do not become real interstitial myofibroblasts (Humphreys et al., 2010). But are the in vitro and in vivo data really contradictory? Actually in vitro studies investigate the molecular mechanism of EMT but do not investigate the basement membrane invading capacity of the transformed cells. On the other hand in vivo experiments investigate the basement membrane invading capacity of the TECs but do not investigate the molecular changes of the TECs during the fibrotic process. So some scientists believe that the aim of the in vitro and in vivo studies is different and thus the results of these studies are not necessarily contradictory.

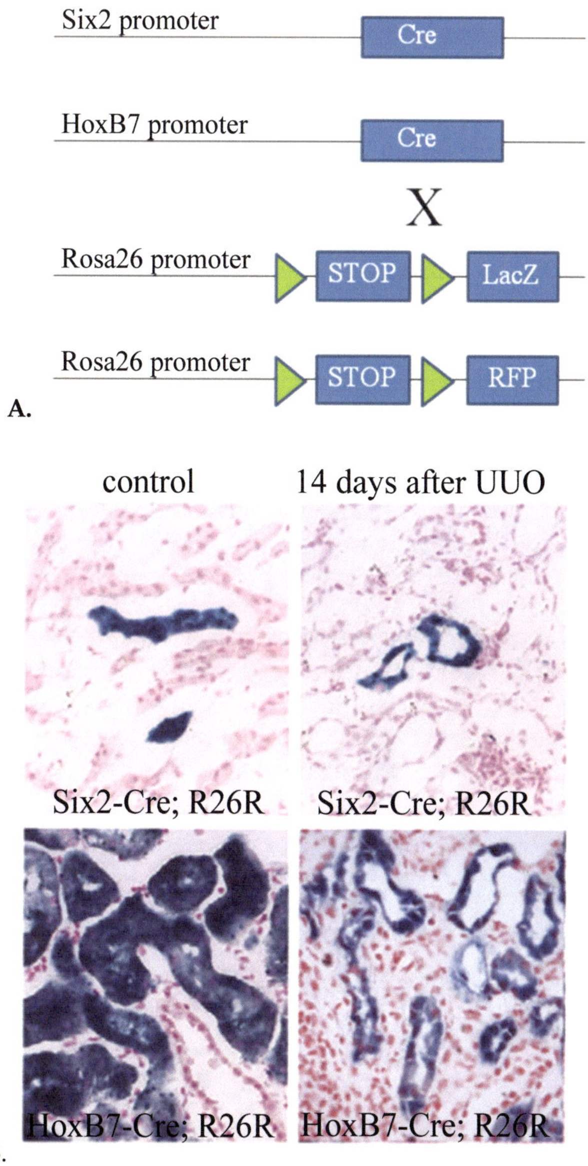

Fig. 4. Control and kidneys 14 days after the UUO from *Six2-GC; R26R* and *HoxB7-Cre; R26R* mice show no evidence for β galactosidase activity in the renal interstitium. A: Double transgen *Six2-GC; R26R* mice activated Cre expression in the cells of the metanephric mesenchyme that are fated to become the cells of the renal tubules. Expression of Cre results in removal of the LoxP-STOP-LoxP sequence in epithelial cells, leading to permanent, heritable expression of β galactosidase in epithelial cells. Similarly in *HoxB7-Cre; R26R* mice activation of Cre expression in the ureteric bud led to the expression of β galactosidase in the epithelial cells of the collecting duct. B: Representative light microscopy images of X-gal stain indicating of β galactosidase activity in the control (left) and in the obstructed (right) kidneys. (After Humphreys et al., 2002)

4.2 Endothelial-mesenchymal transition (EndMT)

EndMT was first described during embryonic heart development, where mesenchymal cells of the endocardial cushion (a tissue that later gives rise to the cardiac septa and valves) arise from endothelial cells of the endocardium. Endothelium is a specialized type of a squamous type epithelium. Thus EndMT is a specific form of EMT. Simirarly to EMT during EndMT endothelial cells (EC) lose their endothelial markers and acquire markers of myofibroblasts. Studies on different organs have demonstrated the relevance of EndMT in the pathomechanism of organ fibrosis. Zeisberg et al. used Tie1 Cre; R26R bigenic mice to fate the EC during cardiac fibrosis (Zeisberg et al., 2007a). They have demonstrated that EC undergo phenotypic conversion and contribute to organ fibrosis. Similarly, Hashimoto et al. using Tie2 Cre; CAG-CAT-LacZ transgenic mice have shown that EC give a significant percent of myofibroblasts in bleomycin induced pulmonary fibrosis (Hashimoto et al., 2010). Recently, the importance of EndMT was suggested in different models of renal fibrosis as well. Zeisberg et al. investigated the contribution of endothelial cells to fibrosis in different animal models of CKD: 1) a mouse model of unilateral obstructive nephropathy; 2) a model of streptozotocin (STZ) induced DN; 3) a mouse model of Alport disease (COL4A3 KO, lack the collagen IV α3 chain). First they investigated the effect of UUO on the population of FSP-1 or αSMA positive myofibroblast. Previously, it has been demonstrated that FSP-1 or αSMA identify distinct population of myofibroblast with a minimal overlap between the different populations (Zeisberg et al., 2007a, 2007b). One week after the ligation of the ureter the number of the FSP-1 or αSMA positive myofibroblast population increased. To investigate the possible endothelial origin of the myofibroblast double immunostaining were performed. The number of the CD31 (marker of the EC) and FSP-1 or CD31 and αSMA positive myofibroblasts were 36% or 25%, respectively (Fig. 5).

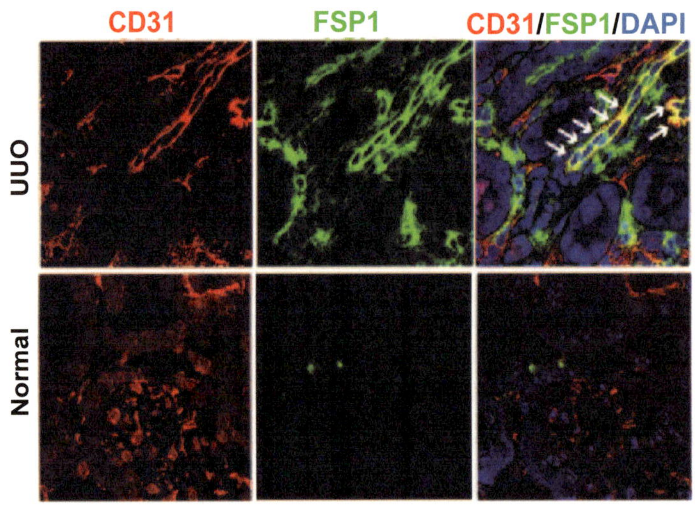

Fig. 5. Immune fluorescent staining to investigate the possible endothelial origin of the myofibroblast. CD31 (red) is a marker of ECs, FSP-1 (green) is that of myofibroblasts. (After work of Zeisberg et al., 2007).

To strengthen the endothelial origin of these double CD31 and FSP-1 or CD31 and αSMA myofibroblast they performed UUO in Tie2-Cre; EYFP double transgenic mice. In these mice cells of endothelial origin express yellow fluorescent protein (YFP). After UUO a substantial portion of FSP-1 or αSMA positive myofibroblast coexpressed YFP, suggesting their endothelial origin. These data strongly suggest that EndMT may account for a considerable percent of myofibroblasts in the mouse model of UUO. Zeisberg et al. also investigated the origin of myofibroblasts in a mouse STZ induced DN. They have demonstrated that 6 moths after the induction diabetes about 50% of the αSMA and 40% of the FSP-1 positive cells were also CD31 positive in the kidney, suggesting the relevance of EndMT in the fibrotic changes in DN. Finally, Zeisberg et al. investigated the origin of myofibroblast in COL4A3 KO mice, in a model of Alport syndrome. In these mice proteinuria, glomerulonephritis and tubulointersitial fibrosis starts at the 8th week of age. In the investigated 22 weeks old mice strong interstitial fibrosis was present as revealed by the Masson Trichrome staining (MTS). In accordance with MTS the number of myofibroblast was elevated in COL4A3 KO compared to wild type mice. To investigate the origin these myofibroblast the coexpression of FSP-1 or αSMA and CD31 was investigated by double immunostaining. They found that about 45% of the αSMA and 60% of the FSP-1 positive myofibroblast were CD31 positive, suggesting the endothelial origin of these cells. In accordance with Zeisberg et al. Li and coworkers revealed the contribution of EndMT in the development of STZ induced renal fibrosis. They developed a Tie2Cre; EGFP mice to trace the localization of the cells with endothelial origin in a mice model of STZ induced DN. Tie2 is a pan endothelial marker which is expressed in EC during embryogenesis and thereafter during adulthood. In the bigenic mice Cre recombinase is expressed under the promoter of Tie2 and mediates the excision of a loxP stop cassette thus activating the expression of EGFP. In accordance with other studies (Schlaeger et al., 1997; Koni et al., 2001; Limbourg et al., 2005) the Cre mediated recombination occurred mainly in the ECs, with only a little activity in other cells. In the normal kidneys of Tie2Cre; EGFP mice CD31 staining colocalized with the EGFP positive cells. However, 1 or 6 months after the induction of STZ induced DN 10.4% or 23.5% of renal αSMA positive interstitial myofibroblasts were EGFP positive, suggesting there endothelial origin. Apparently these studies clearly demonstrate the significant role of EndMT in the pathomechanism of renal fibrosis. However, ECs are specialized squamous epithelium and the similarities between EMT and EndMT is evident suggesting that EndMT is a specific form of EMT. So the question emerges why ECs can invade the basement membrane and become real interstitial myofibroblasts if epithelial cells can not.

4.3 Pericytes, perivascular cells or resident fibroblasts

The definition of pericytes (also known as Rouget cells), perivascular cells or resident fibroblasts in the kidney is still a matter of debate. Pericytes occurs around peritubular capillaries and postcapillary venules in the kidney. Pericytes characteristically line at the outer surface of EC and are covered fully or in part with capillary basement membrane thus fulfilling the major criterias of pericytes. These gaps of capillary basement membrane are frequently colocalise with the projections of pericytes, which are believed to be sites of intercellular communication (Grgic et al., 2011). Some projections of the pericytes also can reach the basement membrane of the TECs, make them similar or identical to the cells called resident fibroblast (Kaissling et al., 1996). Recently it has been suggested that activation of pericytes - which are relatively undifferentiated cells - may led to phenotype transformation of them into myofibroblasts. To investigate the potential role of pericytes as myofibroblast precursors Lin et al. generated a transgenic mice expressing GFP under the promoter of collagen type I, α1 (Lin et al., 2008). In these animals the presence of GFP labels, with high sensitivity, the collagen I, α1 producing cell. In healthy kidney of this, coll1a1-GFP mice peritubular capillaries were lined intermittently with collagen type I, α1 producing cells, which were subendothelial in a direct apposition with CD31 positive ECs and exhibited pedicle like attachment plaques suggesting the direct interaction of collagen type I, α1 producing cells with the ECs. These characteristics define these collagen type I, α1 producing cells as pericytes. In developed, but young, 12 days old animals the majority (98,4%) of these cells also expressed chondroitin sulfate proteoglycan 4 (CSPG4), αSMA and PDGFRβ which are all known markers of pericytes. Later in healthy adult mice renal pericytes lost their CSPG4 and αSMA positivity with time. To investigate the contribution of the pericytes to renal fibrosis Lin et al. induced UUO in these coll1a1-GFP mice. In the kidney of diseased mice pericytes do not lose their CSPG4, αSMA and PDGFRβ positivity, rather their population expands. In this model of renal fibrosis 7 days after ureteral obstruction there was a close but imperfect correlation between the collagen 1, α1producing (GFP+) and αSMA positive interstitial cells. Actually 1% of the GFP producing cell did not express αSMA and 25% of the αSMA producing cells did not express GFP in the renal interstitium. These study of Lin et al. strongly suggest that the main source of the myofibroblasts are the collagen I, α1 producing cells, most likely pericytes in the obstructed kidneys. However, these data also suggest that a remarkable percent of the αSMA producing myofibroblasts may originate from other cells then pericytes. Later this group to strengthen their observations made a genetic fate mapping study to test that pericytes are the primary source of myofibroblasts in the UUO model of fibrosis. Humphreys et al. developed a transgenic Cre driver mice that express bacterial Cre recombinase under the regulation of forkhead box D1 (FoxD1) promoter (Fig.6.) (Humphreys et al., 2010). FoxD1 is a transcriptional factor that is transiently expressed during development in metanephric mesenchyme cells that are fated to become mesangial, vascular smooth muscle cells and pericytes. These transgenic mice were then bred with R26R reporter mice. In the kidney of the FoxD1-Cre; R262 bigenic mice mesangial and vascular smooth muscle cells and many PDGFRβ positive interstitial pericytes were detectable after X-gal staining. Fourteen days after UUO they found a marked expansion of LacZ positive cells in the interstitium of the injured kidneys. These β galactosidase positive cells were αSMA positive and all SMA positive cells exhibited β galactosidase activity as well. Suggesting that there was no significant population of cells becoming myofibroblast, except the previously FoxD1 positive cells. However, following UUO FoxD1 transcripts were detected in the kidney samples of FoxD1-Cre; R262 bigenic mice. This means that not only the cells with the heritable marker of R26R mice, but also the de novo FoxD1 expressing cells are labeled with β galactosidase. To circumvent this problem Humphreys B.D. et al developed FoxD1-GCE transgen mice, in which Cre recombinase is expressed under FoxD1 promoter in a tamoxifen-inducible manner. These mice were then bred with R26R reporter mice. FoxD1-GCE; R26R mice that received tamoxifen during the nephrogenesis had β galactosidase positive cells in the renal interstitium which also expressed PDGFRβ and were negative for αSMA (myofibroblast), CD31 (endothelial cell) or F4/80 (macrophages) defining them as pericytes. However, it should be noted that in FoxD1-GCE; R26R mice approximately 20% of pericytes were labeled with β galactosidase activity. Ten days after UUO all β galactosidase positive interstitial cells remained PDGFRβ positive and acquired expression of αSMA demonstrating that pericytes differentiated into myofibroblast. Nowadays the most accepted theory is the transformation of perycites into myofibroblasts. However, since these experiments are rather new it is still not known how the traditional fibrosis inducing factors like TGFβ-1 or Angiotensin can alter the ECM producing capacity of myofibroblasts derived from perycites.

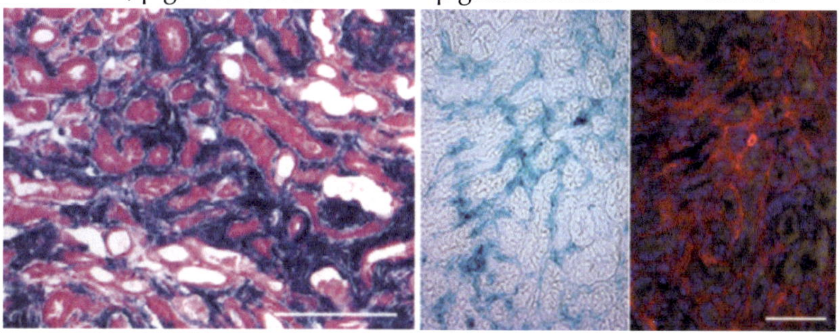

Fig. 6. Fourteen days after UUO a marked expansion of β galactosidase positive cells (blue) was observed in the interstitium of the injured FoxD1-GC; R26R mouse kidneys. Merged light and fluorescence image show the co-expression of β galactosidase (blue) with SMA (red) after UUO day 14. (After Humphreys et al., 2010).

4.4 Bone marrow derived fibrocytes

Fibrocytes are bone marrow (BM) derived mesenchymal cells (Mori et al., 2005; Kisseleva et al., 2006) that express the markers of hematopoietic stem cells, monocytes and fibroblasts (Yang et al., 2002; Mori et al., 2005; Abe et al., 2001). Previously these CD14+ and CD16- fibrocyte precursors were termed as inflammatory monocytes (Gordon & Taylor, 2005). In response to tissue damage these cells are released in high number from the BM and then migrate into the site of the injury. In the tissue most of these inflammatory monocytes then believed to differentiate into macrophages, dendritic cells (Tacke & Randolph, 2006). However, a subpopulation of these CD14+ and CD16- cells can differentiate into other cells types, such as myoblasts, osteoblasts, epithelial, endothelial, neuronal cells (Zhao et al., 2003; Kuwana et al., 2003) or fibrocytes as an intermediate stage of differentiation into mature myofibroblasts. In vitro the co-culture of the CD14+ fibrocyte progenitors with T cells or stimulation of them with TGFβ1, PDGF, IL-4 or IL-13 promotes their maturation into fibrocytes. By contrast aggregated IgG, serum amyloid P, INFγ or IL-12 inhibits the differentiation of CD14+ mononuclear cells into fibrocytes. Fibrocytes express CD34 and CD105 hematopoietic stem cell markers and MHC I and MHC II and the costimulatory molecules CD80 and CD86. Today the presence of CD45, CD34, or other myeloid antigen like CD11b and CD13 is considered to discriminate fibrocytes from leukocytes. Fibrocytes still do not express large amount of ECM (Chesney et al., 1998), however they produce ECM degrading enzymes, such as MMP9 (García-de-Alba et al., 2010). Fibrocytes can differentiate into myofibroblast in vivo (Mori et al., 2005; Schmidt et al., 2003). The further differentiation of the fibrocytes into myofibroblasts is stimulated by TGFβ1 and endothelin-1. The matured myofibroblasts then produce significantly more collagen then fibrocytes and express αSMA. Myofibroblasts also lose the CD34 and CD45 markers of fibrocytes. Despite our huge knowledge about the differentiation of CD14+ mononuclear cells into myofibroblast, the contribution of these BM derived cells to the population of myofibroblast is generally believed to be small. To investigate the contribution of fibrocytes to the population of myofibroblast Iwano M. et al. generated transgenic mice, in which EGFP is expressed under the promoter of FSP-1. In this experiment they used FSP-1 as marker of myofibroblast (Iwano M et al., 2002). The T cell depleted BM of these transgenic mice was intravenously injected into lethally irradiated Balb/c, wild type recipients. Thirty days after the BM transfer the chimeric mice underwent UUO. Finally, 10 days after the UUO the number of FSP-1 and EGFP double positive BM derived cells were counted in the injured and in the collateral, normal kidney samples. By counting several random cortical fields they found that about the 12% of the renal FSP-1 positive cells have BM origin in the normal and about 15% in the injured kidneys. These data suggest that 10 days after UUO only 3% of the FSP-1 positive myofibroblasts are originated from the BM. Others investigating the contribution of fibrocytes to the population of myofibroblast have found similar results. Lin et al. transplanted the BM cells of coll1a1-GFP mice into a lethally irradiated wild type recipient mice. In these chimeric mice all collagen type I, α1 producing cell with BM origin express GFP. To induce renal fibrosis UUO was performed on these chimeric mice. Interestingly, they found that 7 days after UUO only the 0.1% of the myofibroblast expressed the CD34 and CD45 markers of fibrocytes (Abe et al., 2001) in the chimeric mice. Taken together these data suggest that the contribution of CD14+ CD16- BM cells to the population of myofibroblasts is not significant. One week after the UUO only a few percent (0.1-3%) of the myofibroblasts are originated from these CD14+ CD16- BM cells.

5. Summary and concluding remarks

Today there are different theories about the possible origin of the myofibroblasts that are responsible for scar formation in the injured kidney. A hypothesis that recently became popular is the mesenchymal transition of the renal tubular epithelial cells. During EMT epithelial cells undergo phenotypic conversion, which means that they lose their polarity, epithelial adhesion properties and starts the de novo synthesis of αSMA and other mesenchymal factors. This process is already well known in different physiological and pathological processes, notably in embryogenesis and carcinogenesis. In vitro experiments on different epithelial cell lines and on primer epithelial cells strongly suggest the existence of EMT based on their increased expression of αSMA, vimentin and decreased expression of E-cadherin. However, the role of EMT is controversial in renal fibrosis. Recently, Humphreys et al. using double transgenic animals, clearly demonstrated that tubular epithelial cells can not invade the basement membrane, suggesting that EMT does not lead to formation of myofibroblasts, actually not in vivo in the mice model of UUO. Interestingly, the concept of EndMT is widely accepted, despite that the endothelial cells are specialized squamous type epithelial cells suggesting that EndMT is only a specific form of EMT. Actually, the similarities between EMT and EndMT is evident. During the phenotype conversion endothelial or epithelial cells lose their original markers and start to express mesenchymal ones, such as αSMA. However, the question why endothelial cells can invade the basement membrane and epithelial cells can not is still unanswered. Today, perhaps the most accepted theory about the possible origin of myofibroblasts is the transformation of perycites into myofibroblasts. This observation is rather new and it is still not known how the traditional fibrosis inducing factors like TGFβ or angiotensin can alter the ECM producing capacity of myofibroblasts derived from perycites. Finally the contribution of CD14+ CD16- BM cells to the population of myofibroblasts is not significant. These cells are responsible for only 1-2% of the myofibroblast. There estimated number of patients with chronic kidney disease is over 2.5 millions in Europe and the number of patients on chronic renal replacement therapy number is continuously increasing. Thus research in that field has not only scientific impact, but has also important implications on general health and health care systems considering the quality of life in uremia and the socio-economic costs of renal replacement therapies. Actually regardless of the initiating cause (infection, autoimmune response, chemical insult, radiation or tissue injury etc.) fibrosis is the final common pathway for all progressive renal diseases. That is why it is so important to understand the complex interplay among immune cells, myofibroblasts precursors and renal cells. The development of new antifibrotic therapies is getting more and more important, and it requires the understanding of the cellular origin and precise role of myofibroblasts.

6. Acknowledgments

Ádám Vannay is holder of the János Bolyai Research grant; this work was supported by the János Bolyai Research Scholarschip of the Hungarian Academy of Sciences BAROSS GABOR REG_KM_INFRA_09 and OTKA 84087/2010.

7. References

Abe, R., Donnelly, SC., Peng, T., Bucala, R. & Metz CN. (2001). Peripheral blood fibrocytes: differentiation pathway and migration to wound sites. *J Immunol.* 166(12):7556-62.

Allen, AM., Zhuo, J. & Mendelsohn, FA. (2000). Localization and function of angiotensin AT1 receptors. *Am J Hypertens.* 13(1 Pt 2):31S-38S.

Alpers, CE., Seifert, RA., Hudkins, KL., Johnson, RJ. & Bowen-Pope DF. (1993). PDGF-receptor localizes to mesangial, parietal epithelial, and interstitial cells in human and primate kidneys. *Kidney Int.* 43(2):286-94.

Anders, HJ. & Ryu, M. (2011). Renal microenvironments and macrophage phenotypes determine progression or resolution of renal inflammation and fibrosis. *Kidney Int.* 80(9):915-25.

Anders, HJ. (2010) Toll-like receptors and danger signaling in kidney injury. *J Am Soc Nephrol.* 21: 1270–1274.

Andrae, J., Gallini, R. & Betsholtz, C. (2008). Role of platelet-derived growth factors in physiology and medicine. *Genes Dev.* 22(10):1276-312.

Bankl, HC. & Valent, P. (2002). Mast cells, thrombosis, and fibrinolysis: the emerging concept. *Thromb Res* 105:359–365.

Bao, L., Wang, Y., Haas, M. & Quigg RJ. (2011). Distinct roles for C3a and C5a in complement-induced tubulointerstitial injury. *Kidney Int.* 80(5):524-34.

Beaven, MA. & Metzger, H. (1993). Signal transduction by Fc receptors: The Fc epsilon RI case. *Immunol Today* 14: 222–226

Beil, WJ., Füreder, W., Wiener, H., Grossschmidt, K., Maier, U., Schedle, A., Bankl, HC., Lechner, K. & Valent, P. (1998). Phenotypic and functional characterization of mast cells derived from renal tumor tissues. Exp Hematol. 26(2):158-69.

Benigni, A., Cassis, P. & Remuzzi G. (2010). Angiotensin II revisited: new roles in inflammation, immunology and aging. *EMBO Mol Med.* 2(7):247-57.

Blackwell, TS. & Christman, JW. (1997). The role of nuclear factor-kappa B in cytokine gene regulation. *Am J Respir Cell Mol Biol.* 17:3-9.

Bonner, JC. (2004). Regulation of PDGF and its receptors in fibrotic diseases. *Cytokine Growth Factor Rev.* 15(4):255-73.

Boor, P., Konieczny, A., Villa, L., Schult, AL., Bücher, E., Rong, S., Kunter, U., van Roeyen, CR., Polakowski, T., Hawlisch, H., Hillebrandt, S., Lammert, F., Eitner, F., Floege, J. & Ostendorf, T. (2007). Complement C5 mediates experimental tubulointerstitial fibrosis. *J Am Soc Nephrol.* 18(5):1508-15.

Border, WA. & Noble, NA. (1993). Cytokines in kidney disease: the role of transforming growth factor-beta. *Am J Kidney Dis.* 22(1):105-13.

Bradding, P., Walls, AF. & Holgate, ST. (2006). The role of the mast cell in the pathophysiology of asthma. *J Allergy Clin Immunol.* 117:1277–1284.

Bronte, V. & Zanovello, P. (2005). Regulation of immune responses by L-arginine metabolism. *Nat. Rev. Immunol.* 5:641–654.

Brown, KM., Sacks, SH. & Sheerin, NS. (2007). Mechanisms of disease: the complement system in renal injury--new ways of looking at an old foe. *Nat Clin Pract Nephrol.* 3(5):277-86.

Busse, WW. (1998). Leukotrienes and inflammation. *Am J Respir Crit Care Med.* 157(6 Pt 1):S210-3.

Cairns, JA. & Walls, AF. (1997). Mast cell tryptase stimulates the synthesis of type I collagen in human lung fibroblasts. *J Clin Invest* 99: 1313–1321

Cassatella, MA. (1999). Neutrophil-derived proteins: selling cytokines by the pound. *Adv Immunol.* 73:369-509.

Changsirikulchai, S., Hudkins, KL., Goodpaster, TA., Volpone, J., Topouzis, S., Gilbertson, DG. & Alpers, CE. (2002). Platelet-derived growth factor-D expression in developing and mature human kidneys. *Kidney Int.* 62(6):2043-54.

Chen, YT., Chang, FC., Wu, CF., Chou, YH., Hsu, HL., Chiang, WC., Shen, J., Chen, YM., Wu, KD., Tsai, TJ., Duffield, JS. & Lin, SL. (2011). Platelet-derived growth factor receptor signaling activates pericyte-myofibroblast transition in obstructive and post-ischemic kidney fibrosis. *Kidney Int.* [Epub ahead of print]

Chesney, J., Metz, C., Stavitsky, AB., Bacher, M. & Bucala, R. (1998). Regulated production of type I collagen and inflammatory cytokines by peripheral blood fibrocytes. *J Immunol.* 160(1):419-25.

Chowdhury, P., Sacks, SH. & Sheerin, NS. (2010). Endogenous ligands for TLR2 and TLR4 are not involved in renal injury following ureteric obstruction. *Nephron Exp Nephrol.* 115(4):e122-30.

Clarkson, MR., McGinty, A., Godson, C. & Brady, HR. (1998). Leukotrienes and lipoxins: lipoxygenase- derived modulators of leukocyte recruitment and vascular tone in glomerulonephritis. *Nephrol Dial Transplant* 13:3043–3051.

Cochrane, AL., Kett, MM., Samuel, CS., Campanale, NV., Anderson, WP., Hume, DA., Little, MH., Bertram, JF. & Ricardo, SD. (2005). J Renal structural and functional repair in a mouse model of reversal of ureteral obstruction. *Am Soc Nephrol.* 16(12):3623-30.

Cockcroft, JR., O'Kane, KP. & Webb, DJ. (1995). Tissue angiotensin generation and regulation of vascular tone. *Pharmacol Ther.* 65(2):193-213.

Coimbra, TM., Carvalho, J., Fattori, A., Da Silva, CG. & Lachat, JJ. (1996). Transforming growth factor-beta production during the development of renal fibrosis in rats with subtotal renal ablation. *Int J Exp Pathol.* 77(4):167-73.

Colvin, RB., Dvorak, AM. & Dvorak, HF. (1974). Mast cells in the cortical tubular epithelium and interstitium in human renal disease. *Hum Pathol* 5:315–326.

Crisman, JM., Richards, LL., Valach, DP., Franzoni, DF. & Diamond, JR. (2001). Chemokine expression in the obstructed kidney. *Exp Nephrol.* 9:241-248.

De Heer, E., Sijpkens, YW., Verkade, M., den Dulk, M., Langers, A., Schutrups, J., Bruijn, JA. & van Es, LA. (2000). Morphometry of interstitial fibrosis. *Nephrol Dial Transplant.* 15 Suppl 6:72-3.

Del Prete, D., Gambaro, G., Lupo, A., Anglani, F., Brezzi, B., Magistroni, R., Graziotto, R., Furci, L., Modena, F., Bernich, P., Albertazzi, A., D'Angelo, A. & Maschio, G. (2003). Precocious activation of genes of the renin-angiotensin system and the fibrogenic cascade in IgA glomerulonephritis. *Kidney Int.* 64(1):149-59.

Dimitriadou, V., Mecheri, S., Koutsilieris, M., Fraser, W., Al-Daccak, R. & Mourad, W. (1998). Expression of functional major histocompatibility complex class II molecules on HMC-1 human mast cells. *J Leukoc Biol* 64: 791–799

Dong, X., Bachman, LA., Miller, MN., Nath, KA. & Griffin, MD. (2008). Dendritic cells facilitate accumulation of IL-17 T cells in the kidney following acute renal obstruction. *Kidney Int.* 74:1294-1309.

Dudas, PL., Sague, SL., Elloso, MM., Farrell, FX. (2011). Proinflammatory/profibrotic effects of interleukin-17A on human proximal tubule epithelium. *Nephron Exp Nephrol.* 117(4):e114-23.

Duffield, JS., Erwig, LP., Wei, X., Liew, FY., Rees, AJ. & Savill, JS. (2000). Activated macrophages direct apoptosis and suppress mitosis of mesangial cells. *J Immunol.* 164(4):2110-9.

Duffield, JS., Tipping, PG., Kipari, T., Cailhier, JF., Clay, S., Lang, R., Bonventre, JV. & Hughes, J. (2005). Conditional ablation of macrophages halts progression of crescentic glomerulonephritis. *Am J Pathol.* 167(5):1207-19.

Eddy, AA. (1995). Interstitial macrophages as mediators of renal fibrosis. *Exp Nephrol.* 3: 76–79.

Eddy, AA. (2000). Molecular basis of renal fibrosis. *Pediatr Nephrol.* 15(3-4):290-301.

Ehara, T. & Shigematsu, H. (1998). Contribution of mast cells to the tubulointerstitial lesions in IgA nephritis. *Kidney Int.* 54:1675–1683.

Eis, V., Luckow, B., Vielhauer, V., Siveke, JT., Linde, Y., Segerer, S., Perez De Lema, G., Cohen, CD., Kretzler, M., Mack, M., Horuk, R., Murphy, PM., Gao, JL., Hudkins, KL., Alpers, CE., Gröne, HJ., Schlöndorff, D. & Anders, HJ. (2004). Chemokine receptor CCR1 but not CCR5 mediates leukocyte recruitment and subsequent renal fibrosis after unilateral ureteral obstruction. *J Am Soc Nephrol.* 15(2):337-47.

Eitner, F., Bücher, E., van Roeyen, C., Kunter, U., Rong, S., Seikrit, C., Villa, L., Boor, P., Fredriksson, L., Bäckström, G., Eriksson, U., Ostman, A., Floege, J. & Ostendorf, T. (2008). PDGF-C is a proinflammatory cytokine that mediates renal interstitial fibrosis. *J Am Soc Nephrol.* 19(2):281-9.

Eitner, F., Ostendorf, T., Kretzler, M., Cohen, CD., Eriksson, U., Gröne, HJ. & Floege, J; ERCB-Consortium. (2003). PDGF-C expression in the developing and normal adult human kidney and in glomerular diseases. *J Am Soc Nephrol.* 14(5):1145-53.

Eitner, F., Ostendorf, T., Van Roeyen, C., Kitahara, M., Li, X., Aase, K., Gröne, HJ., Eriksson, U. & Floege, J. (2002). Expression of a novel PDGF isoform, PDGF-C, in normal and diseased rat kidney. *J Am Soc Nephrol.* 13(4):910-7.

El-Koraie, AF., Baddour, NM., Adam, AG., El Kashef, EH. & El Nahas, AM. (2001). Role of stem cell factor and mast cells in the progression of chronic glomerulonephritides. *Kidney Int* 60:167–172.

Esteban, V., Rupérez, M., Vita, JR., López, ES., Mezzano, S., Plaza, JJ., Egido, J. & Ruiz-Ortega, M. (2003). Effect of simultaneous blockade of AT1 and AT2 receptors on the NFkappaB pathway and renal inflammatory response. *Kidney Int Suppl.* S33-S38.

Fadok, VA., Bratton, DL., Konowal, A., Freed, PW., Westcott, JY. & Henson, PM. (1998). Macrophages that have ingested apoptotic cells in vitro inhibit proinflammatory cytokine production through autocrine/paracrine mechanisms involving TGF-beta, PGE2, and PAF. *J Clin Invest* 101: 890–898.

Fantone, JC. & Ward, PA. (1985). Polymorphonuclear leukocyte-mediated cell and tissue injury: oxygen metabolites and their relations to human disease. *Hum Pathol.* 16(10):973-8.

Fellström, B., Klareskog, L., Heldin, CH., Larsson, E., Rönnstrand, L., Terracio, L., Tufveson, G., Wahlberg, J. & Rubin, K. (1989). Platelet-derived growth factor receptors in the kidney-upregulated expression in inflammation. Kidney Int. 36(6):1099-102.

Floege, J., Eitner, F. & Alpers, CE. (2008). A new look at platelet-derived growth factor in renal disease. *J Am Soc Nephrol.* 19(1):12-23.

Fukuda, K., Yoshitomi, K., Yanagida, T., Tokumoto, M. & Hirakata, H. (2001). Quantification of TGF-beta1 mRNA along rat nephron in obstructive nephropathy. *Am J Physiol Renal Physiol.* 281(3):F513-21.

Galli, SJ., Kalesnikoff, J., Grimbaldeston, MA., Piliponsky, AM., Williams, CM. & Tsai, M. (2005). Mast cells as "tunable" effector and immunoregulatory cells: recent advances. *Annu Rev Immunol* 23:749–786.

García-de-Alba, C., Becerril, C., Ruiz, V., González, Y., Reyes, S., García-Alvarez, J., Selman, M. & Pardo, A. (2010). Expression of matrix metalloproteases by fibrocytes: possible role in migration and homing. *Am J Respir Crit Care Med.* 182(9):1144-52.

Gibbs, DF., Warner, RL., Weiss, SJ., Johnson, KJ. & Varani, J. (1999). Characterization of matrix metalloproteinases produced by rat alveolar macrophages. *Am J Respir Cell Mol.* 20: 1136–1144.

Godfraind, C., Louahed, J., Faulkner, H., Vink, A., Warnier, G., Grencis, R. & Renauld, JC. (1998). Intraepithelial infiltration by mast cells with both connective tissue-type and mucosal-type characteristics in gut, trachea, and kidneys of IL-9 transgenic mice. J Immunol. 160(8):3989-96.

Goerdt, S. & Orfanos, CE. (1999). Other functions, other genes: alternative activation of antigenpresenting cells. *Immunity* 10: 137–142.

Gordon, S. & Taylor, PR. (2005). Monocyte and macrophage heterogeneity. *Nature Rev Immunol.* 5:953–964.

Gordon, S. (2003). Alternative activation of macrophages. *Nat. Rev. Immunol.* 3:23–35.

Grgic, I., Duffield, JS. & Humphreys, BD. (2011). The origin of interstitial myofibroblasts in chronic kidney disease. *Pediatr Nephrol.* [Epub ahead of print]

Gruber, BL., Marchese, MJ. & Kew, RR. (1994). Transforming growth factor-beta 1 mediates mast cell chemotaxis. *J Immunol.* 152: 5860–5867.

Gurtner, GC., Werner, S., Barrandon, Y. & Longaker, MT. (2008). Wound repair and regeneration. *Nature.* 453(7193):314-21.

Hang, L., Frendéus, B., Godaly, G. & Svanborg, C. (2000). Interleukin-8 receptor knockout mice have subepithelial neutrophil entrapment and renal scarring following acute pyelonephritis. *J Infect Dis.* 182(6):1738-48.

Hashimoto, N., Phan, SH., Imaizumi, K., Matsuo, M., Nakashima, H., Kawabe, T., Shimokata, K. & Hasegawa, Y. (2010). Endothelial-mesenchymal transition in bleomycin-induced pulmonary fibrosis. *Am J Respir Cell Mol Biol.* 43(2):161-72.

He, C., Imai, M., Song, H., Quigg, RJ. & Tomlinson, S. (2005). Complement inhibitors targeted to the proximal tubule prevent injury in experimental nephritic syndrome and demonstrate a key role for C5b-9. *J Immunol.* 174: 5750–5757.

Hellberg, C., Ostman, A. & Heldin, CH. (2010). PDGF and vessel maturation. *Recent Results Cancer Res.* 180:103-14.

Heller, F., Lindenmeyer, MT., Cohen, CD., Brandt, U., Draganovici, D., Fischereder, M., Kretzler, M., Anders, HJ., Sitter, T., Mosberger, I., Kerjaschki, D., Regele, H., Schlöndorff, D. & Segerer, S. (2007). The contribution of B cells to renal interstitial inflammation. *Am J Pathol.* 170(2):457-68.

Herbert, DR., Hölscher, C., Mohrs, M., Arendse, B., Schwegmann, A., Radwanska, M., Leeto, M., Kirsch, R., Hall, P., Mossmann, H., Claussen, B., Förster, I. & Brombacher, F. (2004). Alternative macrophage activation is essential for survival during schistosomiasis and downmodulates T helper 1 responses and immunopathology. *Immunity.* 20(5):623-35.

Hiromura, K., Kurosawa, M., Yano, S. & Naruse, T. (1998). Tubulointerstitial mast cell infiltration in glomerulonephritis. *Am J Kidney Dis.* 32:593–599.

Hochberg, D., Johnson, CW., Chen, J., Cohen, D., Stern, J., Vaughan, ED Jr., Poppas, D. & Felsen, D. (2000). Interstitial fibrosis of unilateral ureteral obstruction is exacerbated in kidneys of mice lacking the gene for inducible nitric oxide synthase. *Lab Invest.* 80(11):1721-8.

Holdsworth, SR. & Summers, SA. (2008). Role of mast cells in progressive renal diseases. *J Am Soc Nephrol.* 19(12):2254-61.

Horton, JK., Davies, M., Topley, N., Thomas, D. & Williams, JD. (1990). Activation of the inflammatory response of neutrophils by Tamm-Horsfall glycoprotein. *Kidney Int.* 37(2):717-26.

Huang, XR., Chen, WY., Truong, LD. & Lan, HY. (2003). Chymase is upregulated in diabetic nephropathy: implications for an alternative pathway of angiotensin II-mediated diabetic renal and vascular disease. *J Am Soc Nephrol.* 14:1738–1747.

Humphreys, BD., Lin, SL., Kobayashi, A., Hudson, TE., Nowlin, BT., Bonventre, JV., Valerius, MT., McMahon, AP. & Duffield, JS. (2010). Fate tracing reveals the pericyte and not epithelial origin of myofibroblasts in kidney fibrosis. *Am J Pathol.* 176(1):85-97.

Ichino, M., Kusaka, M., Kuroyanagi, Y., Mori, T., Morooka, M., Sasaki, H., Shiroki, R., Shishido, S., Kurahashi, H. & Hoshinaga, K. (2010). Urinary neutrophil-gelatinase associated lipocalin is a potential noninvasive marker for renal scarring in patients with vesicoureteral reflux. *J Urol.* 183(5):2001-7.

Isaka, Y., Tsujie, M., Ando, Y., Nakamura, H., Kaneda, Y., Imai, E. & Hori, M. (2000). Transforming growth factor-beta 1 antisense oligodeoxynucleotides block interstitial fibrosis in unilateral ureteral obstruction. *Kidney Int.* 58(5):1885-92.

Ishidoya, S., Morrissey, J., McCracken, R., Reyes, A. & Klahr, S. (1995). Angiotensin II receptor antagonist ameliorates renal tubulointerstitial fibrosis caused by unilateral ureteral obstruction. *Kidney Int.* 47:1285-1294.

Iwano, M., Plieth, D., Danoff, TM,, Xue, C., Okada, H. & Neilson, EG. (2002). Evidence that fibroblasts derive from epithelium during tissue fibrosis. *J Clin Invest.* 110(3):341-50.

Jutel, M., Watanabe, T., Akdis, M., Blaser, K. & Akdis, CA. (2002). Immune regulation by histamine. *Curr Opin Immunol* 14: 735–740

Kaissling, B., Hegyi, I., Loffing, J. & Le Hir, M. (1996). Morphology of interstitial cells in the healthy kidney. *Anat Embryol (Berl).* 193(4):303-18.

Kalluri, R. & Weinberg, RA. (2009). The basics of epithelial-mesenchymal transition. *J Clin Invest.* 119(6):1420-8.

Kaneto, H., Morrissey, J. & Klahr, S. (1993). Increased expression of TGF-beta 1 mRNA in the obstructed kidney of rats with unilateral ureteral ligation. *Kidney Int.* 44: 313–321

Kang, SJ., You, A. & Kwak, MK. (2011). Suppression of Nrf2 signaling by angiotensin II in murine renal epithelial cells. *Arch Pharm Res.* 34(5):829-36.

Kellner, D., Chen, J., Richardson, I., Seshan, SV., El Chaar, M., Vaughan, ED Jr., Poppas, D. & Felsen, D. (2006). Angiotensin receptor blockade decreases fibrosis and fibroblast expression in a rat model of unilateral ureteral obstruction. *J Urol.* 176:806-812.

Ketteler, M., Noble, NA. & Border, WA. (1994). Increased expression of transforming growth factor-beta in renal disease. *Curr Opin Nephrol Hypertens.* 3(4):446-52.

Kim, H., Oda, T., López-Guisa, J., Wing, D., Edwards, DR., Soloway, PD. & Eddy, AA. (2001). TIMP-1 deficiency does not attenuate interstitial fibrosis in obstructive nephropathy. *J Am Soc Nephrol.* 12(4):736-48.

Kim, SM., Jang, HR., Lee, YJ., Lee, JE., Huh, WS., Kim, DJ., Oh, HY. & Kim, YG. (2011). Urinary angiotensinogen levels reflect the severity of renal histopathology in patients with chronic kidney disease. *Clin Nephrol.* 76(2):117-23.

Kisseleva, T., Uchinami, H., Feirt, N., Quintana-Bustamante, O., Segovia, JC., Schwabe, RF. & Brenner, DA. (2006). Bone marrow-derived fibrocytes participate in pathogenesis of liver fibrosis. *J Hepatol.* 45(3):429-38.

Kitagawa, K., Wada, T., Furuichi, K., Hashimoto, H., Ishiwata, Y., Asano, M., Takeya, M., Kuziel, WA., Matsushima, K., Mukaida, N. & Yokoyama, H. (2004). Blockade of CCR2 ameliorates progressive fibrosis in kidney. *Am J Pathol.* 165:237-246.

Kitamoto, K., Machida, Y., Uchida, J., Izumi, Y., Shiota, M., Nakao, T., Iwao, H., Yukimura, T., Nakatani, T. & Miura, K. (2009). Effects of liposome clodronate on renal leukocyte populations and renal fibrosis in murine obstructive nephropathy. *J Pharmacol Sci.* 111:285-292.

Kitamura, Y. (1989). Heterogeneity of mast cells and phenotypic change between subpopulations. *Annu Rev Immunol.* 7: 59–76

Kitching, AR. & Holdsworth, SR. (2011). The emergence of TH17 cells as effectors of renal injury. *J Am Soc Nephrol.* 22(2):235-8.

Kitching, AR., Turner, AL., Wilson, GR., Semple, T., Odobasic, D., Timoshanko, JR., O'Sullivan, KM., Tipping, PG., Takeda, K., Akira, S. & Holdsworth, SR. (2005). IL-12p40 and IL-18 in crescentic glomerulonephritis: IL-12p40 is the key Th1-defining cytokine chain, whereas IL-18 promotes local inflammation and leukocyte recruitment. *J Am Soc Nephrol.* 16(7):2023-33.

Koesters, R., Kaissling, B., Lehir, M., Picard, N., Theilig, F., Gebhardt, R., Glick, AB., Hähnel, B., Hosser, H., Gröne, HJ. & Kriz, W. (2010). Tubular overexpression of transforming growth factor-beta1 induces autophagy and fibrosis but not mesenchymal transition of renal epithelial cells. *Am J Pathol.* 177(2):632-43.

Koni, PA., Joshi, SK., Temann, UA., Olson, D., Burkly, L. & Flavell, RA. (2001). Conditional vascular adhesion molecule 1 deletion in mice; Impaired lymphocyte migration to bone marrow. *J. Exp. Med.* 193: 741-754.

Krausgruber, T., Blazek, K., Smallie, T., Alzabin, S., Lockstone, H., Sahgal, N., Hussell, T., Feldmann, M. & Udalova, IA. (2011). IRF5 promotes inflammatory macrophage polarization and TH1-TH17 responses. *Nat Immunol.* 12(3):231-8.

Kuroiwa, T., Schlimgen, R., Illei, GG., McInnes, IB. & Boumpas, DT. (2000). Distinct T cell/renal tubular epithelial cell interactions define differential chemokine production: implications for tubulointerstitial injury in chronic glomerulonephritides. *J Immunol.* 164(6):3323-9.

Kushiyama, T., Oda, T., Yamada, M., Higashi, K., Yamamoto, K., Sakurai, Y., Miura, S. & Kumagai, H. (2010). Alteration in the Phenotype Macrophages in the Repair of Renal Interstitial Fibrosis in Mice. Nephrology (Carlton). 16(5):522-35.

Kuwana, M., Okazaki, Y., Kodama, H., Izumi, K., Yasuoka, H., Ogawa, Y., Kawakami, Y. & Ikeda, Y. (2003). Human circulating CD14+ monocytes as a source of progenitors that exhibit mesenchymal cell differentiation. *J Leukoc Biol.* 74(5):833-45.

Langenkamp, A., Messi, M., Lanzavecchia, A. & Sallusto, F. (2000). Kinetics of dendritic cell activation: impact on priming of TH1, TH2 and nonpolarized T cells. *Nat Immunol.* 1(4):311-6.

Lesher, AM. & Song, WC. (2010). Complement and its regulatory proteins in kidney diseases. *Nephrology (Carlton).* 15(7):663-75.

Lewis, EJ., Hunsicker, LG., Bain, RP. & Rohde, RD. (1993). The effect of angiotensin-converting-enzyme inhibition on diabetic nephropathy. The Collaborative Study Group. *N Engl J Med.* 329(20):1456-62.

Li, P., Garcia, GE., Xia, Y., Wu, W., Gersch, C., Park, PW., Truong, L., Wilson, CB., Johnson, R. & Feng, L. (2005). Blocking of monocyte chemoattractant protein-1 during tubulointerstitial nephritis resulted in delayed neutrophil clearance. *Am J Pathol.* 167(3):637-49.

Li, Z., Chung, AC., Zhou, L., Huang, XR., Liu, F., Fu, P., Fan, JM., Szalai, AJ. & Lan, HY. (2011). C-reactive protein promotes acute renal inflammation and fibrosis in unilateral ureteral obstructive nephropathy in mice. *Lab Invest.* 91(6):837-51.

Limbourg, FP., Takeshita, K., Radtke, F., Bronson, RT., Chin, MT. & Liao, JK. (2005). Essential role of endothelial Notch 1 in angiogenesis. *Circulation.* 111: 1826-1832.

Lin, SL., Kisseleva, T., Brenner, DA. & Duffield, JS. (2008). Pericytes and perivascular fibroblasts are the primary source of collagen-producing cells in obstructive fibrosis of the kidney. *Am J Pathol.* 173(6):1617-27.

Liu Y. (2010). New insights into epithelial-mesenchymal transition in kidney fibrosis. *J Am Soc Nephrol.* 21(2):212-22.

Liu, L., Rich, BE., Inobe, J., Chen, W. & Weiner, HL. (1998). Induction of Th2 cell differentiation in the primary immune response: dendritic cells isolated from adherent cell culture treated with IL-10 prime naive CD4+ T cells to secrete IL-4. *Int Immunol.* 10(8):1017-26.

Lu, LF., Lind, EF., Gondek, DC., Bennett, KA., Gleeson, MW., Pino-Lagos, K., Scott, ZA., Coyle, AJ., Reed, JL., Van Snick, J., Strom, TB., Zheng, XX. & Noelle, RJ. (2006). Mast cells are essential intermediaries in regulatory T-cell tolerance. Nature. 442(7106):997-1002.

Lutz, J., Yao, Y., Song, E., Antus, B., Hamar, P., Liu, S. & Heemann, U. (2005). Inhibition of matrix metalloproteinases during chronic allograft nephropathy in rats. *Transplantation.* 79: 655–661.

Machida, Y., Kitamoto, K., Izumi, Y., Shiota, M., Uchida, J., Kira, Y., Nakatani, T., Miura, K. (2010). Renal fibrosis in murine obstructive nephropathy is attenuated by depletion of monocyte lineage, not dendritic cells. *J Pharmacol Sci.* 114(4):464-73.

Mallamaci, F., Ruggenenti, P., Perna, A., Leonardis, D., Tripepi, R., Tripepi, G., Remuzzi, G. & Zoccali C. (2011). ACE inhibition is renoprotective among obese patients with proteinuria. *J Am Soc Nephrol.* 22(6):1122-8.

Maloney, CG., Kutchera, WA., Albertine, KH., McIntyre, TM., Prescott, SM. & Zimmerman, GA. (1998). Inflammatory agonists induce cyclooxygenase type 2 expression by human neutrophils. *J Immunol.* 160(3):1402-10.

Mantovani, A., Sica, A., Sozzani, S., Allavena, P., Vecchi, A. & Locati, M. (2004). The chemokine system in diverse forms of macrophage activation and polarization. *Trends Immunol.* 25(12):677-86.
Mantovani, A., Sica, A., Sozzani, S., Allavena, P., Vecchi, A. & Locati, M. (2004). The chemokine system in diverse forms of macrophage activation and polarization. *Trends Immunol.* 25(12):677-86.
Matsuzaki, K. & Okazaki, K. (2006). Transforming growth factor-beta during carcinogenesis: the shift from epithelial to mesenchymal signaling. *J Gastroenterol.* 41(4):295-303.

McCurdy, JD., Lin, TJ. & Marshall, JS. (2001). Toll-like receptor 4-mediated activation of murine mast cells. *J Leukoc Biol.* 70: 977–984

McDonald, B., Pittman, K., Menezes, GB., Hirota, SA., Slaba, I., Waterhouse, CC., Beck, PL., Muruve, DA., Kubes, P. (2010). Intravascular danger signals guide neutrophils to sites of sterile inflammation. *Science.* 330(6002):362-6.

Meng, H., Marchese, MJ., Garlick, JA., Jelaska, A., Korn, JH., Gailit, J., Clark, RA. & Gruber, BL. (1995). Mast cells induce T-cell adhesion to human fibroblasts by regulating intercellular adhesion molecule-1 and vascular cell adhesion molecule-1 expression. *J Invest Dermatol* 105: 789–796

Misseri, R., Meldrum, DR., Dinarello, CA., Dagher, P., Hile, KL., Rink, RC. & Meldrum, KK. (2005). TNF-alpha mediates obstruction-induced renal tubular cell apoptosis and proapoptotic signaling. *Am J Physiol Renal Physiol.* 288:F406-F411.

Miyajima, A., Chen, J., Lawrence, C., Ledbetter, S., Soslow, RA., Stern, J., Jha, S., Pigato, J., Lemer, ML., Poppas, DP., Vaughan, ED. & Felsen, D. (2000). Antibody to transforming growth factor-beta ameliorates tubular apoptosis in unilateral ureteral obstruction. *Kidney Int.* 58(6):2301-13.

Miyazawa, S., Hotta, O., Doi, N., Natori, Y., Nishikawa, K. & Natori, Y. (2004). Role of mast cells in the development of renal fibrosis: use of mast cell-deficient rats. *Kidney Int.* 65(6):2228-37.

Mori, L., Bellini, A., Stacey, MA., Schmidt, M. & Mattoli, S. (2005). Fibrocytes contribute to the myofibroblast population in wounded skin and originate from the bone marrow. *Exp Cell Res.* 304(1):81-90.

Morrissey, JJ., Ishidoya, S., McCracken, R. & Klahr, S. (1996). Nitric oxide generation ameliorates the tubulointerstitial fibrosis of obstructive nephropathy. *J Am Soc Nephrol.* 7(10):2202-12.

Mosser, DM. & Edwards, JP. (2008). Exploring the full spectrum of macrophage activation. *Nat Rev Immunol.* 8: 958–969.

Mu, W., Ouyang, X., Agarwal, A., Zhang, L., Long, DA., Cruz, PE., Roncal, CA., Glushakova, OY., Chiodo, VA., Atkinson, MA., Hauswirth, WW., Flotte, TR., Rodriguez-Iturbe, B. & Johnson, RJ. (2005). IL-10 suppresses chemokines, inflammation, and fibrosis in a model of chronic renal disease. *J Am Soc Nephrol.* 16(12):3651-60.

Muller, DN., Shagdarsuren, E., Park, JK., Dechend, R., Mervaala, E., Hampich, F., Fiebeler, A., Ju, X., Finckenberg, P., Theuer, J., Viedt, C., Kreuzer, J., Heidecke, H., Haller, H., Zenke, M. & Luft, FC. (2002). Immunosuppressive treatment protects against angiotensin II-induced renal damage. *Am J Pathol.* 161(5):1679-93.

Muller, WA. (2009). Mechanisms of transendothelial migration of leukocytes. *Circ Res.* 105: 223–230.

Musial, A., & Eissa, NT. (2001). Inducible nitric-oxide synthase is regulated by the proteasome degradation pathway. *J Biol Chem.* 276:24268-24273.

Nakae, S., Suto, H., Berry, GJ. & Galli, SJ. (2007). Mast cell-derived TNF can promote Th17 celldependent neutrophil recruitment in ovalbumin-challenged OTII mice. *Blood* 109: 3640–3648

Ng, YY., Huang, TP., Yang, WC., Chen, ZP., Yang, AH., Mu, W., Nikolic-Paterson, DJ., Atkins, RC. & Lan, HY. (1998). Tubular epithelial-myofibroblast transdifferentiation in progressive tubulointerstitial fibrosis in 5/6 nephrectomized rats. *Kidney Int.* 54(3):864-76.

Niedermeier, M., Reich, B., Rodriguez Gomez, M., Denzel, A., Schmidbauer, K., Göbel, N., Talke, Y., Schweda, F. & Mack, M. (2009). CD4+ T cells control the differentiation of Gr1+ monocytes into fibrocytes. *Proc Natl Acad Sci U S A.* 106(42):17892-7.

Nishida, M., Fujinaka, H., Matsusaka, T., Price, J., Kon, V., Fogo, AB., Davidson, JM., Linton, MF., Fazio, S., Homma, T., Yoshida, H. & Ichikawa, I. (2002). Absence of angiotensin II type 1 receptor in bone marrow-derived cells is detrimental in the evolution of renal fibrosis. *J Clin Invest.* 110:1859-1868.

Nishida, M., Okumura, Y., Ozawa, S., Shiraishi, I., Itoi, T. & Hamaoka, K. (2007). MMP-2 inhibition reduces renal macrophage infiltration with increased fibrosis in UUO. *Biochem Biophys Res Commun.* 354(1):133-9.

Ostendorf, T., Eitner, F. & Floege, J. (2011). The PDGF family in renal fibrosis. *Pediatr Nephrol.* [Epub ahead of print]

Ouyang, X., Le, TH., Roncal, C., Gersch, C., Herrera-Acosta, J., Rodriguez-Iturbe, B., Coffman, TM., Johnson, RJ. & Mu, W. (2005). Th1 inflammatory response with altered expression of profibrotic and vasoactive mediators in AT1A and AT1B double-knockout mice. *Am J Physiol Renal Physiol.* 289(4):F902-10.

Ozes, ON., Mayo, LD., Gustin, JA., Pfeffer, SR., Pfeffer, LM. & Donner, DB. (1999). NFkappaB activation by tumour necrosis factor requires the Akt serinethreonine kinase. *Nature.* 401:82-85.

Pavone-Macaluso, M. (1960). Tissue mast cells in renal diseases. *Acta Pathol Microbiol Scand* 50:337–346.

Payne, V. & Kam, PC. (2004). Mast cell tryptase: a review of its physiology and clinical significance. *Anaesthesia* 59:695–703.

Peng, C. (2003). The TGF-beta superfamily and its roles in the human ovary and placenta. *J Obstet Gynaecol Can.* 25(10):834-44.

Peters, H., Noble, NA. & Border, WA. (1997). Transforming growth factor-beta in human glomerular injury. *Curr Opin Nephrol Hypertens.* 6(4):389-93.

Pohlers, D., Brenmoehl, J., Löffler, I., Müller, CK., Leipner, C., Schultze-Mosgau, S., Stallmach, A., Kinne, RW., Wolf, G.. (2009). TGF-beta and fibrosis in different organs - molecular pathway imprints. *Biochim Biophys Acta.* 1792(8):746-56.

Prodeus, AP., Zhou, X., Maurer, M., Galli, SJ. & Carroll, MC. (1997). Impaired mast cell-dependent natural immunity in complement C3-deficient mice. *Nature* 390: 172–175

Raissian, Y., Nasr, SH., Larsen, CP., Colvin, RB., Smyrk, TC., Takahashi, N., Bhalodia, A., Sohani, AR., Zhang, L., Chari, S., Sethi, S., Fidler, ME. & Cornell, LD. (2011). Diagnosis of IgG4-related tubulointerstitial nephritis. *Am Soc Nephrol.* 22(7):1343-52.

Rampoldi, L., Scolari, F., Amoroso, A., Ghiggeri, G. & Devuyst, O. (2011). The rediscovery of uromodulin (Tamm-Horsfall protein): from tubulointerstitial nephropathy to chronic kidney disease. *Kidney Int.* 80(4):338-47.

Ravetch, JV. & Bolland, S. (2001). IgG Fc receptors. *Annu Rev Immunol.* 19:275–290.

Ren, Z., Liang, W., Chen, C., Yang, H., Singhal, PC. & Ding, G. (2011). Angiotensin II induces nephrin dephosphorylation and podocyte injury: Role of caveolin-1. *Cell Signal.* [Epub ahead of print]

Ricardo, SD., van Goor, H. & Eddy, AA. (2008). Macrophage diversity in renal injury and repair. *J Clin Invest.* 118(11):3522-30.

Ronco, P. & Chatziantoniou, C. (2008). Matrix metalloproteinases and matrix receptors in progression and reversal of kidney disease: therapeutic perspectives. *Kidney Int.* 74: 873–878.

Rüster, C. & Wolf, G. (2011). Angiotensin II as a morphogenic cytokine stimulating renal fibrogenesis. *J Am Soc Nephrol.* 22(7):1189-99.

Saeki, T., Saito, A., Yamazaki, H., Emura, I., Imai, N., Ueno, M., Nishi, S., Miyamura, S. & Gejyo, F. (2007). Tubulointerstitial nephritis associated with IgG4-related systemic disease. *Clin Exp Nephrol.* 11(2):168-73.

Sawyer, DW., Donowitz, GR. & Mandell, GL. (1989). Polymorphonuclear neutrophils: an effective antimicrobial force. *Rev Infect Dis.* 11 Suppl 7:S1532-44.

Schlaeger, TM., Bartunkova, S., Lawitts, JA., Teichmann, G., Risau, W., Deutsch, U. & Sato, TN. (1997). Uniform vascular-endothelial-cell-specific gene expression in both embryonic and adult transgenic mice. *Proc Natl Acad Sci U S A.* 94(7):3058-63.

Schmidt, M., Sun, G., Stacey, MA., Mori, L. & Mattoli, S. (2003) Identification of circulating fibrocytes as precursors of bronchial myofibroblasts in asthma. *J Immunol.* 171(1):380-9.

Scudamore, CL., Jepson, MA., Hirst, BH. & Miller, HR. (1998). The rat mucosal mast cell chymase, RMCP-II, alters epithelial cell monolayer permeability in association with altered distribution of the tight junction proteins ZO-1 and occludin. *Eur J Cell Biol.* 75: 321–330.

Seifert, RA., Alpers, CE. & Bowen-Pope, DF. (1998) Expression of platelet-derived growth factor and its receptors in the developing and adult mouse kidney. *Kidney Int.* 54(3):731-46.

Sharma, AK., Mauer, SM., Kim, Y. & Michael, AF. (1995). Altered expression of matrix metalloproteinase-2, TIMP, and TIMP-2 in obstructive nephropathy. *J Lab Clin Med.* 125(6):754-61.

Siragy, HM. (2004). AT1 and AT2 receptor in the kidney: role in health and disease. *Semin Nephrol.* 24(2):93-100.

Song, E., Ouyang, N., Horbelt, M., Antus, B., Wang, M. & Exton, MS. (2000). Influence of alternatively and classically activated macrophages on fibrogenic activities of human fibroblasts. *Cell Immunol.* 204: 19–28.

Sorokin, L. (2010). The impact of the extracellular matrix on inflammation. *Nat Rev Immunol.* 10: 712–723.

Steinmetz, OM., Sadaghiani, S., Panzer, U., Krebs, C., Meyer-Schwesinger, C., Streichert, T., Fehr, S., Hamming, I., van Goor, H., Stahl, RA. & Wenzel, U. (2007). Antihypertensive therapy induces compartment-specific chemokine expression and a Th1 immune response in the clipped kidney of Goldblatt hypertensive rats. *Am J Physiol Renal Physiol.* 292(2):F876-87.

Strutz, F. & Neilson, EG. (1994). The role of lymphocytes in the progression of interstitial disease. *Kidney Int.* Suppl. 45:S106-10. 37.

Supajatura, V., Ushio, H., Nakao, A., Akira, S., Okumura, K., Ra, C. & Ogawa, H. (2002). Differential responses of mast cell Toll-like receptors 2 and 4 in allergy and innate immunity. *J Clin Invest.* 109: 1351–1359

Suzuki, Y., Ruiz-Ortega, M., Lorenzo, O., Ruperez, M., Esteban, V. & Egido J. (2003). Inflammation and angiotensin II. *Int J Biochem Cell Biol.* 35(6):881-900.

Swaminathan, S. & Griffin, MD. (2008). First responders: understanding monocyte-lineage traffic in the acutely injured kidney. *Kidney In.t* 74: 1509–1511.

Tacke, F. & Randolph, GJ. (2006). Migratory fate and differentiation of blood monocyte subsets. *Immunobiology* 211:609–618.

Tang, WW., Ulich, TR., Lacey, DL., Hill, DC., Qi, M., Kaufman, SA, Van, GY., Tarpley, JE. & Yee, JS. (1996). Platelet derived growth factor-BB induces renal tubulointerstitial myofibroblastmformation and tubulointerstitial fibrosis. *Am J Pathol.* 148:1169-1180.

Tapmeier, TT., Fearn, A., Brown, K., Chowdhury, P., Sacks, SH., Sheerin, NS. & Wong, W. (2010). Pivotal role of CD4+ T cells in renal fibrosis following ureteric obstruction. Kidney Int. 78(4):351-62.

Thiery, JP. & Sleeman, JP. (2006). Complex networks orchestrate epithelial-mesenchymal transitions. *Nat Rev Mol Cell Biol.* 7(2):131-42.

Topley, N., Steadman, R. & Williams JD. (2005). Neutrophil activation and renal scarring. *Kidney Int.* 67(6):2504

Trojanowska, M. (2008). Role of PDGF in fibrotic diseases and systemic sclerosis. *Rheumatology (Oxford).* 47 Suppl 5:v2-4.

Tsuda, Y., Takahashi, H., Kobayashi, M., Hanafusa, T., Herndon, DN. & Suzuki, F. (2004). Three different neutrophil subsets exhibited in mice with different susceptibilities to infection by methicillin-resistant Staphylococcus aureus. *Immunity.* 21(2):215-26.

Tucci, M., Ciavarella, S., Strippoli, S., Dammacco, F. & Silvestris, F. (2009). Oversecretion of cytokines and chemokines in lupus nephritis is regulated by intraparenchymal dendritic cells: a review. *Ann N Y Acad Sci.* 1173:449-57.

Tucci, M., Quatraro, C., Lombardi, L., Pellegrino, C., Dammacco, F. & Silvestris, F. (2008). Glomerular accumulation of plasmacytoid dendritic cells in active lupus nephritis: role of interleukin-18. *Arthritis Rheum.* 58(1):251-62.

Turner, JE., Paust, HJ., Steinmetz, OM. & Panzer, U. (2010). The Th17 immune response in renal inflammation. *Kidney Int.* 77(12):1070-5.

Verkade, MA., van Druningen, CJ., Vaessen, LM., Hesselink, DA., Weimar, W. & Betjes, MG. (2007). Functional impairment of monocyte-derived dendritic cells in patients with severe chronic kidney disease. Nephrol Dial Transplant. 22(1):128-38.

Vielhauer, V., Anders, HJ., Mack, M., Cihak, J., Strutz, F., Stangassinger, M., Luckow, B., Gröne, HJ. & Schlöndorff, D. (2001). Obstructive nephropathy in the mouse: progressive fibrosis correlates with tubulointerstitial chemokine expression and accumulation of CC chemokine receptor 2- and 5-positive leukocytes. *J Am Soc Nephrol.* 12(6):1173-87.

Wada, T., Furuichi, K., Sakai, N., Iwata, Y., Kitagawa, K., Ishida, Y., Kondo, T., Hashimoto, H., Ishiwata, Y., Mukaida, N., Tomosugi, N., Matsushima, K., Egashira, K. & Yokoyama, H. (2004). Gene therapy via blockade of monocyte chemoattractant protein-1 for renal fibrosis. *J Am Soc Nephrol.* 15: 940–948.

Wajant, H., Pfizenmaier, K. & Scheurich, P. (2003). Tumor necrosis factor signaling. *Cell Death Differ.* 10: 45–65.

Weidner, S., Carl, M., Riess, R. & Rupprecht, HD. (2004). Histologic analysis of renal leukocyte infiltration in antineutrophil cytoplasmic antibody-associated vasculitis: importance of monocyte and neutrophil infiltration in tissue damage. *Arthritis Rheum.* 50(11):3651-7.

Winkler, EA., Bell, RD. & Zlokovic, BV. (2010). Pericyte-specific expression of PDGF beta receptor in mouse models with normal and deficient PDGF beta receptor signaling. *Mol Neurodegener.* 5:32.

Wu, K., Zhou, T., Sun, G., Wang, W., Zhang, Y., Zhang, Y., Hao, L. & Chen, N. (2006). Valsartan inhibited the accumulation of dendritic cells in rat fibrotic renal tissue. *Cell Mol Immunol.* 3(3):213-20.

Wynn, TA. (2004). Fibrotic disease and the T(H)1/T(H)2 paradigm. *Nat Rev Immunol.* 4: 583–594.

Xu, H., He, X., Sun, J., Shi, D., Zhu, Y. & Zhang, X. (2009). The expression of B-cell activating factor belonging to tumor necrosis factor superfamily (BAFF) significantly correlated with C4D in kidney allograft rejection. *Transplant Proc.* 41(1):112-6.

Yamagishi, H., Yokoo, T., Imasawa, T., Shen, JS., Hisada, Y., Eto, Y., Kawamura, T. & Hosoya, T. (2001). Genetically modified bone marrow-derived vehicle cells site specifically deliver an anti-inflammatory cytokine to inflamed interstitium of obstructive nephropathy. *J Immunol.* 166:609-616.

Yang, J. & Liu, Y. (2001). Dissection of key events in tubular epithelial to myofibroblast transition and its implications in renal interstitial fibrosis. *Am J Pathol.* 159(4):1465-75.

Yang, L., Scott, PG., Giuffre, J., Shankowsky, HA., Ghahary, A. & Tredget EE. (2002). Peripheral blood fibrocytes from burn patients: identification and quantification of fibrocytes in adherent cells cultured from peripheral blood mononuclear cells. *Lab Invest.* 82(9):1183-92.

Zeisberg, EM., Potenta, S., Xie, L., Zeisberg, M. & Kalluri, R. (2007b). Discovery of endothelial to mesenchymal transition as a source for carcinomaassociated fibroblasts. *Cancer Res.* 67:10123–10128,

Zeisberg, EM., Potenta, SE., Sugimoto, H., Zeisberg, M. & Kalluri, R. (2008). Fibroblasts in kidney fibrosis emerge via endothelial-to-mesenchymal transition. *J Am Soc Nephrol.* 19(12):2282-7.

Zeisberg, EM., Tarnavski, O., Zeisberg, M., Dorfman, AL., McMullen, JR., Gustafsson, E., Chandraker, A., Yuan, X., Pu, WT., Roberts, AB., Neilson, EG., Sayegh, MH., Izumo, S. & Kalluri, R. (2007a). Endothelial-to-mesenchymal transition contributes to cardiac fibrosis. *Nat Med.* 13(8):952-61.

Zeisberg, M., Khurana, M., Rao, VH., Cosgrove, D., Rougier, JP., Werner, MC., Shield, CF., Werb, Z. & Kalluri, R. (2006). Stage-specific action of matrix metalloproteinases influences progressive hereditary kidney disease. PLoS Med. 3(4):e100.

Zhang, JL., Sun, DJ., Hou, CM., Wei, YL., Li, XY., Yu, ZY., Feng, JN., Shen, BF., Li, Y. & Xiao, H. (2010). CD3 mAb treatment ameliorated the severity of the cGVHD-induced lupus nephritis in mice by up-regulation of Foxp3+ regulatory T cells in the target tissue: kidney. *Transpl Immunol.* 24(1):17-25.

Zhao, Y., Glesne, D. & Huberman, E. (2003). A human peripheral blood monocytederived subset acts as pluripotent stem cells. *Proc Natl Acad Sci USA.* 100:2426–2431.

Zhou, T., Li, X., Zou, J., Cai, M., Sun, G., Zhang, Y., Zhao, Y., Zhang, M., Zhang, Y. & Chen, N. (2009). Effects of DC-SIGN expression on renal tubulointerstitial fibrosis in nephritis. *Front Biosci.* 14:3814-24.

5

Effects of Maternal Renal Dysfunction on Fetal Development

Toshiya Okada[1], Yoko Kitano-Amahori[1], Masaki Mino[1], Tomohiro Kondo[1], Ai Takeshita[1] and Ken-Takeshi Kusakabe[2]
[1]Osaka Prefecture University, Izumi-Sano, Osaka
[2]Yamaguchi University, Yamaguchi
Japan

1. Introduction

Maternal conditions affect the growth of the fetal kidney, which begins to secrete urine during late gestation (Bakala et al., 1985; Schaeverbeke & Cheignon, 1980). For example, during pregnancy, the maternal kidney undergoes various changes such as an increase in glomerular filtration rate (Baylis, 1994; Atherton & Pirie, 1981) and an alteration in tubular function (Dafnis & Sabatini, 1992). Furthermore, maternal undernutrition by the restriction of protein intake induces low fetal birth and leads to renal morphological and physiological changes (Mesquita et al., 2010). Maternal bilateral ligation of the uterine artery, protein restriction, smoking, nephrotoxic medication as well as salt loading cause intrauterine growth retardation (IUGR) to fetuses (Bentz & Amann, 2010), inducing fetal programing of renal function. Previously, we investigated the development of the fetal kidney during maternal renal dysfunction induced by bilateral ureteral ligation (Okada et al., 1997) and uninephrectomy (Okada et al., 2000, 2006), and we found that the development of the fetal kidney is accelerated by the operations. Furthermore, we found that maternal bilateral ureteral ligation (Okada & Morikawa, 1988) and uninephrectomy (Okada et al., 1998) decrease fetal body weight. In this chapter, we present a summary of the changes that occur in the fetal kidney after maternal bilateral ureteral ligation, uninephrectomy, and subtotal (5/6) nephrectomy, in addition to a summary of the changes that occur in the remaining kidney after uninephrectomy and 5/6 nephrectomy. Although 5/6 nephrectomy produces a bigger functional demand to maternal and fetal kidneys than the other two operations, little information is available on fetal development of the kidney when the maternal kidney is 5/6th removed. Therefore, we focused on studying the remaining kidney of unilateral and 5/6 nephrectomy and the fetal kidney under maternal renal dysfunction.

2. Effects of nehrectomy on remaining kidney

Nephrectomy can be used for research on renal growth and renal failure. Specifically uninephrectomy can be performed for research on the biology of compensatory renal growth (Fine, 1986) and subtotal nephrectomy for renal failure. In studies of subtotal nephrectomy, 3/4 nephrectomy (Friedman & Pityer, 1986) and 5/6 nephrectomy

(Manotham et al., 2004) have been performed. In this section, effects of uninephrectomy and 5/6 nephrectomy on the remaining kidney are discussed.

2.1 Effects of uninephrectomy on the cell proliferation and EGF in the remaining kidney

Compensatory renal growth after unilateral nephrectomy has been intensely investigated (Dicker & Shirley, 1971; Johnson & Vera Roman, 1966; Mok et al., 2003) and includes cellular hypertrophy, hyperplasia, and apoptosis (Wang et al., 1997). In the adult kidney, differentiated nephrons are relatively quiescent, with few cells undergoing mitosis (Girardi et al., 2002). Compensatory response after renal mass ablation shows increase in both cell size and cellular protein content without any increase in cell number (Girardi et al., 2002). The compensatory renal growth largely occurs by hypertrophy rather than hyperplasia of the remaining nephrons (Chen et al., 2005). Kanda et al. (1993) have observed that 24 h after uninephrectomy of an adult mouse kidney, there was an initiation of the proliferation of cortical tubular cells in the remaining kidney stained with anti-BrdU antibody. On the other hand, it has been seen that the compensatory response to uninephrectomy is stronger in immature animals than in adult ones (Fine, 1986) and the removal of the contralateral kidney induces an evident increase in cell proliferation, especially in proximal tubules, in young uninephrectomized rats (Girardi et al., 2002). Furthermore, we have recently reported that in the remaining kidney of uninephrectomized immature (3-week-old) rats few proliferatiomg cell nuclear antigen (PCNA)-positive cells in distal tubules were little observed and that a significant increase in the PCNA-positive cell ratios was observed in the proximal convoluted and straight tubules (Okada et al., 2010). Moreover, we have reported that in the immature rats 1 and 3 days after uninephrectomy there were significant increases in renal weight and the PCNA-positive cell ratios of the glomerulus and proximal convoluted and straight tubules (Okada et al., 2010). Kanda et al. (1993) have also reported that in immature rats, the increase in kidney mass immediately after nephrectomy is mainly due to hyperplasia, whereas 2 weeks after nephrectomy both hyperplasia and hypertrophy processes equally participate. Therefore, we concluded that there is an increase in proliferative activity in the proximal tubules during the early stage of compensatory renal growth in immature rats. Thus, the compensatory reaction of immature animals is different from that of adult animals, in terms of proliferative activity but is similar with regard to an increase in proliferating cells during the 24 h after uninephrectomy.

Considering the relationship of epidermal growth factor (EGF) to the elevated proliferating activity of nephrectomized immature animals, we examined the immunolocalization of EGF (Okada et al., 2010). Although Toubeau et al. (1994) and Jung et al. (2005) have observed the immunolocalizations of EGF in distal convoluted tubules and the thick ascending limb of Henle's loop of adult rat kidneys, our results revealed that EGF-positive cells localized to the proximal and the distal tubules in the kidney of immature rats indicating the difference of immunolocalization of EGF in the kidney between adult and immature animals (Okada et al., 2010). There are controversial reports on the involvement of EGF on the proliferative activity of the adult kidney. For example, Pugh et al. (1995) have found that the addition of EGF to renal organ culture medium increases uptake of BrdU while Toubeau et al. (1994) have found that cell proliferation occurs immediately after the decrease of renal EGF and its receptor (EGFR) in the rat experimentally subjected to acute renal failure. Further, in the unilaterally ureter obstructed rat model, the administration of EGF causes a decrease in proliferative activity in the contralateral kidney (Chevalier, 1999). Moreover, EGF expression and the role of EGF in the developing kidney is also controversial as follows: in the developing kidney, EGF expression appears as nephrons mature (Nouwen et al., 1994); exogenous EGF delays the development of the loop of Henle by reducing both apoptosis and cell proliferation (Lee et al., 2004); robust EGF synthesis is clearly a characteristic of the mature kidney rather than that of a rapidly-growing fetal organ (Goodyer et al., 1991a); renal EGF is undetectable in the human fetus (Goodyer, et al., 1991b) and renal EGF content is increased from days 6 to 21 after birth in mice (Gattone et al., 1992).

We have recently observed that on the first post-operative day, the proximal tubular cells showed a weaker reaction to EGF antibody in uninephrectomized rats than in sham-operated rats and that the degree of reactivity to EGF was the same in both groups on the third post-operative day and that the level of expression of preproEGF mRNA was significantly lower in uninephrectomized rats than in sham-operated rats at the first post-operative day (Okada et al., 2010). These findings reveal that unilateral nephrectomy in immature rats causes an increased proliferative activity and a decreased expression of EGF in the remaining kidney during the early period of compensatory renal growth.

2.2 Effects of subtotal (5/6) nephrectomy on the remaining kidney: Growth factor and protein restriction

Subtotal (5/6) nephrectomy has been performed on laboratory animals to achieve a model for chronic renal failure (Manotham et al., 2004; Zhang et al., 1999). After the reduction of renal mass, remnant renal tissue was less able to maintain stability of blood flow and filtration rate during variations in renal perfusion pressure (Brown et al., 1995), and various pathological changes are observed. In the remaining kidney, glomerular sclerosis is observed following increased proliferative activity in glomeruli (Floege et al., 1992), and renal fibrosis is accompanied with apoptotic cells (Li et al., 2004). The remaining kidney of 5/6 nephrectomized animals was utilized as a model for renal fibrosis (Johnson et al., 1997; Nangaku et al., 2002; Yang et al., 2001) and a model for glomerular sclerosis (Floege et al., 1992; Griffin et al., 1994). Since in immature rats as well as adult animals, 5/6 nephrectomy induces significant increases in BUN, glomerular sclerosis index (GSI), and interstitial fibrosis score (IFS), compared with sham-oprated ones (Mino et al., 2007), 5/6 nephrectomized immature animals are useful as animal model for renal failure.

In adult animals, it has been reported that a low protein diet reduces uremic toxicity in experimentally-induced uremia (Sterner et al, 1994) and that in the 5/6 nephrectomized renal failure model, the restriction of protein intake improves renal failure (Heller et al., 1994). It has been reported that a low protein intake improves survival over normal protein intake in 3/4 nephrectomized immature rats (Friedman & Pityer, 1986). Further, Mino et al. (2007) have reported that a low protein diet induces a significant decrease in BUN, GSI, and IFS in 5/6 nephrectomized immature rats. These findings suggest that protein intake restriction is effective in preventing renal failure in immature animals, which is in accord with the results in adult rats.

Increased glomerular hydraulic pressure and the ultrafiltration plasma proteins contribute to the onset and progression of chronic renal damage (Remuzzi et al., 2005). Inhibitor of angiotensin converting enzyme (ACE) and angiotensin type II receptor antagonists can be used in combination to maximize renin-angiotensin-aldosterone system (RAAS) inhibition and more effectively reduce proteinuria and GFR decline in diabetic and non-diabetic renal disease (Remuzzi et al., 2005; Klein et al., 2003). Since activation of RAAS induces decreased level of endothelial nitric oxide synthase (eNOS) expression (Zhao et al., 2005), it is thought that NO also plays an important role in the progression of renal failure. Therefore, in 5/6 nephrectomized animals, factors, including RAAS and NO, relating to the progression of renal failure and effects of protein restriction are discussed.

We have previously reported that in the normal developing kidney in perinatal rats, EGF plays an important role in proliferative activity (Okada et al., 2001) and apoptosis (Okada et al., 2003). Further, chronic renal failure caused by 5/6 nephrectomy is improved by extrinsic EGF (Moskowitz et al., 1992), and EGF accelerates the regeneration of tubular cells and ameliorates renal failure (Humes et al., 1989). Furthermore, in 5/6 nephrectomized immature rats, the incidence of TUNEL positive cells in distal tubules was lowered and more EGF-positive cells in the segments were observed after protein restriction (Mino et al., 2007). These findings reveal that protein restriction is effective in preventing renal tubular scarring in immature rats and that EGF is involved in the process of this prevention.

Transforming growth factor-β (TGF-β) suppresses proliferative activity of the cells (Cheng & Grande, 2002) and converts renal tubular epithelial cells to fibroblasts (Stahl & Felsen, 2001). The fibroblast cells induce fibrosis of the renal tubular interstitium (Blobe et al., 2002; Iwano et al., 2002). TGF-β is also related to the infiltration of macrophages (Wahl et al., 1987). Feeding of a low protein (6% protein) diet to 5/6 nephrectomized immature rats induces decreased immunoreactivity of TGF-β (Fig. 1) and ED1 (Fig. 2). The increased expression of TGF-β in the distal tubules of the kidney is involved in the damage of the remaining kidney of 5/6 nephrectomized animals and protein restriction suppresses the elevation of TGF-β expression and the progression of renal failure.

The expression of NO is increased in the kidney of animals with renal failure, and increased expression of NO is involved in the process of renal failure (Matubara et al., 2000). In the developing kidney, NO plays an important role in maintaining normal physiological function (Solhaug et al., 1996) and in regulating renal homodynamics (Han et al., 2005). Maintenance of adequate NO is an additional mechanism for the preservation of vasculature in progressive renal diseases (Kang et al., 2002). Inhibition of inducible NO synthase (iNOS) provides a mechanism against the developing ischemic renal injury and inflammation in the adult rat kidney (Mark et al., 2005). Nuclear factor-kappa B (NF-κB) is known to be involved in the induction of the human iNOS gene (Taylor et al., 1998). Furthermore, elevation in renin-angiotensin system (RAS) activity and DNA-binding activity of NF-κB are involved in the progression of renal failure in the remnant kidney of 5/6 nephrectomized rats (Ots et al., 1998; Fujihara et al., 2007). On the other hand, decreased expression levels of eNOS in the glomerulus are often seen in rats with renal disease (Bremer et al., 1997). In the remnant kidney model, inhibition of NO synthesis with L-NAME resulted in a decline of renal function and severe glomerulosclerosis (Kang, et al., 2002). In the current model for endotoxin-induced thrombotic microangiopathy, which accompanies glomerular injury, endothelial injury is associated with decreased eNOS expression levels (Shao et al., 2001). NO produced by eNOS confers antioxidant properties on vascular cells (Walford & Loscalzo, 2003), and the endogenous low steady state levels of NO produced by eNOS dynamically regulates mitochondrial respiration. This regulation thus provides protection against H_2O_2 mediated injury and death (Paxinou et al., 2001).

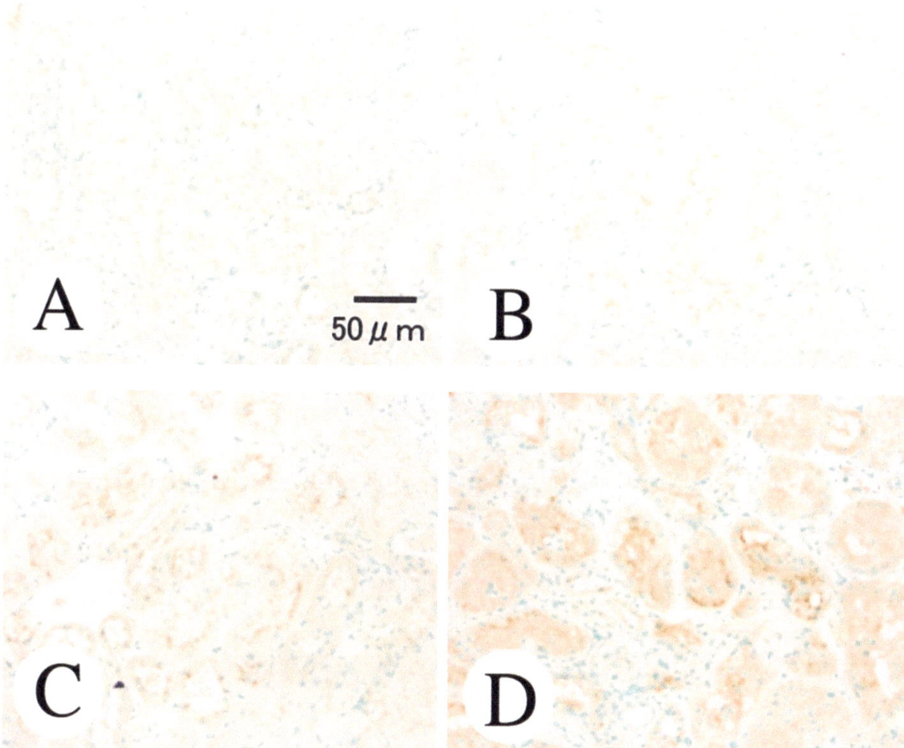

Fig. 1. Kidneys of 5/6 nephrectomized immature rats stained with an anti-TGF-β antibody. bar = 50 μm. **A**, low protein group 4 weeks after the operation. TGF-β positive cells are seen in the distal tubules. **B**, normal protein group 4 weeks after the operation. TGF-β positive cells are seen in the distal tubules and the reaction activity to TGF-β antibody is stronger compared to that in the age-matched low protein group in figure 1A. **C**, low protein group 8 weeks after the operation. The reaction activity to TGF-β antibody is stronger when compared with those in the low protein group 4 weeks after the operation in figure 1A. **D**, normal protein group 8 weeks after the operation. The reaction activity to TGF-β is stronger compared to those in the age-matched low protein group in figure 1C and is stronger compared to that in the normal protein group 4 weeks after the operation in figure 1B.

Thus, eNOS has a protective role in glomerulonephritis (Shao et al., 2001; Heering et al., 2002), and RAS is involved in changes in eNOS expression (Zhao et al., 2005; Varziri et al., 2002). As shown in figure 3, the eNOS positive cells were observed in the glomerulus in the rats of every group at 4 and 8 weeks after the operation in 5/6 nephrectomized immature rats (Fig. 3B and D). The positive reaction to the anti-eNOS antibody was stronger in the 4-week postoperative rats than in the 8-week postoperative rats, and the reaction was stronger in the protein-restricted rats than in the control rats 4 weeks after the operation (Fig. 3).

Mino et al. (2010) have observed that the remaining kidney of 5/6 nephrectomized and protein-restricted immature rats exhibits an elevated levels of the endothelial eNOS protein expression and a decrement in iNOS positive cells in the distal tubules and in the expression of renin mRNA. They also concluded that protein-restriction is effective in preventing renal failure of immature rats and that the changes in the expression levels of renin, eNOS, and iNOS are involved in the process of this prevention.

A

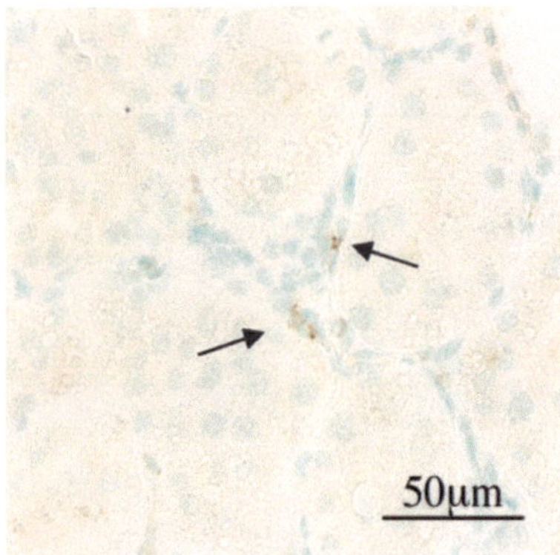

B

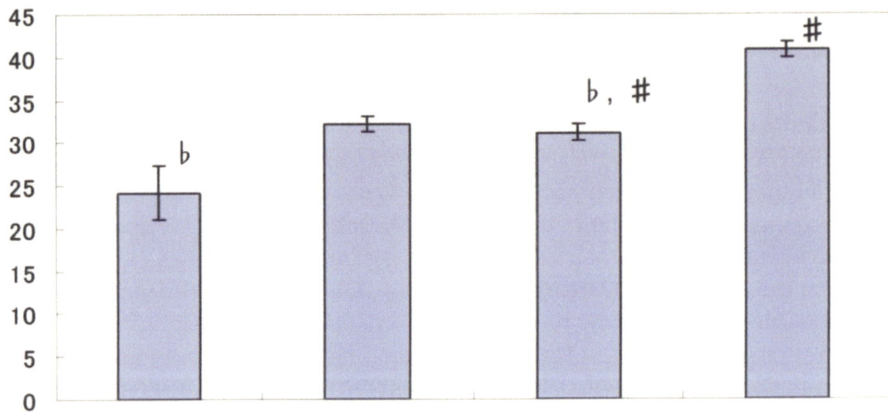

Fig. 2. **A**, Kidney stained with anti-ED1 antibody. ED1 positive cells (arrows) are observed in the interstitium. **B**, Changes in number of ED1 positive cells per area (300 x 400 μm) (Means±SEM) in the kidney of 5/6 nephrectomized rats.
Lp (4Ws), low protein group 4 weeks after the operation.
Np (4Ws), normal protein group 4 weeks after the operation.
Lp (8Ws), low protein group 8 weeks after the operation.
Np (8Ws), normal protein group 8 weeks after the operation.
b, Significantly different from age-matched normal protein group ($p<0.05$).
#, Significantly different from same group 4weeks after the operation ($p<0.05$)

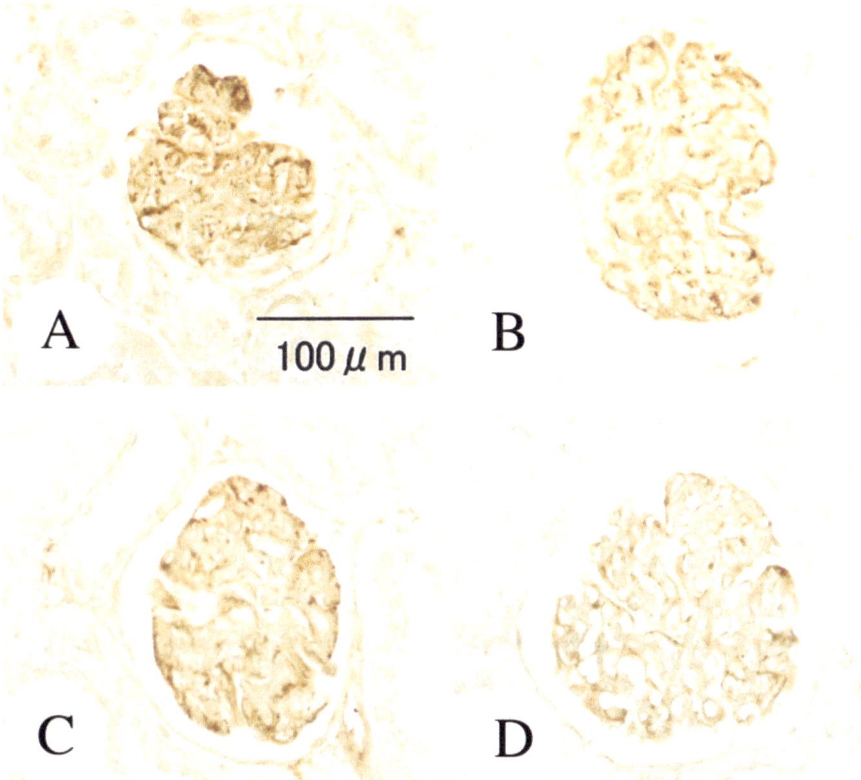

Fig. 3. Kidneys of 5/6 nephrectomized immature rats stained with an anti-eNOS antibody. bar = 100 μm. **A**, Low protein diet fed rats 4weeks after the operation. The eNOS positive cells are seen in the glomerulus. **B**, Normal protein diet fed rats 4 weeks after the operation. The reaction activity to eNOS antibody is weaker compared to that in age-matched low protein diet fed rats in figure 1A. **C**, Low protein diet fed rats 8 weeks after the operation. The reaction activity to the eNOS antibody is weaker when compared with those in the low protein diet fed rats 4 weeks after the operation in figure 1A. **D**, Normal protein diet fed rats 8 weeks after the operation. The reaction activity to the eNOS antibody is slightly weaker when compared with that in the normal protein diet fed rats 4 weeks after the operation in figure 1B and is slightly weaker compared to that in the age-matched low protein diet fed rats in figure 1C.

3. Effects of maternal renal dysfunction on the development of fetal kidney

The concentrations of many substances are known to change physiologically in pregnancy relative to the length of gestation (Kelly et al., 1978). The study of renal physiology during pregnancy has been mainly related to glomerular function (Studd, 1971; MacLean et al., 1972). In humans, glomerular filtration rate (GFR) reaches a peak of 40-50% higher than nonpregnant values between 9 and 11 weeks of pregnancy and is sustained until at least the 36th week (Dafnis & Sabatini, 1992). Atherton & Pirie (1981) have reported that GFR and salt and water reabsorption significantly elevate in early pregnancy. Furthermore, maternal renal function elevates during pregnancy in rats (Churchill et al., 1982). Throughout gestation, fetal waste products are primarily excreted by maternal kidneys through placental circulation (Liggins, 1972) and fetal kidneys start secreting urine during the final days of gestation (Bakala et al., 1985). This implies that an increase of fetal waste products in circulation, indicative of the latter gestational period, stimulates fetal kidneys to start urine production. Therefore, development of the fetal kidney is thought to be stimulated by functional demands associated with maternal renal dysfunction.

3.1 Effects of ligation of maternal ureters on the development of the fetal kidney

When pregnant rats are subjected to bilateral ureteral ligation for one day, the BUN level is elevated 5 to 8 times of control values, and BUN passes through the placenta into the fetal circulation to stimulate fetal kidney urine production (Matsuo et al., 1986). Fetal urine production is thereby stimulated by maternal ureteral ligation (Wells, 1946). We observed that in the kidney of fetuses of fetal days 20 and 22 from bilaterally ureter ligated mothers apical vacuoles in the proximal tubular cells are increased by the ligation (Okada & Morikawa, 1990). Furthermore, the surface area of the glomerular basement membrane and the length of the glomerular capillary per unit volume of glomerulus are increased (Okada & Morikawa, 1993) and shortening of the time for filtration of HRP through the glomerular basement membrane is observed in the fetuses from the ligated mothers (Okada et al., 1997). Therefore, the maternal bilateral ligation causes an elevation of BUN concentration, acceleration of the growth and differentiation of the proximal tubules, accelerated formation of fetal glomerular basement membrane, and stimulated glomerular function in the filtration in the fetal rat kidney when the fetal kidney is functional in urine production.

3.2 Effects of maternal uninephrectomy on the development of fetal kidney

In uninephrectomized pregnant rats on day 5 of gestation, BUN concentration is significantly increased 1 day after the operation and remained high at term (Okada et al., 1998). Previously, we have reported that glomerular volume (Okada et al., 1994) and proximal tubular length (Okada et al., 1995) are larger in pups from uninephrectomized mothers than in those from sham-operated ones, suggesting the accelerated renal development was influenced by maternal uninephrectomy. By the electron microscopic observation on distribution of cationized ferritin (CF) in fetal glomerulus after CF injection, we found that the formation of anionic sites in the glomerular basement membrane of fetuses is accelerated by uninephrectomy (Okada et al., 1998). Furthermore, we previously reported that maternal uninephrectomy induces lowered proliferative activity in mature glomerulus and enhanced positive reactions to both EGF and EGFR antibodies in proximal tubular cells in the fetal kidney (Okada et al., 2000). Recently, we have revealed that an increase in apoptosis in the collecting ducts of fetal kidney is induced by maternal uninephrectomy and that the increase is related to the decreased expression of *bcl-2*, an apoptotic suppressor gene (Okada et al., 2006).

3.3 Effects of maternal subtotal nephrectomy on the development of fetal kidney

3.3.1 Aim of study

Fetal waste products are primarily excreted by maternal kidneys through placental circulation (Liggins, 1972). During the final days of gestation, fetal kidneys start secreting urine (Bakala et al., 1985). This implies that an increase of fetal waste products in circulation, indicative of the latter gestational period, stimulates fetal kidneys to start urine production. Therefore, development of the fetal kidney is thought to be stimulated by functional demands associated with maternal renal dysfunction. Bilateral ureteral ligation for 1 day (Matsuo et al., 1986) and uninephrectomy (Okada et al., 1998) induce an elevation in BUN, 5 to 8 times of control values and 1.5 times of control values, respectively. In a preliminary study, rats died in the third day after bilateral ureteral ligation; we therefore concluded that bilateral ureteral ligation cannot be used as a model for chronic renal failure. Similarly, uninephrectomy cannot be used as a model of renal failure because it does not cause pathological changes in the remaining kidney. Therefore, 5/6 nephrectomy, which induces renal fibrosis (Nangaku et al., 2002; Yang et al., 2001) and glomerular sclerosis (Griffin et al., 1994), is used for to model chronic renal failure (Manotham et al., 2004). There have been several reports on the development of the fetus from 5/6 nephrectomized mothers. Gibson et al. (2007) have examined changes in growth and urine volume of fetal sheep with maternal 5/6 nephrectomy. Salas et al. (2003) have examined fetal body weight and placental weight with maternal 5/6 nephrectomy. However, neither groups studied the kidney from the 5/6 nephrectomized mothers. Brandon et al. (2009) have determined the plasma renin level of offspring from 5/6 nephrectomized mothers and reported that in the neonates there is an impaired ability to regulate glomerular filtration independent of arterial pressure. In this section, experiments were designed to investigate the development of the fetal kidney under maternal renal dysfunction by 5/6 nephrectomy.

3.3.2 Materials & methods

Animals and tissue processing: Wistar strain rats were reared under ordinary conditions (24 ± 1°C, 14 hrs light and 10 hrs dark) and were given both a commercial diet (CE-2, Clea, Osaka, Japan) and water *ad libitum*. The day following an overnight mating was determined as day 1 of gestation. To make maternal renal dysfunction conditions, 5/6 nephrectomy was performed. Under isoflurane anesthesia, on day 5 of gestation 2/3 of the left kidney were excised and on day 12 of gestation the right kidney was removed. The body weights of 5/6 nephrectomized or sham-operated mothers were measured on days 3, 5, 7, 10, 12, 14, 18, 20, and 22 of gestation. BUN levels of 5/6 nephrectomized or sham-operated mothers were measured. Under isoflurane anesthesia, blood was drawn from the plexus ophthalamicus with a capillary glass tube at days 3, 7, 10, 14, 18, 20, and 22 of gestation. BUN concentration was determined with an automatic dry chemistry analyzer system (Spotchem SP-4410, Kyoto Daiichi-Kagaku Kyoto, Japan). On day 22 of gestation, fetuses were removed from the uterus under isoflurane anesthesia. Under the anesthesia, fetal kidneys were removed and fixed in methanol-Carnoy's solution [a mixture of methanol, chloroform, acetic acid (6:3:1)] or 10 % neutral buffered formalin. The kidneys were dehydrated in a graded series of alcohol, embedded in Tissue Prep (Fisher Scientific, Fair Lawn, NJ, USA), and sectioned at 6 μm. The sections from methanol-Carnoy fixed material were treated with PCNA, TGF-β, and TGF-β receptors (TGF-βRI and TGF-βRII) antibodies. The sections from formalin fixed material were treated with TUNEL method.

Detection of apoptotic cells and immunohistochemical procedures: After deparaffinization with xylene, the sections were transferred to distilled water through a degraded series of ethanol and were rinsed in phosphate buffered saline. The apoptotic cells were detected by TUNEL methods, using an in situ apoptosis detection kit (Takara, Kyoto, Japan). Briefly, the sections were incubated with the TdT enzyme and FITC-labeled dUTP at 37 °C for 90 min, further incubated with an anti-FITC HRP conjugate at 37 °C for 30 min, and finally incubated with DAB for 5 min. Negative controls were produced by omitting the TdT enzyme. Immunostaining for PCNA was performed by incubating with mouse anti-human PCNA antibody (19A2, Coulter Immunology, Hialeah, FL, USA, 1:160) at 4 °C overnight, after which the sections were incubated with biotinylated rabbit anti-mouse immunoglobulins antibody (BioGenex Laboratories, San Roman, CA, USA, 1:50) and streptavidin conjugated peroxidase (Zymed Laboratories, South San Francisco, CA, USA, 1:50) for 30 min, respectively. The TGF-β and the TGF-βRI immunostainings were performed as follows: The sections were incubated with rabbit anti-human TGF-βRI antibody (Santa Cruz Biotech, Santa Cruz, CA, USA, 1:100) at 4 °C overnight or rabbit anti-porcine TGF-β antibody (R&D Systems, Minneapolis, MN, USA, 1:100) at 4 °C for 3 nights. Then, the sections were incubated with biotinylated goat anti-rabbit IgG antibody (1:200) and avidin-biotin peroxidase complex (1:200) for 30 minutes, respectively. Last, the sections were incubated with DAB for 5 min. Negative controls were produced by omitting the primary antibody in immunohistochemical procedure. No positive immunoreactivity was recognized when antibody was preincubated with an excess of antigen (25µg/ml human TGF-βRI peptide, Santa Cruz Biotech, Santa Cruz, CA, USA; TGFβ antibody, 1mg/ml human TGFβ King Brewing, Kakogawa, Japan).

Determination of PCNA positive cell ratio: To determine the PCNA positive ratio in the glomerulus, 10 glomeruli were used. To determine the ratio in the proximal tubules, more than 500 nuclei were used in the proximal convoluted and straight tubules respectively. The nuclei positive and negative to PCNA were counted and the ratio of positive nuclei to total nuclei was expressed as a percentage.

3.3.3 Results & discussion

The result that a 5/6 nephrectomy operation on pregnant rats induced a significant decrease in body weight on day 14 of gestation and thereafter (Fig. 4) indicates that the operation has applied a burden to the mother. A slightly but significant increment in BUN concentration was induced after removing 2/3 of the left kidney, an intense increase in BUN was induced after removing the right kidney, and gradual decrease in BUN was observed on day 14 and thereafter (Fig. 5). The elevation in BUN concentration of nephrectomized mothers implies the elevation in functional demand to remaining kidney. Since the fetal kidney becomes functional during the late gestation period (Bakala et al., 1985), the decrease in BUN from day 14 to 22 of gestation reflects the instigation of fetal urine production. On day 22 of gestation, the concentration of urea nitrogen (UN) in maternal blood, fetal blood, and amniotic fluid were significantly higher in 5/6 nephrectomized pregnant rats than in sham-operated ones (Fig. 6). This finding suggests that increased UN in 5/6 nephrectomized mother passes through placenta to fetal blood circulation and that fetal kidney secretes the UN to the amniotic fluid. This notion is well in-line with the reports by Matsuo et al. (1986) which suggest that increased maternal BUN induces the elevation in fetal BUN and by Garcia et al. (1988) that found that an increase in fetal renal function induces the elevation in urea nitrogen levels of the amniotic fluid.

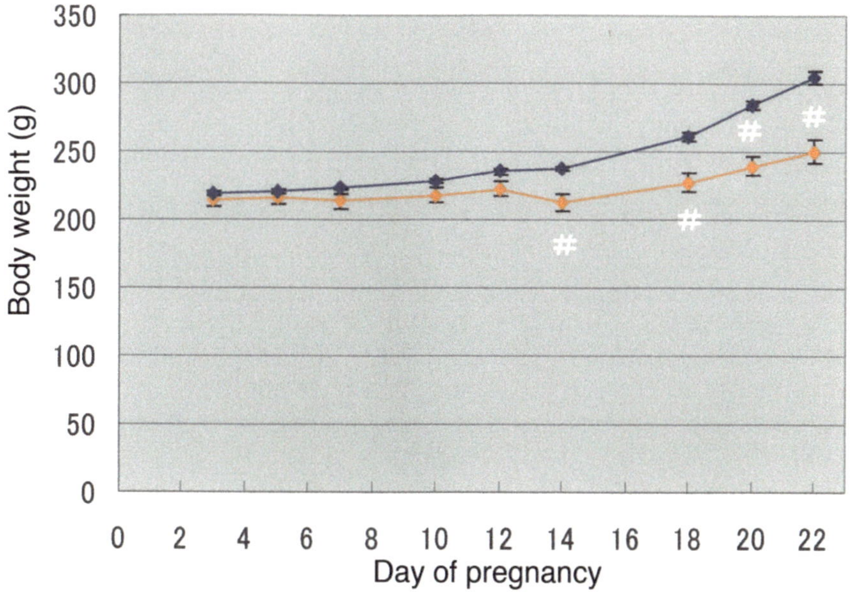

Fig. 4. Changes in body weights (Means±SEM) of 5/6 nephrectomized (orange line) and sham-operated (blue line) mothers

#, Significantly different from age-matched sham-operated mothers ($p<0.05$)

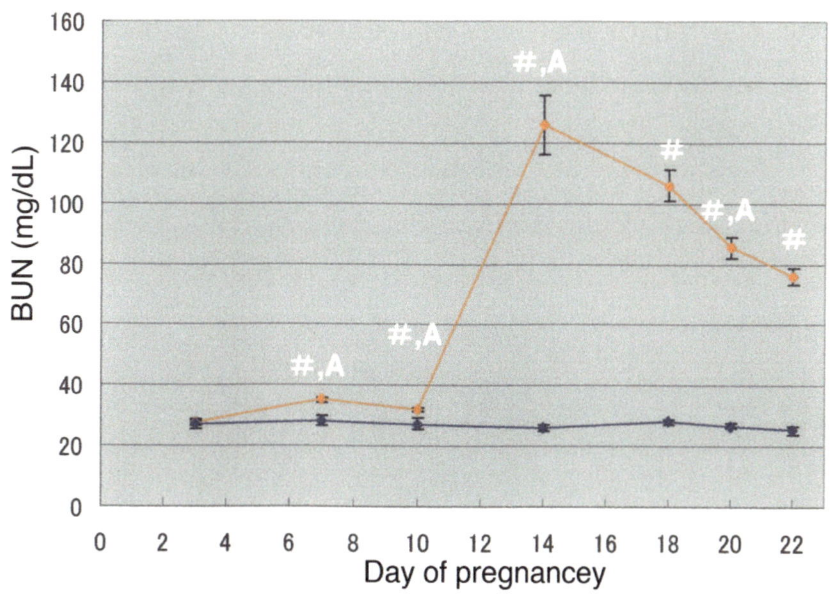

Fig. 5. Changes in BUN concentration (Means±SEM) of 5/6 nephrectomized (orange line) and sham-operated (blue line) mothers

#, Significantly different from age-matched sham-operated mothers ($p<0.05$)

A, Significantly different from preceding age group ($p<0.05$)

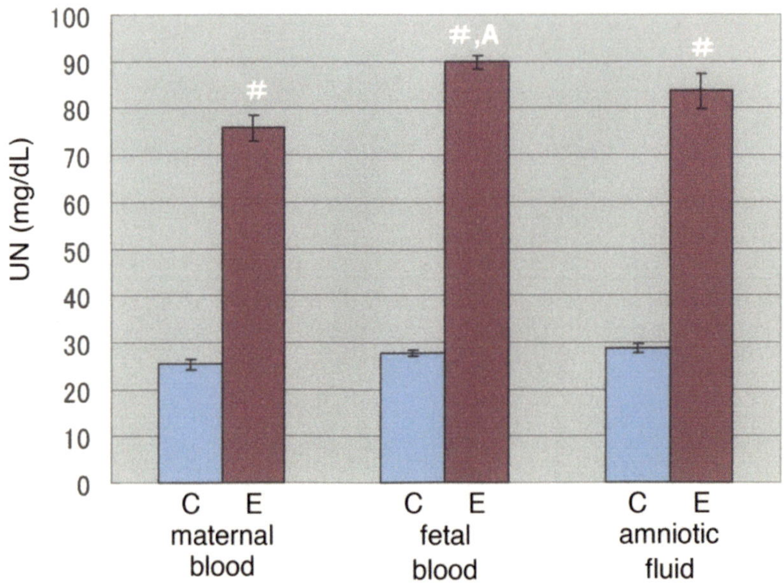

Fig. 6. The concentration of urea nitrogen in maternal blood, fetal blood, and amniotic fluid (Means±SEM) of 5/6 nephrectomized (E) and sham-operated (C) pregnant rats on day 22 of gestation.
#, Significantly different from sham-operated group (p<0.05)
A, Significantly different from maternal blood, in the same group (p<0.05)

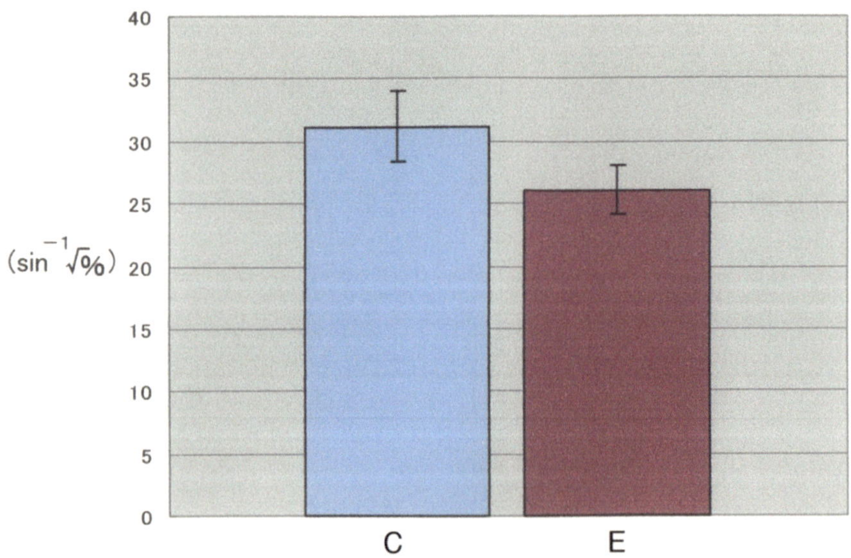

Fig. 7. PCNA positive cell ratio (Means±SEM) in the kidneys of fetuses from 5/6 nephrectomized (E) and sham-operated (C) mothers.
An insiginficant difference is observed between the 2 groups.

The PCNA positive cell ratio in the kidney of fetuses from 5/6 nephrectomized mothers was slightly lower than that of fetuses from sham-operated mothers but not significant (Fig. 7). We previously reported that the more the glomerulus develops, the lower the PCNA positive cell ratio in the kidney of perinatal rats (Okada et al., 2001); therefore, the slight decrease in the ratio of fetal glomerulus with maternal 5/6 nephrectomy reflects nonsuppressive effect on renal development by the operation.

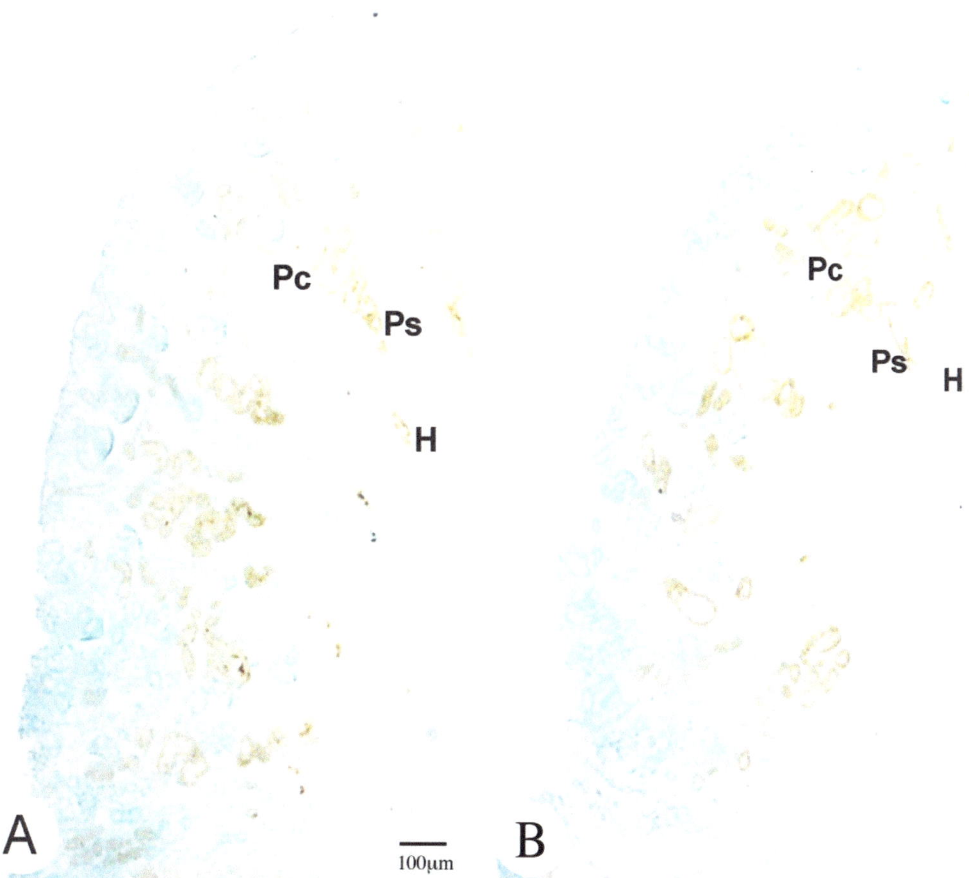

Fig. 8. Fetal kidneys stained with an anti-TGF-β antibody. bar = 100μm. **A**, fetus from sham-operated mothers. **B**, fetus from 5/6 nephrectomized mothers. In both fetuses, positive reactions are observed in the proximal tubules and the loop of Henle and no remarkable difference is observed between the fetuses. Ps, proximal straight tubules; Pc, proximal convoluted tubules; H. loop of Henle.

TGF-β was mainly localized in the distal tubule and insignificant differences in immunoreactivity of TGF-β between fetuses from 5/6 nephrectomized and sham-operated mothers were observed (Fig. 8). The stronger immunoreactivity of the TGF-βRI in collecting tubules was noted in fetuses from 5/6 nephrectomized mothers (Fig. 9). Addition of TGF-β to the culture medium induces an inhibition of the differentiation from the metanephric

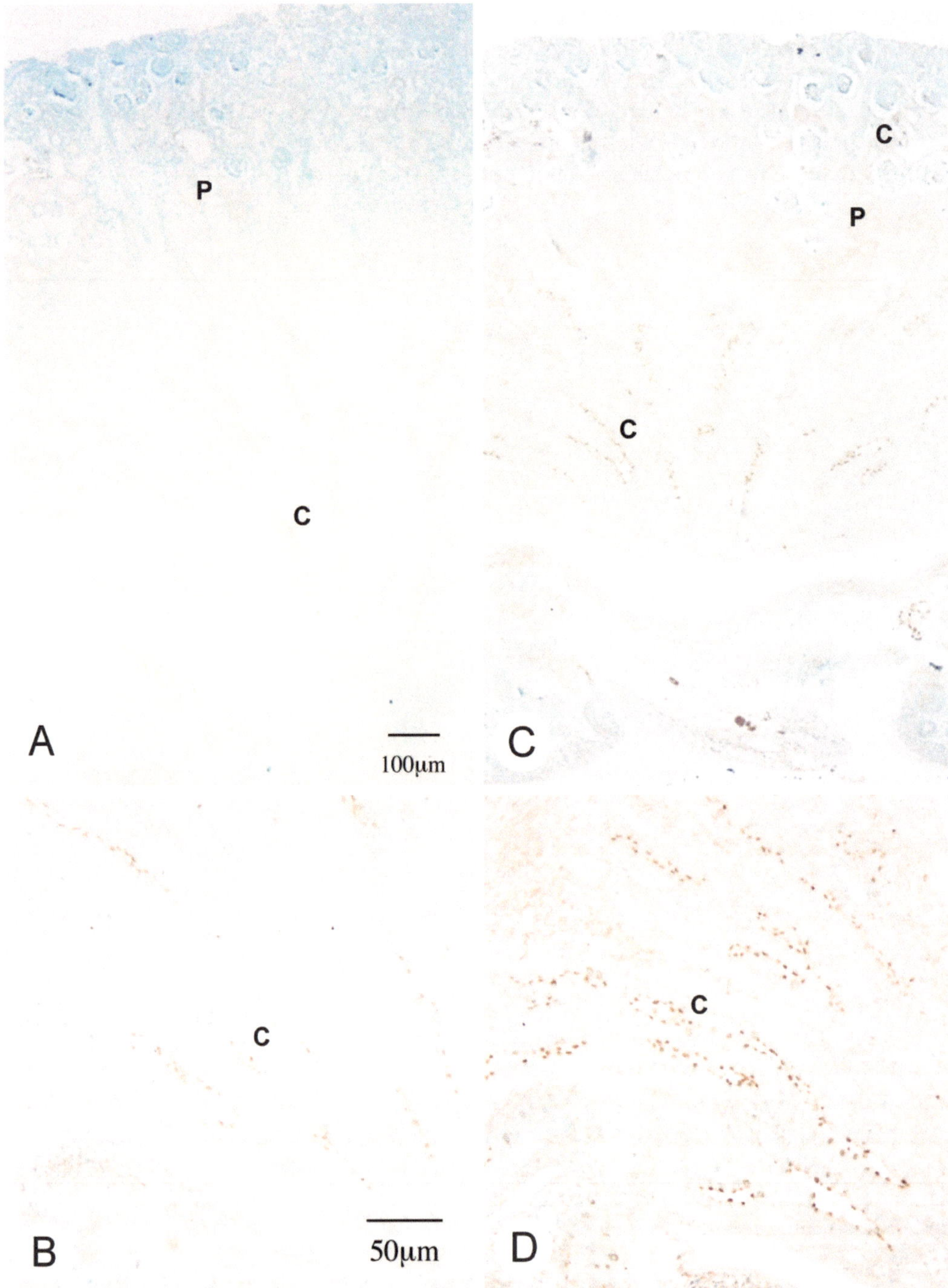

Fig. 9. Fetal kidneys stained with an anti-TGF-βRI antibody. **A** and **B**, fetus from sham-operated mothers. **C** and **D**, fetus of from 5/6 nephrectomized mothers. More TGF-βRI positive cells of the collecting ducts in the medullary zone are seen in the fetus from 5/6 nephrectomized mothers than in sham-operated ones. P, proximal tubules, C, collecting ducts.

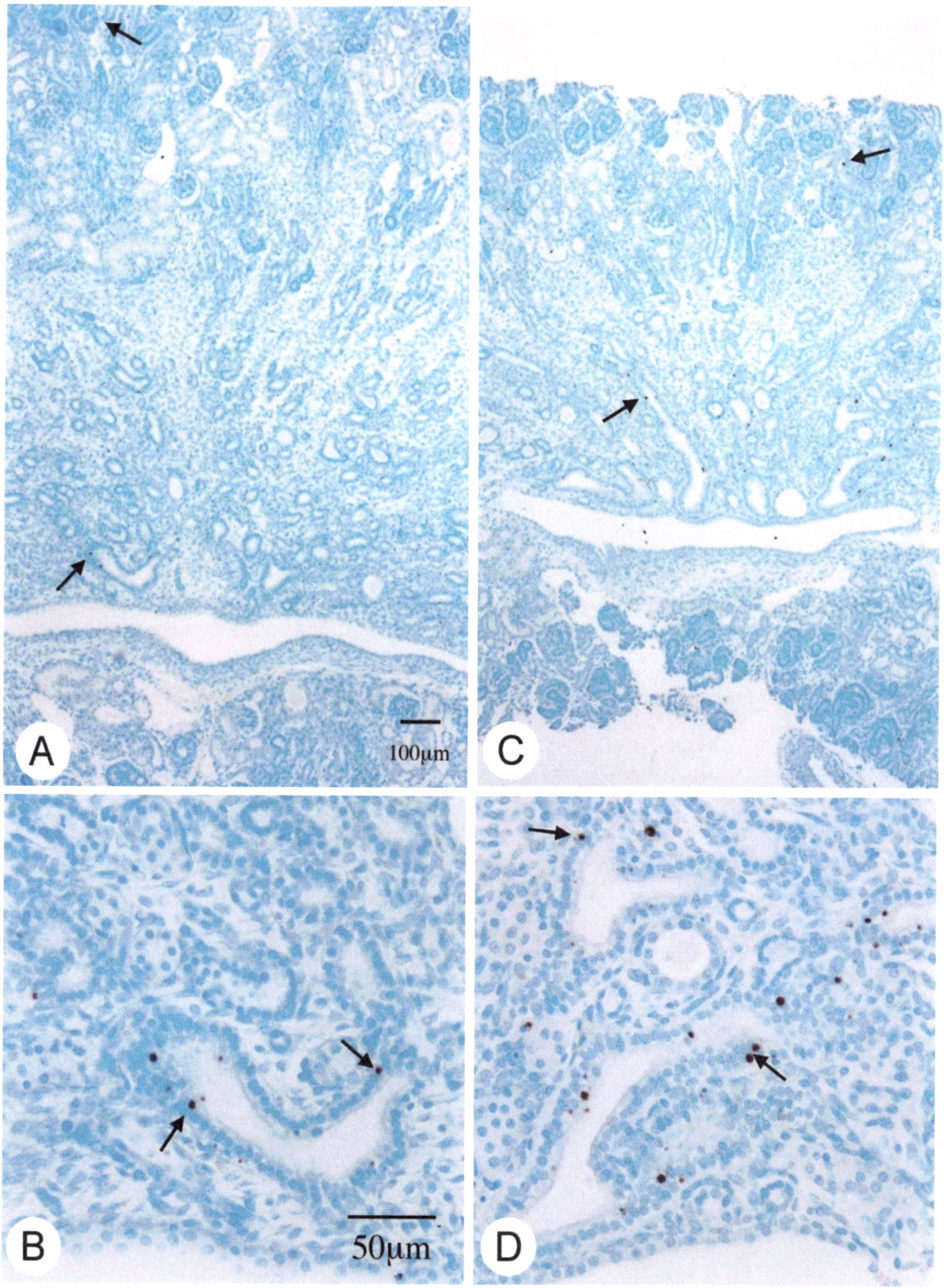

Fig. 10. Fetal kidneys stained with TUNEL methods from sham-operated mothers (**A** and **B**), and 5/6 nephrectomized mothers (**C** and **D**). More TUNEL positive cells (arrows) are seen in the fetus from 5/6 nephrectomized mothers than in that from sham-operated mothers, especially in the collecting ducts in the medulla.

blastema to the nephron and addition of neutral antibody to TGF-β causes the acceleration in nephron formation (Rogers et al., 1993). The changes in TGF-βRI of the fetal kidney by maternal 5/6 nephrectomy may be related to the differentiation of collecting tubules, especially apoptosis in the tubules, because more TUNEL positive cells were observed in the kidney of fetuses from 5/6 nephrectomized mothers than in the kidney of fetuses from sham-operated ones (Fig. 10). Kim et al. (1996) has reported on the developing kidney of the rat and found that intercalated cells show an apoptotic feature and are removed by neighboring principal cells or inner medullary collecting duct (IMCD) cells, resulting in the differentiation of the collecting ducts. Lee et al. (2004) have observed a delayed elimination of type A intercalated cells in the medullary collecting duct with a decreased apoptotic index in the collecting duct of the renal medulla and concluded that apoptosis plays an important role in the morphogenesis of the renal papilla during kidney development. Therefore, the result that the number of TUNEL positive cells in the collecting ducts per unit area (1mm^2) of the kidney was significantly larger in fetuses from 5/6 nephrectomized mothers than in fetuses from sham-operated ones (Fig. 11) indicates that 5/6 nephrectomy of pregnant rats causes the acceleration of the differentiation of the collecting ducts in the fetal kidney. These results suggest that maternal renal dysfunction induces apoptosis in the fetal kidney and that the development of collecting ducts is largely involved in the elevated expression of TGF-β receptor.

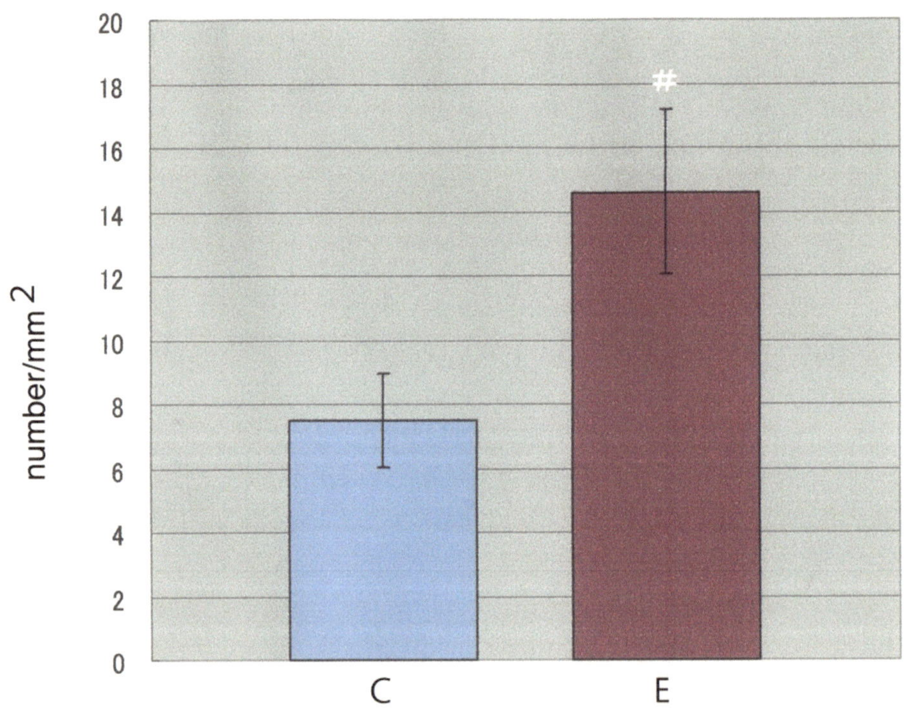

Fig. 11. The number of TUNEL positive cells per unit area (1mm^2) (Means±SEM) of the kidney of fetuses from 5/6 nephrectomeized (E) and sham-operated (C) mothers.
#, Significantly different from fetuses from sham-operated mothers.

4. Effects of the maternal renal dysfunction on the fetus

Infants who are born small have been reported to have higher blood pressure in adulthood (Woods & Weeks, 2004). Furthermore, a clear relation between low birth weight and adverse renal outcome is evident as early as during childhood (Dötsch et al., 2011). The Intrauterine Growth Retardation (IUGR) is very important health problem with a prevalence estimated at ~10% in the general population (Gardosi, 2011). The IUGR model can be produced by bilateral ligation of uterine artery, protein restriction, smoking, nephrotoxic medication as well as salt loading (Bentz & Amann, 2010). Exposure to maternal low protein diet in utero induces IUGR and increases expression of glomerular AT1 receptors and reduces AT2 receptor expression in young rat (Battista et al., 2002; Sahajpal & Ashton, 2005). A low protein diet of the mother is associated with lower birth weight and higher blood pressure in offspring, due to the suppression of renin mRNA and the decrease in the angiotensin II levels in the newborn rat kidney (Woods et al., 2001; Zimmerman & Dunham, 1997).

As described in the above sections, the development of the fetal kidney is accelerated by maternal bilateral ureteral ligation and maternal uninephrectomy. However, the operations induce the suppression of fetal growth in terms of the body and renal weights in Table 1. Maternal 5/6 nephrectomy also induces low body and renal weight in fetuses. Therefore, maternal 5/6 nephrectomy may be one of the means for producing an IUGR model. Thus, to clarify whether maternal 5/6 nephrectomy is a good model for IUGR, further studies including investigation of changes renin-angiotensin system will be need.

Groups	Body weight (g)	Renal weight (mg)	Reference
Bilateral ureterar ligated group	5.00±0.11*	27.17±0.84	Okada and Morikawa, 1988
Sham-operated group	5.56±0.14	30.31±1.40	
Uninephrectomized group	5.29±0.10*	25.42±0.79	Okada et al., 1998
Sham-operated group	5.73±0.12	26.23±0.85	
5/6 nephrectomized group	4.36±0.14*	18.74±0.62*	The present study
Sham-operated group	4.90±0.14	20.59±0.91	

Table 1. Body weight and renal weight (Means±SEM) of fetuses on fetal day 22 from bilateral ureter ligated, uninephrectomized, 5/6 nephrectomized, and sham-operated mothers.
*, significantly different from sham-operated group ($p<0.05$).

5. Conclusion

Detrimental maternal conditions such as renal failure, have various influences on the offspring. Maternal uninephrectomy induces changes in fetal renal development, including an increase in the glomerular volume and proximal tubular length, suggesting the accelerated renal development is influenced by maternal uninephrectomy. Acceleration of development of the fetal kidney is also seen 24 hours after maternal bilateral ureteral ligation, which is a model of acute renal failure. 5/6 nephrectomy to immature and adult animals induces renal fibrosis and glomerular sclerosis and leads to renal failure, and the progression of renal failure is suppressed by protein intake restriction. The 5/6 nephrectomy to pregnant rats (as a model of pregnant renal failure) induced a significant decrease in body weight and a significant increase in BUN concentration. By maternal 5/6 nephrectomy, however, the immunoreactivity of TGF-βRI is strengthened and TUNEL positive cells are increased in the collecting ducts of the kidney of fetuses, suggesting the acceleration of fetal development of the kidney. Based upon these findings, maternal renal dysfunction induces various desirable effects on fetuses, while a phenomenon similar to IUGR is also seen.

6. References

Atherton, J. C. & Pirie, S. C. (1981) The effect of pregnancy on glomerular filtration rate and salt and water reabsorption in the rat. *J Physiol* 319: 153-164.

Bakala, H., Geloso-Meyer, A., Cheignon, M. & Schaeverbeke, J. (1985) Differentiation of the glomerular filtration barrior in the rat fetus: possible role of collagen. *Connect Tissue Res* 13: 283-290.

Battista, M.-C., Geloso-Meyer, A., Lopez-Casillas, F. & Massague, J. (2002) Intrauterine growth restriction in rats is associated with hypertension and renal dyafunction in adulthood. *Am J Physiol,* 283: E124-E131.

Baylis, C. (1994) Glomerular filtration and volume regulation in gravid animal models. *Baillieres Clin Obstet Gynaecol,* 8: 235-264.

Bentz, K. & Amann, K. (2010) Maternal nutrition, low nephrons number and arterial hypertension in later life. *Biochem Biophy Acta,* 1802: 1309-1317.

Blobe, G. C., Schiemann, W. P. & Lodish, H. F. (2002) Role of transforming growth factor β in human disease. *N Engl J Med,* 342: 1350-1358.

Brandon, A. E., Boyce, A. C., Lumbers, E. R. & Gibson, K. J. (2009) Maternal renal dysfunction in sheep is associated with salt insensitivity in female offspring. *J Phyiol,* 587: 261-270.

Bremer, V., Tojo, A., Kimura, K., Hirata, Y., Goto, A., Nagamatsu, T., Suzuki, Y. & Omata, M. (1997) Role of nitric oxide in rat nephrotoxic nephritis: comparison between inducible and constitutive nitric oxide synthase. *J Am Soc Nephrol,* 8: 1712-1721.

Brown, S. T., Finco, D. R. & Navar, G. (1995) Impaired renal autoregulatory ability in dogs with reduced renal mass. *J Am Soc Nephrol,* 5: 1768-1774.

Chen, J.-K., Chen, J., Neilson, E. G., & Harris, R. C. (2005) Role of mammalian target of rapamycin signaling in compensatory renal hypertrophy. *J Am Soc Nephrol,* 16: 1384-1391.

Cheng, J. & Grande, J. P. (2002) Transforming growth factor-beta signal transduction and progressive renal disease. *Exp Biol Med,* 227: 943-956.

Chevalier, R. L. (1999) Molecular and cellular pathophysiology of obstructive nephropathy. *Pediatr Nephrol,* 13: 612-619.

Churchill, S. E., Bengele, H. H. & Alexander, E. A. (1982) Renal function in the term pregnant rat: a micropuncture study. *Renal Physiol,* 5: 1-9.

Dafnis, E. & Sabatini, S. (1992) The effect of pregnancy on renal function: Physiology and pathology. *Am J Med Sci*, 303:184-205.

Dicker, S. E. & Shirley, D. G. (1971) Mechanism of compensatory renal hypertrophy. *J Physiol*, 219: 507-523.

Dötsch, J., Plank, C. & Amann, K. (2011) Fetal programing of renal function. *Pediatr Nephrol*, DOI 10.1007/s00467-011-1781-5.

Fine, L. (1986) The biology of renal hypertrophy. *Kidney Int*, 29: 619-634.

Floege, J., Burns, M. W., Alpers, C. E., Yoshimura, A., Pritzl, P., Gordon, K., Seifert, R. A., Bowen-Pope, D. F., Couser, W. G. & Johnson, R. J. (1992) Glomerular cell proliferation and PDGF expression precede glomerulosclerosis in remnant rat kidney model. *Kidney Int*, 41: 297-309.

Friedman, A. L. & Pityer, R. (1986) Beneficial effect of moderate protein restriction on growth, renal function and survival in young rats with chronic renal failure. *J Nutr*, 116: 2466-2477.

Fujihara CK, Antunes GR, Mattar AL, Malheiros DM, Viera Jr JM, & Zatz, R. (2007) Chronic inhibition of nuclear factor-{kappa}-B attenuates renal injury in the 5/6 renal ablation model. *Am J Physiol Renal Physiol*, 292: F92-F99.

Garcia, M. V., Martin-Barrientos, J. & Medina J. M. (1988) Maternal-fetal relationship in ammonia metabolism during late gestation period in the rat. *Biol Neonate* 53: 315-320.

Gardosi, J. (2011) Clinical strategies for improving the detection of fetal growth restriction. *Clin Perinol*, 38: 21-31.

Gattone, II. V. H., Sherman, D. A., Hinton, D. A, Niu, F. W., Topham, R. T., & Klein, R. M. (1992) Epidermal growth factor in the neonatal mouse salivary gland and kidney. *Biol Neonate*, 61: 54-67.

Gibson, K. J., Boyce, A. C., Karime, B. M. & R. Lumbers, E. R. (2007) Maternal renal insufficiency alters plasma composition and renal function in the fetal sheep. *Am J Physiol Regul Integr Comp Physiol*, 292: R1204 - R1211.

Girardi, A. C. C., Rocha, R. O., Britto, L. R. G. & Rebouças, N. A. (2002) Upregulation of NHE3 is associated with compensatory cell growth response in young uninephrectomized rats. *Am J Physiol Renal Physiol*, 283: F1296-F1303.

Goodyer, P. R., Fata, J., Goodyer, C. G., & Guyda, H. (1991a) Transforming growth factor-alpha and the ontogeny of epidermal growth factor receptors in rat kidney. *Growth Regul*, 1: 105-109.

Goodyer, P. R., Fata, J., Mulligan, L., Fisher, D., Fagan, R., Guyda, H. J., & Goodyer, C. G. (1991b) Expression of transforming growth factor-alpha and epidermal growth factor receptor in human fetal kidneys. *Mol Cell Endocrinol*, 77: 199-206.

Griffin, K. A., Picken, M. & Bidani, A. K. (1994) Method of renal mass reduction is a critical modulator of subsequent hypertension and glomerular injury. *J Am Soc Nephrol*, 4: 2023-2031.

Han, K.-H., Lim, J.-M., Kim, W.-Y., Kim, H., Madsen, K. M., & Kim, J. (2005) Expression of endothelial nitric oxide synthase in developing rat kidney. *Am J Physiol Renal Physiol*, 288: F694-702.

Heering, O., Steenbergen, E. & van Goor, H. (2002) A protective role for endothelial nitric oxide synthase in glomerulonephritis. *Kidney int*, 61: 822-825.

Heller. J., Cervenka. L. & Hellerova, S. (1994) The effect of a low-protein diet and certain pharmaceutical agents on the course of ablation nephropathy in rats. *Cas Lek Cesk,* 133: 429-433.

Humes, H. D., Cieslinski, D. A., Coimbra, T. M., Messana, J. M. & Galvao, C. (1989) Epidermal growth factor enhances renal tubule cell regeneration and repair and accelerates the recovery of renal function in postischemic acute renal failure. *J Clin Invest,* 84: 1757-1761.

Iwano, M., Plieth, D., Danoff, T. M., Xue, C., Okada, H. & Neilson, E. G. (2002) Evidence that fibroblasts derive from epithelium during tissue fibrosis. *J Cli Invest,* 110: 341-350.

Johnson, H. A. & Vera Roman, J. M. (1966) Compensatory renal enlargement. Hypertrophy versus hyperplasia. *Am J Pathol,* 49: 1-13.

Johnson, T. S., Griffin, M., Thomas, G.L., Skill, J., Cox, A., Yang, B., Nicholas, B., Brickbichler, P. J., Muchaneta-Kubara, C. & El Nahas, A. M. (1997) The role of transglutaminase in the rat subtotal nephrectomy model of renal fibrosis. *J Clin Invest,* 99: 2950-2960.

Jung, J. Y., Song, J. H., Li, C., Yang, C. W., Kang, T. C., Won, M. H., Jeong, Y. G., Han, K. H., Choi, K. B., Lee, S. H. & Kim, J. (2005) Expression of epidermal growth factor in the developing rat kidney. *Am J Physiol Renal Physiol,* 288: F227-F235.

Kanda, S., Hisamatsu, H., Igawa, T., Eguchi, J., Taide, M., Sakai, H., Kanetake, H., Saito, Y., Yoshitake, Y. & Nishikawa, K. (1993) Peritubular endothelial cell proliferation in mice during compensatory renal growth after unilateral nephrectomy. *Am J Physiol Renal Physiol,* 265: F712-F716.

Kang, D.-H., Nakagawa, T., Feng, L. & Johnson, R. J. (2002) Nitric oxide modulates vascular disease in the remnant kidney model. *Am J Pathol,* 161: 239-248

Kelly, A. M., McNay, M. B. & McEwan, H. P. (1978) Renal tubular function in normal pregnancy. *Br J Obstet Gynecol,* 85: 190-196.

Kim, J., Cha, J.-H., Tisher, C. C. & Madsen, K. M. (1996) Role of apoptotic and non apoptotic cell death in removal intercalated cells from developing rat kidney. *Am J Physiol,* 270: F575-F592.

Klein, I. H., Ligtenberg, G., Oey, P. L., Koomans, H.A. & Blamkestijn, P. J. (2003) Enalapril and losartan reduce sympathetic hyperactivity in patients with chronic renal failure. *J Am Soc Nephrol,* 14: 425-430.

Lee, S. H., Jung, J. Y., Han, K. H., Yang, C. W., Choi, K. B. & Kim, J. (2004) Effect of epidermal growth factor on the developing rat renal papilla. *Am J Nephrol,* 24: 212-220.

Li, C., Lim, S., Sun, B., Choi, B., Glowacka, S., Cox, A. J., Kelly, D. J., Kim, Y., Kim, J., Bang, B. & Yang, C. (2004) Expression of apoptosis-related factors in chronic cyclosporine nephrotoxicity after cyclosporine withdrawal. *Acta Pharmacol Sin,* 25: 401-411.

Liggins, G. C. (1972) The fetus and birth. pp.77-109, C. R. and Short, R. V. eds) Cambridge Univ. Press, London.

MacLean, P. R., Paterson, W. G., Smart, G. E., Petrie, J. J., Robson, J. S. & Thomson, D. (1972) Proteinuria in toxaemia and abruptio placentae. *J Obstet Gynaecol Br Comm,* 79: 321-326.

Manotham, K., Tanaka, T., Matsumoto, M., Ohse, T., Miyata, T., Inagi, R., Kurokawa, K., Fujita, T. & Nangaku, M. (2004) Evidence of tubular hypoxia in the early phase in the remnant kidney model. *J Am Soc Nephrol,* 15: 1277-1288.

Mark, L. A., Robinson, A. V. & Schulak, J. A. (2005) Inhibition of nitric oxide synthase reduces renal ischemia/reperfusion injury. *J Surg Res*, 129: 236-241

Matsubara, H., Moriguchi, Y., Moti, Y., Masaki, H., Tsutsumi, Y., Shibasaki, Y., Uchiyama-Tanaka, Y., Fujiyama, S., Koyama, Y., Nose-Fujiyama, A., Iba, S., Tateishi, E. & Iwasaki, T. (2000) Transactivation of EGF receptor induced by angiotensin II regulates fibronectin and TGF-β gene epression via transcriptional and posttranscriptional mechanisms. *Mol Cel Biochem*, 212: 187-201.

Matsuo, M., Morikawa, Y., Hashimoto, Y. & Baraz, R. S. (1986) Changes in blood urea nitrogen (BUN) concentration. during pregnancy in rat with or without obstructive uremia. *Exp Pathol*, 30:203-208.

Mesquita, F. F., Gontijo, J. A. R. & Boer, P. A. (2010) Maternal undernutrition and the offspring kidney: from fetal to adult life. *Braz J Med Biol Res*, 43: 1010-1018.

Mino, M., Nakamura, J., Nakamuta, N., Morioka, H., Morikawa, Y. & Okada, T. (2007) Effects of low protein intake on the development of the remaining kidney in subtotally nephrectomized immature rats: apoptosis and epidermal growth factor. *J Vet Med Sci*, 69: 247-252.

Mino, M., Ihara, H., Kozaki, S., Kondo, T., Takeshita, A., Kusakabe, K.T., & Okada, T. (2010) Effects of low protein intake on the development of the remaining kidney in subtotally nephrectomized immature rats: Expression of inducible and endothelial NO synthase. *Med Mol Morphol*, 43: 116-122.

Mok, K. Y., Sandberg, K., Sweeny, J. M., Zheng, W., Lee, S. & Mulroney, S. E. (2003) Growth hormone regulation of glomerular AT_1 angiotensin receptors in adult uninephrectomized male rats. *Am J Physiol Renal Physiol*, 285: F1085-F1091.

Moskowitz, D. W., Schneider, A. N., Lane, P. H., Schmitz, P. G. & Gillespie, K. N. (1992) Effect of epidermal growth factor in the rat 5/6 renal ablation model. *J Am Soc Nephrol*, 3: 1113-1118.

Nangaku, M., Pippin, J. & Couser, W. G. (2002) C6 mediates chronic progression of tubulointerstitial damage in rats with remnant kidney. *J Am Soc Nephrol*, 13: 928-936.

Nouwen, E. J., Verstrepen, W. A. & Broe, M. E. (1994) Epidermal growth factor in acute renal failure. *Ren Fail*, 16: 49-60.

Okada, T. & Morikawa, Y. (1988) Effects of maternal bilateral ureteral ligation on the development of fetal kidney in rats: histometrical study. *Jpn J Vet Sci*, 50: 985-989.

Okada, T. & Morikawa, Y. (1990) Effects of maternal bilateral ureteral ligation on the development of the proximal tubule of the kidney in fetal rats: morphometry and lectrom microscopic study. *Anat Rec*, 228: 456-460.

Okada, T. & Morikawa, Y. (1993) Effects of maternal bilateral ureteral ligation on the development of kidney in Rats: morphometrical changes in glomerular components. *Anat Rec*, 236: 563-567.

Okada, T., Iwamoto, A., Kusakabe, K., Mukamoto, M., Kiso, Y., Morioka, H., Sasaki, F. & Morikawa, Y. (2001) Perinatal development of the rat kidney: proliferative activity and epidermal growth factor. *Biol Neonate*, 79: 46-53.

Okada, T., Iwamoto, A., Nakamura, J., Kusakabe, K., Kiso, Y., Morioka, H., Sasaki, F. & Morikawa, Y. (2003) Perinatal development of the rat kidney: apoptosis and epidermal growth factor. *Congenit Anom Kyoto*, 43: 161-167.

Okada, T., Mitsuoka, K., Mino, M., Mukamoto, M., Nakamura, J., Morioka, H., & Morikawa, Y. (2006) Effects of maternal uninephrectomy on the development of fetal rat kidney: apoptosis and the expression of oncogenes, *Congenit Anom Kyoto,* 46:43-47.

Okada, T., Mitsuoka, K., Mukamoto, M., Nakamura, J., Morioka, H. & Morikawa, Y. (2000) Effects of maternal uninephrectomy on the development of fetal rat kidney with special reference to the proliferative activity and epidermal growth factor (EGF), *Congenit Anom Kyoto,* 40: 275-281.

Okada, T., Morikawa, Y. Kiso, Y. & Sasaki, F. (1997) Effects of maternal bilateral ureteral ligation on the glomerular basement mambrane in fetal rat kidney. *Anat Rec,* 249:181-186.

Okada, T., Yamagishi, T. & Morikawa, Y. (1994) Morphometry of the kidney in rat pups from uninephrectomized mothers. *Anat Rec,* 240:120-124.

Okada, T., Yamagishi, T. & Morikawa, Y. (1998) Effects of maternal uninephrectomy on the development of fetal rat kidney: Numeric and volumetric changes of glomerulus and formation of the anionic site in the glomerular basement membrane. *J Morphol,* 238: 337-342.

Okada, T., Yamagishi, T., Kiso, Y., Morikawa, Y. & Sasaki, F. (1995) Morphometry on proximal tubule of the kidney in rat pups from uninephrectomized mothers. *J Vet Med Sci,* 57: 415-417.

Okada, T., Omoto-Kitao, M., Mukamoto, M., Nakamura, J., Mino, M., Kondo, T., Takeshita, A., Kusakabe, K.-T., and Kato, K. (2010) Compensatory renal growth in uninephrectomized immature rats: proliferative activity and epidermal growth factor. *J Vet Med Sci,* 72: 975-980.

Ots, M., Mackenzie, H. S., Troy, J. L., Rennke, H. G. & Brenner, B. M. (1998) Effects of combination therapy with enalaprill and losartan on the rate of progression of renal injury in rats with 5/6 renal mass. *J Am Soc Nephrol,* 9: 224-230.

Paxinou, E., Weisse, M., Chen, Q., Souza, J. M., Hertkorn, C., Selak, M., Daikhin, E., Yudkoff, M., Sowa, G., Sessa, W. C. & Ischiropoulos, H. (2001) Dynamic regulation of metabolism and respiration by endogeneously produced nitric oxide protects against oxidative stress. *PNAS,* 98: 11575-11580.

Pugh, J. L., Sweeney, Jr. W. E. & Avner, E. D. (1995) Tyrosine kinase activity of the EGF receptor in murine metanephric organ culture. *Kidney Int,* 47: 774-781.

Remuzzi, G., Perico, N., Macia, M. & Ruggeneti, P. (2005) The role of renin-angiotensin-aldosterone system in the progression of chronic kidney disease. *Kiney int,* 99: S57-65.

Rogers, S. A., Ryan, G., Purchio, A. F. & Hammerman, M. C. (1993) Metanephric transforming growth factor-β1 regulates nephrogenesis in vitro. *Am J Physiol,* 264: F996-F1002.

Sahajpal, V. & Ashton, N. (2005) Increased glomerular angiotensin II binding in rats exposed to a maternal low protein diet in utero. *J Physiol,* 563:193-201.

Salas, S. P., Giacaman, A. & Vío, C. P. (2003) Pregnant rats with 5/6 nephrectomy have normal volume expansion despite lower renin and kallikrein. *Hypertension,* 42: 744 - 748.

Schaeverbeke, J. & Cheignon, M. (1980) Differentiation of glomerular filter and tubular reabsorption apparatus during foetal development . *J Embryol Exp Morphol,* 58: 157-175.

Shao, J., Miyata, T., Yamada, K., Hanafusa, N., Wada, T., Gordon, K. L., Inagi, R., Kurokawa, K., Fujita, T., Johonson, R. J. & Nangaku, M. (2001) Protective role of nitric oxide in a model of thrombotic microangiopathy in rats. *J Am Soc Nephrol,* 12: 2088-2097

Solhaug, M. J., Ballervre, L. D., Guignard, J. P., Granger, J. P. & Adelman, R. D. (1996) Nitric Oxide in the developing kidney. *Pediatr Nephrol,* 10: 529-539.

Stahl, P. J. & Felsen, D. (2001) Transforming growth factor-β, basement membrane, and epithelial-mesenchymal transdifferentiation: implications for fibrosis in kidney disease. *Am J Pathol,* 159: 1187-1192.

Sterner, N. G., Diemer, H., Magnusson, I. K. & Wennberg, A. K. (1994) Low nitrogen diets preserve nutritional status but not residual renal function in rats with severe renal failure. *J Nutr,* 124: 1065-1071.

Studd, J. W. (1971) Immunoglobulins in normal pregnancy, pre-eclampsia and pregnancy complicated by the nephrotic syndrome. *J Obstet Gynaecol Br Comm,* 78: 786-790.

Taylor, B. S., de Vera, M. E., Ganster, R. W., Wang, Q., Shapiro, R. A., Morris, S. M. Jr., Billiar, T. R. & Geller, D. A. (1998) Multiple NF–κB enhancer elements regulate cytokine induction of the human inducible nitric oxide synthase gene. *J Biol Chem,* 273: 15148-15156

Toubeau, G., Nonclercq, D., Zanen, J., Laurent, G., Schaudies, P. R. & Heuson-Stiennon, J. A. (1994) Renal tissue expression of EGF and EGF receptor after ischaemic tubular injury: an immunohistochemical study. *Exp Nephrol,* 2: 229-239.

Varziri, N. D., Wang, X. Q., Ni, Z., Kivlighn, S. & Shahinfar, S. (2002) Effects of aging and AT-1 receptor blockade on NO synthase expression and renal function in SHR. *Biochim Biophys Acta,* 1592: 153-161.

Wahl, S. M., Hunt, D. A., Wakefield, L. M., McCartney-Francis, N., Wahl, L. M., Roberts, A. B. & Sporn, M. B. (1987) Transforming growth factor type beta induces monocyte chemotaxis and growth factor production. *Proc Nat Acad Sci USA,* 84: 5788-5792.

Walford, G. & Loscalzo, J. (2003) Nitric oxide in vascular biology. *J Thromb Haemost,* 1: 2112-2118.

Wang, X., Gu, F., & Yang, B. (1997) Apoptosis in the early stage of compensatory renal growth following uninephrectomy in the young and old rats. *Chung Hua Tsa Chih,* 77: 742-744.

Wells, L. J. (1946) Observations on secretion of urine by kidneys of fetal rats. *Anat Rec,* 95: 504.

Woods, L. L. & Weeks, D. A. (2004) Naturally occurring intrauterine growth retardation and adult blood pressure in rats. *Pediatr Res,* 56: 763-767.

Woods, L. L., Ingelfinger, J. R., Nyengaard, J. R., & Rasch, R. (2001) Maternal protein restriction suppresses the newborn renin-angiotensin system and programs adult hypertension and kidney disease. *Peditr Res,* 49: 460-467.

Yang, B., Johnson, T. S., Thomas, G. L., Watson, P. F., Wagner, B., Skill, N. J., Haylor, J. L. & EI Nahas, A. M. (2001) Expression of apoptosis-related genes and proteins in experimental chronic renal scarring. *J Am Soc Nephrol,* 12: 275-288.

Zhang, H., Wada, J., Kanwar, Y. S., Tsuchiyama, Y., Hiragushi, K., Hida, K., Shikata, K. & Makino, H. (1999) Screening for genes up-regulated in 5/6 nephrectomized mouse kidney. *Kidney Int,* 56: 549-558.

Zhao, X., Li, X., Trusa, S. & Olson, S. C. (2005) Angiotensin type 1 receptor is linked to inhibition of nitric oxide production in pulmonary endothelial cells. *Regul Pept,* 132: 113-122.

Zimmerman, B. G. & Dunham, E. W. (1997) Tissue renin-angiotensin system: a site of drug action? *Annu Rev Pharmacol Txicol,* 37: 53-69.

6

Proteomic Biomarkers for the Early Detection of Acute Kidney Injury

Stefan Herget-Rosenthal[1,#], Jochen Metzger[2], Amaya Albalat[3,*], Vasiliki Bitsika[4,*] and Harald Mischak[2,3,#,*]

[1]*Department of Medicine and Nephrology, Rotes Kreuz Krankenhaus, Bremen,*
[2]*Mosaiques Diagnostics GmbH, Hannover,*
[3]*BHF Glasgow Cardiovascular Research Centre, University of Glasgow, Glasgow,*
[4]*Biomedical Research Foundation Academy of Athens,*
[1,2]*Germany*
[3]*UK*
[4]*Greece*

1. Introduction

Acute kidney injury (AKI), previously termed acute renal failure, is a frequent clinical condition in critically ill patients, especially in intensive care units (ICU). It is characterized by a rapid decline or loss of renal function. Its incidence varies from 1-7 % of all hospitalized patients to 30-50 % of patients in ICU [29,69]. Clinical manifestations include a rapid decrease (oliguria) or cessation (anuria) of urine output and of glomerular filtration rate (GFR) below 10 mL/min within hours to days. AKI is further indicated by accumulation of nitrogenous-waste substances in blood resulting in elevated serum levels of creatinine and blood urea nitrogen (BUN). It is important to differentiate AKI from chronic kidney disease (CKD), as AKI has the potential to be reversible. AKI and CKD can be differentiated by the dynamics nitrogenous-waste substances increase in the serum and urinary output decreases.

Irrespective of the progress being made in the understanding of the pathophysiology of AKI and its underlying processes and the advances in critical care medicine, mortality rate associated with AKI remains high especially in ICU patients at more than 50 % [97]. In addition, a significant proportion of surviving patients (20 %) develops CKD and end-stage renal disease, requiring chronic renal replacement therapy [8,32]. Long-term outcome is worse for patients after recovery from AKI [45,14], further impacting health care cost and quality of life [10].

Advances in our understanding, prevention and treatment of AKI have been hampered especially by two factors. Firstly, until recently there was a lack of uniform criteria for definition and classification of AKI. Secondly, there is still an incomplete understanding of the pathogenesis of AKI [72]. The risk to develop AKI is determined by patient's

---

[*] Members of EuroKUP
[#] Members of EUTox

susceptibility and exposure or causative factors. Patient susceptibility in developing countries varies from that of the developed countries. In developing countries, AKI is more common in young and pediatric patients, while in developed countries elderly patients are predominant [95,34]. However, it is difficult to differentiate demographic variables which directly contribute to the risk of developing AKI from those that are more attributed to the underlying disease [72]. Conditions known to cause AKI in susceptible populations include sepsis, ischemia, heart failure, liver disease, major surgery (especially vascular and cardiac), rhabdomyolysis, urinary tract obstruction and various nephrotoxic drugs and radiocontrast agents [80]. In critically ill patients the most common cause of AKI is sepsis, accounting for 50 % of all cases [2,4,5].

2. Diagnostic problem

In order to standardize and detect AKI, two different sets of definition criteria have been recently established. The Acute Dialysis Quality Initiative developed the RIFLE criteria for the diagnosis of acute renal failure in critically ill patients [6] and the Acute Kidney Injury Network developed the AKIN criteria for the diagnosis of AKI [51]. Both criteria (**Figure 1**) for diagnosis are mainly based on measurements of urine output and serum creatinine. In clinical practice, however, AKI is predominantly detected by changes in serum creatinine [51].

RIFLE criteria (Bellomo et al., Crit Care 2004, [6])

Stage	Serum creatinine ↑ or GFR ↓	Urine output ↓
Risk	150 % or > 25 – 50 %	< 0.5 mL/kg/h for 6 h
Injury	200 % or > 50 – 75 %	< 0.5 mL/kg/h for 12 h
Failure	300 % or ≥ 4 mg/dL or > 75 %	< 0.3 mL/kg/h for 24 h or anuria for 12 h
Loss	Persistent AKI = Complete loss of renal funktion > 4 wk	
ESRD	End-stage renal disease = Complete loss of renal function > 3 mo	

AKIN criteria (Mehta et al., Crit Care 2007, [51])

Stage	Serum creatinine ↑	Urine output ↓
1	≥ 0.3 mg/dL or 150 – 200 %	< 0.5 mL/kg/h within 6 – 12 h
2	201 – 300 %	< 0.5 mL/kg/h for > 12 h
3	> 300 % or dialysis	< 0.3 mL/kg/h for > 24 h or anuria for > 12 h

Fig. 1. AKI staging according to the RIFLE and AKIN criteria.

Creatinine is a 113 Dalton molecule derived from creatine metabolism after creatinine's release from the muscle. As creatinine is freely filtered by the glomerulus and excreted without significant metabolic changes or reabsorption by the kidney, this molecule has been a useful indicator of kidney function. However, serum creatinine has important limitations as a tool for assessing GFR. Firstly, creatinine levels are affected by a variety of non-renal factors such as age, gender, muscle mass, diet and nutritional status [76]. Although equations have been developed to correct for some of these factors, these are only applicable for CKD but not for AKI as they require stable creatinine metabolism [41]. Secondly, serum creatinine concentration and its value is influenced by its volume of distribution that can be substantially affected by volume overload, a common situation in AKI [75]. Finally, and probably most importantly, serum creatinine increases only after substantial loss of GFR resulting in a lag phase in the temporal relationship between serum creatinine increase and loss of GFR. As a result, current clinical diagnosis of AKI based on creatinine limits its early detection in clinical routine as well as the early implementation of preventive measures. Therefore, the development of new AKI biomarkers have had high priority in the nephrological community during the last years with the aim to identify markers that are superior to serum creatinine in the early detection of AKI. In the following part we will shortly summarise the most promising single biomarkers for AKI.

3. Single biomarkers for AKI

New biomarkers for AKI can be categorized as inflammatory mediators, excreted tubular proteins and surrogate markers indicative for tubular damage (albumin, α 1-microglobulin, β 2-glycoprotein, plasma retinol binding protein, N-acetyl-β-D-glucosaminidase (NAG)) and liver-type fatty acid binding protein (L-FABP) [90,18]. The most promising of the AKI biomarker candidates, namely neutrophil gelatinase-associated lipocalin (NGAL), kidney injury molecule-1 (KIM-1), interleukin-18 (IL-18) and cystatin C (CysC) will be presented in more detail:

3.1 Neutrophil gelatinase-associated lipocalin (NGAL)

Function: NGAL, also known as lipocalin-2, is a 25-kDa protein strongly up-regulated by interleukin-1 during inflammation. NGAL has the ability of sequestering siderophores, microbial iron-chelating agents required for bacterial growth, and prevents urinary tract infection.

Diagnostic evidence: NGAL has been presented as biomarker for early detection of AKI and for AKI prognosis [68]. The first study that pointed out the association of NGAL with AKI development was performed by Mishra and colleagues in 2005 [55]. In this prospective study urine and plasma NGAL rose significantly in children developing AKI after cardiac surgery within 2 h postoperatively. However, the classification performance of NGAL decreased in similar studies performed in adults also having cardiac surgery [21] possibly due to confounding variables and comorbid conditions that accumulate with age. Other positive results have been obtained when NGAL has been tested as a biomarker of AKI in kidney transplantation and the subsequent development of delayed graft function [56]. Among other, NGAL was tested in hemolytic uremic syndrome [78], urinary tract infections [96], critically ill children and adults [91,70] and also CKD [20]. Taken together, NGAL is the most promising novel renal biomarker in urine and also in plasma. However, as pointed out by Chawla and Kellum [9], NGAL is expressed in multiple organs affording further studies to understand how non-kidney sources of NGAL have an impact on urinary NGAL. As a consequence, prospective multicenter studies are urgently required to determine the performance of plasma and urinary NGAL in unselected ICU patient populations including patients with preexisting CKD [53,50]. Since the reported cut-off values for NGAL differ across a wide range it seems reasonable to speculate, that each clinical setting may require different cut-off values [57].

3.2 Interleukin-18 (IL-18)

Function: IL-18 is an 18-kDa proinflammatory cytokine secreted by macrophages and other antigen presenting cells. It has the ability to induce interferon γ production in type-1 T helper cells and is a sensitive mediator of ischemic injury in different organs such as heart, brain and kidney [73].

Diagnostic evidence: A first evidence for IL-18's role in ischemic AKI was given by animal studies [52,26]. Later studies in humans suggested that urinary IL-18 may serve as marker of AKI development after cardiac surgery, of graft function after kidney allograft transplantation, and of mortality in acute respiratory distress syndrome [61,62,89]. Siew et al. [71] reported that urinary IL-18, when measured within 48 h of AKI development, could not reliably predict AKI in a broadly selected, critically ill adult patients cohort. Despite this negative result, urinary IL-18 remained predictive in this study for worse clinical outcome such as death and acute dialysis within 28 days of ascertainment independently of other factors [71]. A matter of concern is that IL-18 increases in a variety of pathophysiological conditions, such as sepsis, inflammatory arthritis, inflammatory bowel disease, systemic lupus erythematosus, psoriasis, hepatitis and multiple sclerosis. This property significantly limits its application, due to reduced sensitivity and specificity [81].

3.3 Kidney injury molecule-1 (KIM-1)

Function: KIM-1 is a type 1 transmembrane glycoprotein that is undetectable in normal kidneys but highly expressed by proximal tubules epithelial cells after ischemic or toxic injury [31,25] with the ectodomain being shedded into the tubular lumen [100]. It functions as a phosphatidyl-serine receptor and confers a phagocytic phenotype on epithelial cells, most likely to clear cellular debris during enhanced apoptosis [30].

Diagnostic evidence: In previous studies in adults, KIM-1 was able to discriminate patients with acute tubular necrosis from those without, and predicted AKI in adults undergoing cardiac surgery [24,82,87]. In another prospective study on 201 hospital patients with AKI, an increase of urinary KIM-1 was associated with increased mortality or dialysis requirement [44]. Its potential use as an early marker is based so far on limited data: a rise in its urinary levels was detectable before the increase of BUN and creatinine in plasma during cadmium-induced renal damage [64] as well as its expression in biopsy sections of kidney allograft recipients before histological signs of acute tubular necrosis became evident [99].

3.4 Cystatin C (CysC)

Function: CysC is a cysteine protease inhibitor that is synthesized and continuously released into the blood by nucleated cells. Its levels are not significantly affected by age, gender, infection, liver disease or muscle mass in contrast to serum creatinine. This molecule is freely filtered by the glomerulus but, unlike creatinine, reabsorbed and metabolized by the proximal tubule. Therefore, elevated levels of CysC in serum correlate inversely with GFR while increased urinary CysC indicates renal tubular damage [40] and in fact the diagnostic accuracy of serum CysC to reflect GFR has been shown to be superior compared to serum creatinine since its levels are less influenced by inflammation, infection, body mass, diet and drugs [65].

Diagnostic evidence: Serum CysC is not a biomarker of AKI since its levels are not a direct marker of renal injury, and rather serves as GFR marker [73]. Several studies have focused on the diagnostic accuracy of CysC in predicting AKI. Unfortunately, results have been conflicting. In high-risk patients serum CysC detected AKI 1-2 days earlier than serum creatinine [27]. However, in a mixed heterogeneous, multicenter ICU population serum and urinary CysC were poor predictors of AKI and the need for renal replacement therapy [66]. In a meta-analysis performed by Zhang et al. [101] using the data of 19 studies from 11 countries and 3,336 patients, it was found that serum CysC could be used as reliable marker with an odds ratio of 23.5 in the prediction of AKI whereas urinary CysC showed only moderate diagnostic accuracy with an odds ratio of only 2.6.

Endre et al. [17] in a recent prospective observational study of 529 ICU patients and Lameire et al. [38] in a commentary on this work came to a sobering conclusion on the diagnostic and prognostic performance of these single AKI markers. In the study of Endre et al. [17] none of these markers reached an AUC value above 0.7 for the prediction of AKI on ICU entry and of death in 7 days, while urinary NGAL, CysC and IL-18 predicted dialysis in 7 days with AUC's of 0.79, 0.71 and 0.73, respectively. This is in contrast to some previous studies with AUC values above 0.9 [47,55] which was attributed by their selection of homogeneous study populations [38]. In conclusion, the single AKI markers performed well in selected, predominantly homogenous patient cohorts, whereas they failed for the most part in multicenter, heterogenous cohorts which rather represent clinical routine (see **Table 1** for a listing of clinical studies). Due to this, multimarker patterns were suggested by experts in this field for which proteomic technologies are predestined.

4. Proteomic approaches and biomarkers profiles for AKI

The main rationale for the application of proteome analysis in the context of AKI is that AKI is a multifactorial and heterogeneous process. Due to the diversity of pathological processes leading to AKI, it is highly unlikely that one single diagnostic marker may serve as reliable predictor for all AKI forms. A broadly applicable, multimarker diagnostic model will avoid this. The advantage of such a multimarker strategy is that it allows compensation for potential biological, pre-analytical and analytical variances of single biomarkers.

Mass spectrometry combined with chromatographic separation techniques has advanced exceptionally in recent years and has become a valuable tool for profiling of human proteomes and a systematic search of protein and peptide markers indicative for various renal and non-renal diseases without the need for a hypothesis-driven propagation process [54,19,1,93].

While proteome analysis aiming at biomarkers for renal disease can be focused on urine, plasma, or serum, urine seems to be the most attractive body fluid for several reasons. Firstly, urine can be obtained in large quantities in a non-invasive manner. Secondly, the

Reference	Marker	Clinical setting	No. of patients/ AKI cases	AUC	Time point of sample collection
Koyner et al., 2008 [35]	uCysC	Post-cardiac surgery	72/34	0.724	6 h after ICU admission
Liangos et al., 2009 [42]	uCysC	CPB	103/13	0.50	2 h after CPB
Koyner et al., 2010 [36]	uCysC	Post-cardiac surgery	123/46	0.72	ICU admission
Royakkers et al., 2011 [66]	uCysC	Mixed ICU	151/91	0.72	2 d before AKI diagnosis
Endre et al., 2011 [17]	uCysC/uCr	Mixed ICU	529/229	0.67	ICU admission
Endre et al., 2011 [17]	uCysC/uCr	Mixed ICU with eGFR <60 ml/min	24/3	0.69	Within 6 h after ICU admission
Endre et al., 2011 [17]	uCysC/uCr	Mixed ICU with eGFR <60 ml/min	12/8	0.88	Within 12-36 h after ICU admission
Endre et al., 2011 [17]	uCysC/uCr	Mixed ICU with eGFR ≥60 ml/min	153/34	0.68	Within 6 h after ICU admission
Endre et al., 2011 [17]	uCysC/uCr	Mixed ICU with eGFR ≥60 ml/min	104/41	0.77	Within 6-12 h after ICU admission
Wald et al., 2010 [88]	pCysC	CPB	150/47	0.68	2 h after CPB
Nejat et al., 2010 [58]	pCysC	Mixed ICU	444/198	0.80	Within 12 h after ICU admission
Herget-Rosenthal et al., 2004 [27]	sCysC	Mixed ICU	85/44	0.82	2 d before AKI diagnosis
Herget-Rosenthal et al., 2004 [27]	sCysC	Mixed ICU	85/44	0.97	1 d before AKI diagnosis
Haase-Fielitz et al., 2009 [23]	sCysC	Post-cardiac surgery	100/23	0.83	ICU admission
Haase et al., 2009 [22]	sCysC	Post-cardiac surgery	100/46	0.76	Immediately after surgery
Chung et al., 2010 [11]	sCysC	Liver cirrhosis	53/9	0.735	Admission
Krawczeski et al., 2010 [37]	sCysC	CPB-children	374/119	0.81	12 h after CPB
Soto et al., 2010 [74]	sCysC	Nonsurgical ED	616/130	0.87	Admission
Mishra et al., 2005 [55]	uNGAL	CPB-children	71/20	0.998	2 h after CPB
Zappitelli et al., 2007 [97]	uNGAL	Mixed ICU - children	140/106	0.78	ICU admission
Koyner et al., 2008 [35]	uNGAL	Post-cardiac surgery	72/34	0.705	ICU admission
Xin et al., 2008 [93]	uNGAL	Post-cardiac surgery	33/9	0.883	2 h after surgery
Wagener et al., 2008 [85]	uNGAL	Post-cardiac surgery	426/80	0.603	3 h after surgery
Bennett et al., 2008 [7]	uNGAL	CPB	196/99	0.95	2 h after CPB
Liangos et al., 2009 [42]	uNGAL	CPB	103/13	0.50	2 h after CPB
Tuladhar et al., 2009 [79]	uNGAL	CPB	50/9	0.96	2 h after CPB
Makris et al., 2009 [47]	uNGAL	Multi-trauma patients in ICU	31/11	0.977	Within 12 h after ICU admission
Siew et al., 2009 [70]	uNGAL	Mixed ICU	451/86	0.64	Within 12 h after ICU admission
Han et al., 2009 [24]	uNGAL	Post-cardiac surgery	90/36	0.59	Immediately after surgery
Han et al., 2009 [24]	uNGAL, NAG & uKIM-1	Post-cardiac surgery	90/36	0.75	Immediately after surgery

Reference	Marker	Clinical setting	No. of patients/ AKI cases	AUC	Time point of sample collection
Koyner et al., 2010 [36]	uNGAL	Post-cardiac surgery	123/46	0.72	6 h after ICU admission
McIlroy et al., 2010 [50]	uNGAL	Post-cardiac surgery, pre-op. eGFR 60-90 ml/min	142/35	0.66	3 h after surgery
McIlroy et al., 2010 [50]	uNGAL	Post-cardiac surgery, pre-op. eGFR 90-120 ml/min	109/13	0.88	24 h after surgery
Metzger et al., 2010 [53]	uNGAL	Mixed ICU	30/16	0.54	3.4±1.0 d before AKI diagnosis
Wagener et al., 2011 [86]	uNGAL/uCr	Liver transplantation	92/37	0.8	3 h after transplantation
Doi et al., 2011 [16]	uNGAL	Mixed ICU	339/131	0.70	Within 12 h after ICU admission
Endre et al., 2011 [17]	uNGAL/uCr	Mixed ICU	529/229	0.66	ICU admission
Endre et al., 2011 [17]	uNGAL/uCr	Mixed ICU with eGFR <60ml/min	12/8	0.85	Within 12-36 h after ICU admission
Endre et al., 2011 [17]	uNGAL/uCr	Mixed ICU with eGFR ≥60 ml/min	153/34	0.68	Within 6 h after ICU admission
Endre et al., 2011 [17]	uNGAL/uCr	Mixed ICU with eGFR ≥60 ml/min	83/17	0.69	Within 6-12 h after ICU admission
Endre et al., 2011 [17]	uNGAL/uCr	Mixed ICU with eGFR ≥60 ml/min	104/41	0.71	Within 12-36 h after ICU admission
Haase et al., 2009 [22]	pNGAL	Post-cardiac surgery	100/46	0.77	Immediately after surgery
Haase-Fielitz et al., 2009 [23]	pNGAL	Post-cardiac surgery	100/23	0.8	ICU admission
Tuladhar et al., 2009 [79]	pNGAL	CPB	50/9	0.80	2 h after CPB
Cruz et al., 2010 [13]	pNGAL	Mixed ICU	301/133	0.78	2 d before AKI diagnosis
Constantin et al., 2010 [12]	pNGAL	Mixed ICU	88/52	0.92	ICU admission
Wheeler et al., 2008 [91]	sNGAL	children with SIRS or septic shock in ICU	143/22	0.677	ICU admission
Koyner et al., 2008 [36]	uKIM-1	Post-cardiac surgery	123/46	0.67	6 h after ICU admission
Han et al., 2009 [24]	uKIM-1	Post-cardiac surgery	90/36	0.68	Immediately after surgery
Liangos et al., 2009 [42]	uKIM-1	CPB	103/13	0.78	2 h after CPB
Metzger et al., 2010 [53]	uKIM-1	Mixed ICU	30/16	0.71	3.4±1.0 d before AKI diagnosis
Endre et al., 2011 [17]	uKIM-1/uCr	Mixed ICU	529/229	0.66	ICU admission
Endre et al., 2011 [17]	uKIM-1/uCr	Mixed ICU with eGFR <60 ml/min	24/3	0.73	Within 6 h after ICU admission
Endre et al., 2011 [17]	uKIM-1/uCr	Mixed ICU with eGFR ≥60 ml/min	83/17	0.72	Within 6-12 h after ICU admission
Endre et al., 2011 [17]	uKIM-1/uCr	Mixed ICU with eGFR ≥60 ml/min	104/41	0.66	Within 12-36 h after ICU admission
Parikh et al., 2006 [62]	uIL-18	CPB-children	71/20	0.75	12 h after CPB
Xin et al., 2008 [93]	uIL-18	Post-cardiac surgery	33/9	0.894	2 h after surgery

Reference	Marker	Clinical setting	No. of patients/ AKI cases	AUC	Time point of sample collection
Liangos et al., 2009 [42]	uIL-18	CPB	103/13	0.66	2 h after CPB
Metzger et al., 2010 [53]	uIL-18	Mixed ICU	30/16	0.57	3.4±1.0 d before AKI diagnosis
Siew et al., 2010 [71]	uIL-18	Mixed ICU	451/86	0.62	Within 24 h after ICU admission
Doi et al., 2011 [16]	uIL-18	Mixed ICU	339/131	0.69	Within 12 h after ICU admission
Endre et al., 2011 [17]	uIL-18/uCr	Mixed ICU	529/229	0.62	ICU admission
Endre et al., 2011 [17]	uIL-18/uCr	Mixed ICU with eGFR <60 ml/min	12/8	0.94	Within 12-36 h after ICU admission
Endre et al., 2011 [17]	uIL-18/uCr	Mixed ICU with eGFR ≥60 ml/min	83/17	0.72	Within 6-12 h after ICU admission
Liangos et al., 2009 [43]	pIL-8	CPB	143/59	0.62	2 h after CPB
Han et al., 2009 [24]	uNAG	Post-cardiac surgery	90/36	0.61	Immediately after surgery
Liangos et al., 2009 [42]	uNAG	CPB	103/13	0.62	2 h after CPB
Doi et al., 2011 [16]	uNAG	Mixed ICU	339/131	0.62	Within 12 h after ICU admission
Portilla et al., 2007 [63]	uL-FABP	Post-cardiac surgery - children	40/21	0.81	4 h after surgery
Doi et al., 2011 [16]	uL-FABP	Mixed ICU	339/131	0.75	Within 12 h after ICU admission
Matsui et al., 2012 [49]	uL-FABP	Post-cardiac surgery	85/48	0.86	Immediately after surgery
Katagiri et al., 2012 [33]	uL-FABP & uNAG	CPB	77/28	0.81	2 h after CPB

Abbreviations: AKI, acute kidney injury; AUC, area under the curve; CPB, cardiopulmonary bypass; Cr, creatinine; CysC, Cystatin C; ED, emergency department; eGFR, estimated glomerular filtration rate; IL-18, Interleukin-18; KIM-1, Kidney injury molecule-1; L-FABP, Liver-type fatty acid-binding protein; NAG, N-acetyl-β-D-glucosaminidase; NGAL, Neutrophil gelatinase-associated lipocalin; p, plasma; s, serum; u, urinary.

Table 1. Diagnostic performance of different single biomarkers of AKI in different clinical settings

urinary proteome is relative stable since it is retained in the bladder for several hours, providing sufficient time for complete proteolytic processing by endogenous proteases. The low molecular weight proteome of the urine does not undergo any significant change if urine is stored for up to 3 days at 4°C or 6 h at room temperature [67,77].

For these reasons, several groups have embraced the search for urinary proteomic biomarkers for the early detection of AKI using different analytical platforms. In an early study conducted in 2005, Nguyen et al. [59] identified 4 proteins with a mass-to-charge ratio (m/z) of 6.4, 28.5, 43 and 66 kDa, being increased at baseline and at 2 and 6 h post-operation in the urine of children that developed ischemic kidney injury 2-3 days after cardiopulmonary bypass (CPB). These proteins in combination allowed detection of AKI in this small patient cohort with 100 % sensitivity and specificity. One of these proteins (m/z 6.4) was later identified as aprotinin [60], a very basic polypeptide with serine protease inhibitory activity, negatively affecting both coagulation and fibrinolysis [48]. The other 3 peaks were identified as acute-phase proteins α 1-microglobulin (28.5 kDa), α 1-acid glycoprotein (43 kDa) and albumin (66 kDa) [15].

Using the same analytical platform Ho and colleagues identified, besides known up-regulated tubular injury markers, two novel peptide peaks at 2.43 and 2.78 kDa that were significantly increased in patients after CPB surgery not developing AKI [28]. The authors were able to resolve one of these peptides as hepcidin-25, the active form of hepcidin, which is secreted by the liver to maintain iron homeostasis and which is up-regulated during acute phase response [83].

Metzger et al. [53] used capillary electrophoresis mass spectrometry to identify urinary peptide markers predictive for AKI in urine samples obtained from ICU patients who later developed AKI defined by a serum creatinine increase ≥ 50 % in ≤ 48 hours (maximum 5 days prior AKI) or remained normal in kidney function. The 20 statistically most significant peptide markers in a comparative group analysis (**Figure 2**) were combined to a support vector machine-based classifier, which allowed classification of a blinded test set of ICU patient samples (n=20, 9 case and 11 controls) with 89 % sensitivity and 82 % specificity. In order to evaluate general applicability, this classifier was further applied to the classification of urine samples from hematopoietic stem cell transplanted patients of whom 13 developed AKI after transplantation and 16 did not. AUC in this validation set was 0.90 with sensitivity and specificity values of 94 and 82 %, respectively. The 20 polypeptides were identified by amino acid sequencing as degradation products of 6 proteins. Fragments of albumin, α 1-antitrypsin and β 2-microglobulin were up-regulated, fibrinogen α chain, collagen 1 α(I) and collagen 1 α(III) were down-regulated in AKI. The alterations of these polypeptides identified in the urine may be attributed to differences in production rates, increased assembly into filaments, increased proteolysis in the plasma or urine, abnormal renal function, or a combination of the above, and may be relevant at different points of the disease process as outlined in **figure 3**.

A recent study of Maddens et al. [46] using LTQ-OrbiTRAP for mass spectrometry analysis identified urinary NGAL, thioredoxin, gelsolin, chitinase 3-like protein 1 and 3 and acidic mammalian chitinase as being the most discriminating markers for experimental sepsis-induced AKI in mice. Differential expression was verified by immunoblot analysis in urine, plasma and renal tissue homogenates. In a small set of human septic patients the authors detected possible differences in excretion levels of the human homologue of chitinase 3-like protein 1 and acidic mammalian chitinase protein between patients with compared to those without AKI. However, the study was too small to draw any conclusions. The potential use of chitinase proteins as sensitive markers for diagnosis of septic-induced AKI is limited, as the authors stated, mostly by the fact that increased levels are also detectable during inflammatory responses, such as asthma or inflammatory bowel disease, liver fibrosis and also for non-AKI patients of the AKI study group without recognizable comorbidities.

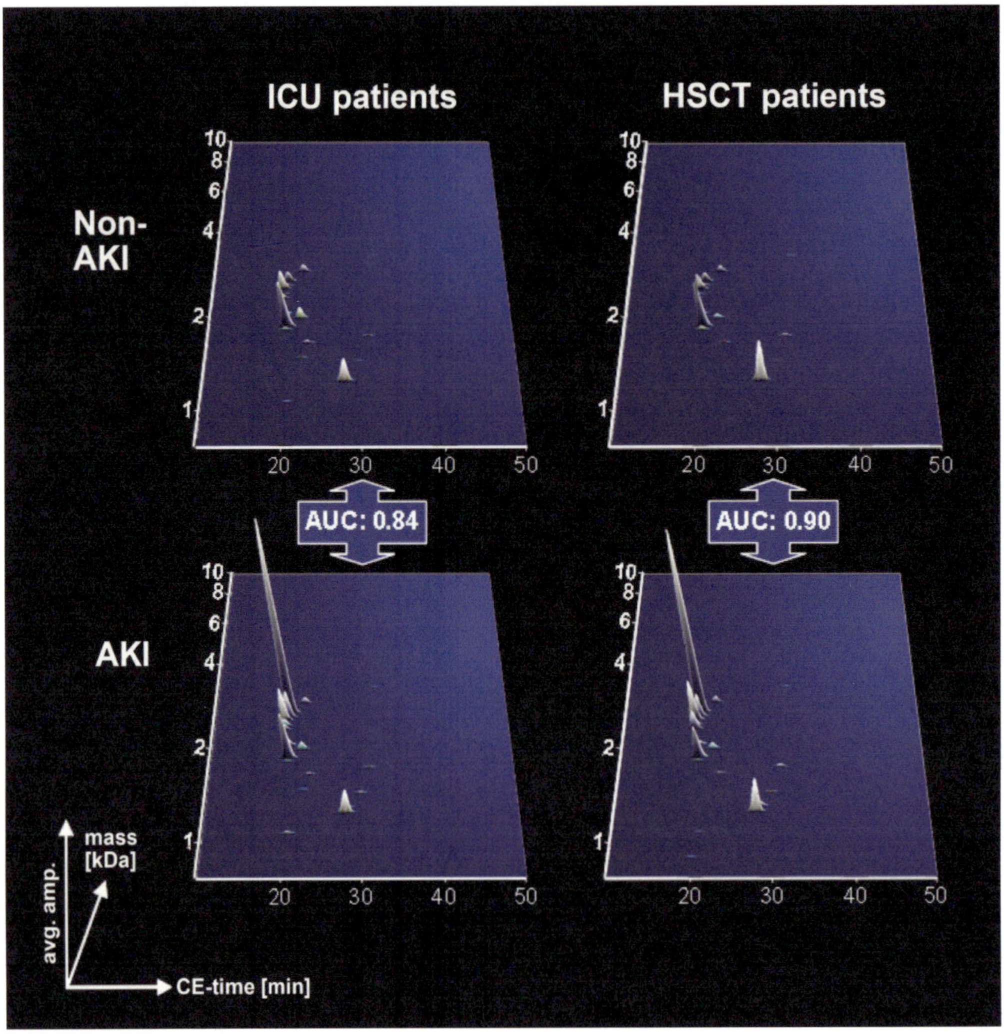

Fig. 2. Distribution of urinary peptides included in the AKI-specific biomarker panel of Metzger et al., 2010 [53]. AUC's for ROC comparison of AKI and non-AKI within the ICU and HSCT patient groups are shown in the insets. Abbreviations: AKI, acute kidney injury; AUC, area under the curve; HSCT, hematopoietic stem cell transplantation; ICU, intensive care unit; ROC, receiver operating characteristics. Modified from data shown in Metzger et al., 2010 [53].

Gel-based proteomics has also been tested as a platform in the search for biomarkers of AKI. Using this methodological approach, Aregger et al [3] identified 3 proteins in a cohort of 36 patients undergoing CPB to be differentially regulated between patients who developed AKI and those who not. The identified proteins were albumin, being upregulated, and zinc α 2-glycoprotein and adrenomedullin-binding protein, both down-regulated. Limiting the results of the study, only zinc α 2-glycoprotein was applied to a validation set of 22 patients with AKI and 46 patients without to test its diagnostic performance in immunoblot and ELISA. An AUC value of 0.68 revealed that zinc α 2-glycoprotein is only a weak predictor of AKI.

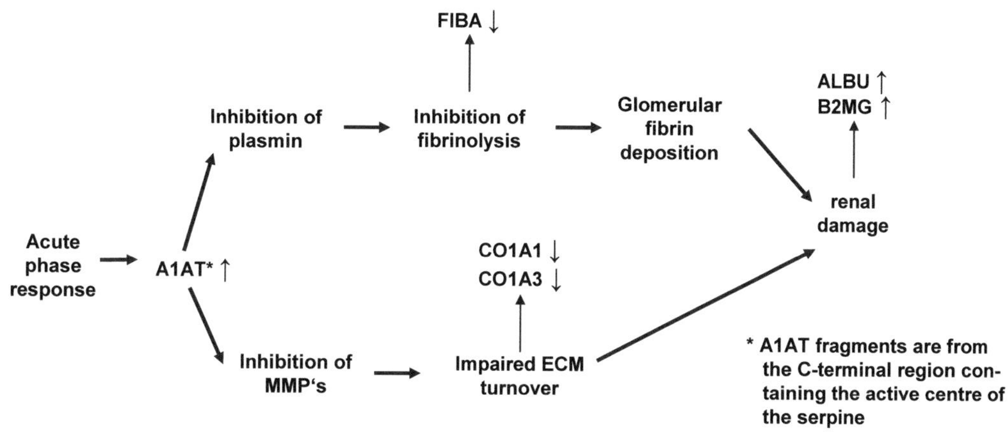

Fig. 3. Pathophysiological relevance of parent proteins from the peptides included in the AKI-specific proteomic biomarker model of Metzger et al., 2010 [53].
Abbreviations: A1AT, α 1-antitrypsin; ALBU, albumin; B2MG, β 2-microglobulin; CO1A1, collagen 1 α(I) chain; CO1A3, collagen 1 α(III) chain; ECM, extracellular matrix; FIBA, fibrinogen α chain; MMP, matrix metallopeptidases.

5. Conclusion

It is evident that an effective prevention or intervention strategy for patients particularly in the ICU (with the possible therapeutic options depicted in **figure 4**) relies on accurate and early detection of AKI. Considering the heterogeneity and complexity of AKI, a multiple marker approach seems to be more favourable over single markers. A multimarker approach will not rely on particular, single aspects of AKI, i.e. tubular damage, fibrosis, inflammation, necrosis or apoptosis, but combine the significant findings indicative of specific etiologies, ideally enabling detection of AKI independent of the underlying cause.

Irrespective of the approach, large, prospective, multicentre clinical trials on unselected patient populations are required to validate the different proposed biomarkers or classifiers. In analogy to a recent editorial by Vlahou [84], such a large study would best be performed in a way that allows testing all the biomarkers currently proposed. Unfortunately, neither industry, nor government agencies currently see the need for such a large trial.

Once suitable biomarkers and classifiers for accurate, early detection of AKI have been identified, it is essential to design an easy-to-apply analytical test based on these markers that is suitable for routine laboratory use ideally as a point of care device in intensive care units. One promising approach is the application of MALDI-MS as a robust and fast platform for efficient analysis of urinary biomarkers, which has been demonstrated feasible in CKD [39].

Common intervention	Therapeutic intervention
• Correct hypovolemia	• Administration of vasodilator agents
• Early goal directed therapy for sepsis and shock treatment	• In shock states: noradrenalin as preferred vasoconstrictor
• Avoid nephrotoxic antimicrobials	• Volume substitution prior and post indicated radio contrast
• Avoid radio contrast	• Rather cristalloids than colloids. If hydroxyethyl starch, only limited amount, low rather than high-molecular weight one.

Fig. 4. Intervention aiming at AKI prevention.

6. Acknowledgement

This work was supported in part by grant G1000791/1 from the MRC to HM. VB was supported by grant GA 251368 (Protoclin) from the FP7-PEOPLE-2009-IAPP program. HM was supported in part by EU Funding through SysKID (HEALTH–F2–2009–241544).

7. References

[1] Albalat A, Mischak H and Mullen W. Urinary proteomics in clinical applications: technologies, principal considerations and clinical implementation. Prilozi. 2011; 32(1): 13-44.

[2] Ali T, Khan I, Simpson W et al. Incidence and outcomes in acute kidney injury: a comprehensive population-based study. J Am Soc Nephrol. 2007; 18: 1292-1298.

[3] Aregger F, Pilop C, Uehlinger DE et al. Urinary proteomics before and after extracorporeal circulation in patients with and without acute kidney injury. J Thorac Cardiovasc Surg. 2010; 139(3): 692-700.

[4] Bagshaw SM, George C, Bellomo R et al. Early acute kidney injury and sepsis: a multicentre evaluation. Crit Care. 2008; 12(2): R47.

[5] Bagshaw SM, Uchino S, Bellomo R et al. Septic Acute Kidney Injury in Critically Ill Patients: Clinical Characteristics and Outcomes. Clin J Am Soc Nephrol. 2007; 2(3): 431-439.
[6] Bellomo R, Ronco C, Kellum JA et al. Acute renal failure - definition, outcome measures, animal models, fluid therapy and information technology needs: the Second International Consensus Conference of the Acute Dialysis Quality Initiative (ADQI) Group. Crit Care. 2004; 8(4): R204-R212.
[7] Bennett M, Dent CL, Ma Q et al. Urine NGAL predicts severity of acute kidney injury after cardiac surgery: a prospective study. Clin J Am Soc Nephrol. 2008; 3(3): 665-673.
[8] Chawla LS, Amdur RL, Amodeo S et al. The severity of acute kidney injury predicts progression to chronic kidney disease. Kidney Int. 2011; 79(12): 1361-1369.
[9] Chawla LS and Kellum JA. Biomarkers are transforming our understanding of AKI. Nat Rev. 2012; 8: 68-70.
[10] Chertow GM, Burdick E, Honour M et al. Acute Kidney Injury, Mortality, Length of Stay, and Costs in Hospitalized Patients. J Am Soc Nephrol. 2005; 16(11): 3365-3370.
[11] Chung MY, Jun DW and Sung SA. Diagnosis value of cystatin C for predicting acute kidney injury in patients with liver cirrhosis. Korean J Hepatol. 2010; 16(3): 301-307.
[12] Constantin JM, Futier E, Perbet S et al. Plasma neutrophil gelatinase-associated lipocalin is an early marker of acute kidney injury in adult critically ill patients: A prospective study. J Crit Care. 2010;25(1):176.e1-6.
[13] Cruz DN, de Cal M, Garzotto F et al. Plasma neutrophil gelatinase-associated lipocalin is an early biomarker for acute kidney injury in an adult ICU population. Intensive Care Med. 2010; 36(3): 444-451.
[14] Dasta JF, Kane-Gill SL, Durtschi AJ et al. Costs and outcomes of acute kidney injury (AKI) following cardiac surgery. Nephrol Dial Transpl. 2008; 23(6): 1970-1974.
[15] Devarajan P, Krawczeski CD, Nguyen MT et al. Proteomic identification of early biomarkers of acute kidney injury after cardiac surgery in children. Am J Kidney Dis. 2010; 56(4): 632-642.
[16] Doi K, Negishi K, Katagiri D et al. Evaluation of new acute kidney injury biomarkers in a mixed intensive care unit. Crit Care Med. 2011; 39(11): 2646-2649.
[17] Endre ZH, Pickering JW, Walker RJ et al. Improved performance of urinary biomarkers of acute kidney injury in the critically ill by stratification for injury duration and baseline renal function. Kidney Int. 2011; 79: 1119-1130.
[18] Ferguson MA and Waikar SS. Established and emerging markers of kidney function. J Crit Care. 2010;25(1):176.e1-6.
[19] Frantzi M, Bitsika V, Charonis A et al. Proteomics approaches in the quest of kidney disease biomarkers. Prilozi. 2011; 32(2): 33-51.
[20] Goldstein SL and Devarajan P. Progression form acute kidney injury to chronic kidney disease: a pediatric perspective. Adv Chronic Kidney Dis. 2008; 15: 278-283.
[21] Haase M, Bellomo R, Devarajan P et al. Accuracy of neutrophil gelatinase-associated lipocalin (NGAL) in diagnosis and prognosis in acute kidney injury: a systematic review and meta-analysis. Am J Kidney Dis. 2009; 54: 1012-1024.
[22] Haase M, Bellomo R, Devarajan P et al. Novel Biomarkers Early Predict the Severity of Acute Kidney Injury After Cardiac Surgery in Adults. Ann Thorac Surg. 2009; 88(1): 124-130.

[23] Haase-Fielitz A, Bellomo R, Devarajan P et al. Novel and conventional serum biomarkers predicting acute kidney injury in adult cardiac surgery-a prospective cohort study. Crit Care Med. 2009; 37(2): 553-560.

[24] Han WK, Wagener G, Zhu Y et al. Urinary biomarkers in the early detection of acute kidney injury after cardiac surgery. Clin J Am Soc Nephrol. 2009; 4: 873-882.

[25] Han WK, Bailly V, Abichandani R et al. Kidney Injury Molecule-1 (KIM-1): A novel biomarker for human renal proximal tubule injury. Kidney Int. 2002; 62(1): 237-244.

[26] He Z, Lu L, Altmann C et al. Interleukin-18 binding protein transgenic mice are protected against ischemic acute kidney injury. Am J Physiol - Ren Physiol. 2008; 295(5): F1414-F1421.

[27] Herget-Rosenthal S, Marggraf G, Husing J et al. Early detection of acute renal failure by serum cystatin C. Kidney Int. 2004; 66: 1115-1122.

[28] Ho J, Lucy M, Krokhin O et al. Mass spectrometry-based proteomic analysis of urine in acute kidney injury following cardiopulmonary bypass: a nested case-control study. Am J Kidney Dis. 2009; 53: 584-595.

[29] Hou SH, Bushinsky DA, Wish JB et al. Hospital-acquired renal insufficiency: A prospective study. Am J Med. 1983; 74(2): 243-248.

[30] Ichimura T, Asseldonk EJ, Humphreys BD et al. Kidney injury molecule-1 is a phosphatidylserine receptor that confers a phagocytic phenotype on epithelial cells. J Clin Invest. 2008; 118(5): 1657-1668.

[31] Ichimura T, Bonventre JV, Bailly V et al. Kidney Injury Molecule-1 (KIM-1), a Putative Epithelial Cell Adhesion Molecule Containing a Novel Immunoglobulin Domain, Is Up-regulated in Renal Cells after Injury. J Biol Chem. 1998; 273(7): 4135-4142.

[32] Ishani A, Xue JL, Himmelfarb J et al. Acute kidney injury increases risk of ESRD among elderly. J Am Soc Nephrol. 2009; 20: 223-228.

[33] Katagiri D, Doi K, Honda K et al. Combination of Two Urinary Biomarkers Predicts Acute Kidney Injury After Adult Cardiac Surgery. Ann Thorac Surg. 2012; 93(2): 577-583.

[34] Kohli HS, Bhat A, Jairam A et al. Predictors of Mortality in Acute Renal Failure in a Developing Country: A Prospective Study. Ren Fail. 2007; 29(4): 463-469.

[35] Koyner JL, Bennett MR, Worcester EM et al. Urinary cystatin C as an early biomarker of acute kidney injury following adult cardiothoracic surgery. Kidney Int. 2008; 74: 1059-1069.

[36] Koyner JL, Vaidya VS, Bennett MR et al. Urinary biomarkers in the clinical prognosis and early detection of acute kidney injury. Clin J Am Soc Nephrol. 2010; 5(12): 2154-2165.

[37] Krawczeski CD, Vandevoorde RG, Kathman T et al. Serum cystatin C is an early predictive biomarker of acute kidney injury after pediatric cardiopulmonary bypass. Clin J Am Soc Nephrol. 2010; 5(9): 1552-1557.

[38] Lameire NH, Vanholder RC and Van Biesen WA. How to use biomarkers efficiently in acute kidney injury. Kidney Int. 2011; 79(10): 1047-1050.

[39] Lapolla A, Molin L, Sechi A et al. A further investigation on a MALDI-based method for evaluation of markers of renal damage. J Mass Spectrom. 2009; 44(12): 1754-1760.

[40] Laterza OF, Price CP and Scott MG. Cystatin C: an improved estimator of glomerular filtration rate? Clin Chem. 2002; 48: 699-707.

[41] Levey AS, Bosch JP, Lewis JB et al. A more accurate method to estimate glomerular filtration rate from serum creatinine: a new prediction equation. Modification of Diet in Renal Disease Study Group. Ann Intern Med. 1999; 130: 461-470.
[42] Liangos O, Tighiouart H, Perianayagam MC et al. Comparative analysis of urinary biomarkers for early detection of acute kidney injury following cardiopulmonary bypass. Biomarkers. 2009; 14: 423-431.
[43] Liangos O, Kolyada A, Tighiouart H et al. Interleukin-8 and acute kidney injury following cardiopulmonary bypass: a prospective cohort study. Nephron Clin Pract. 2009; 113: c148-c154.
[44] Liangos O, Perianayagam MC, Vaidya VS et al. Urinary N-Acetyl-+¦-(D)-Glucosaminidase Activity and Kidney Injury Molecule-1 Level Are Associated with Adverse Outcomes in Acute Renal Failure. J Am Soc Nephrol. 2007; 18(3): 904-912.
[45] Loef BG, Epema AH, Smilde TD et al. Immediate Postoperative Renal Function Deterioration in Cardiac Surgical Patients Predicts In-Hospital Mortality and Long-Term Survival. J Am Soc Nephrol. 2005; 16(1): 195-200.
[46] Maddens B, Ghesquiere B, Vanholder R et al. Chitinase-like proteins are candidate biomarkers for sepsis-induced acute kidney injury. Mol Cell Proteomics. 2012; Epub ahead of print.
[47] Makris K, Markou N, Evodia E et al. Urinary neutrophil gelatinase-associated lipocalin (NGAL) as an early marker of acute kidney injury in critically ill multiple trauma patients. Clin Chem Lab Med. 2009; 47: 79-82.
[48] Mannucci PM. Hemostatic drugs. N Engl J Med. 1998; 339(4): 245-253.
[49] Matsui K, Kamijo-Ikemori A, Sugaya T et al. Usefulness of Urinary Biomarkers in Early Detection of Acute Kidney Injury After Cardiac Surgery in Adults. Circ J. 2012; 76(1): 213-220.
[50] McIlroy DR, Wagener G and Lee HT. Neutrophil gelatinase-associated lipocalin and acute kidney injury after cardiac surgery: the effect of baseline renal function on diagnostic performance. Clin J Am Soc Nephrol. 2010; 5: 211-219.
[51] Mehta RL, Kellum JA, Shah SV et al. Acute Kidney Injury Network: report of an initiative to improve outcomes in acute kidney injury. Crit Care. 2007;11(2):R13.
[52] Melnikov VY, Faubel S, Siegmund B et al. Neutrophil-independent mechanisms of caspase-1- and IL-18-mediated ischemic acute tubular necrosis in mice. J Clin Invest. 2002; 110(8): 1083-1091.
[53] Metzger J, Kirsch T, Schiffer E et al. Urinary excretion of twenty peptides forms an early and accurate diagnostic pattern of acute kidney injury. Kidney Int. 2010; 78: 1252-1262.
[54] Metzger J, Luppa PB, Good DM et al. Adapting mass spectrometry-based platforms for clinical proteomics applications: The capillary electrophoresis coupled mass spectrometry paradigm. Crit Rev Clin Lab Sci. 2009; 46(3): 129-152.
[55] Mishra J, Dent C, and Tarabishi R. Neutrophil gelatinase-associated lipocalin (NGAL) as a biomarker for acute renal injury after cardiac surgery. Lancet. 2005; 365: 1231-1238.
[56] Mishra J, Ma K, Kelly C et al. Kidney NGAL is a novel early marker of acute injury following transplantation. Pediatr Nephrol. 2006; 21: 856-863.
[57] Moore E, Bellomo R and Nichol A. Biomarkers of acute kidney injury in anesthesia, intensive care and major surgery: from the bench to clinical practice. Minerva Anestesiol. 2010; 76(6): 425-440.

[58] Nejat M, Pickering JW, Walker RJ et al. Rapid detection of acute kidney injury by plasma cystatin C in the intensive care unit. Nephrol Dial Transplant. 2010;25(10):3283-3289.

[59] Nguyen MT, Ross GF, Dent CL et al. Early prediction of acute renal injury using urinary proteomics. Am J Nephrol. 2005; 25: 318-326.

[60] Nguyen MT, Dent CL, Ross GF et al. Urinary aprotinin as a predictor of acute kidney injury after cardiac surgery in children receiving aprotinin therapy. Pediatr Nephrol. 2008; 23(8): 1317-1326.

[61] Parikh CR, Abraham E, Ancukiewicz M et al. Urine IL-18 is an early diagnostic marker for acute kidney injury and predicts mortality in the intensive care unit. J Am Soc Nephrol. 2005; 16: 3046-3052.

[62] Parikh CR, Mishra J, Thiessen-Philbrook H et al. Urinary IL-18 is an early predictive biomarker of acute kidney injury after cardiac surgery. Kidney Int. 2006; 70(1): 199-203.

[63] Portilla D, Dent C, Sugaya T et al. Liver fatty acid-binding protein as a biomarker of acute kidney injury after cardiac surgery. Kidney Int. 2007; 73(4): 465-472.

[64] Prozialeck WC, Edwards JR, Lamar PC et al. Expression of kidney injury molecule-1 (Kim-1) in relation to necrosis and apoptosis during the early stages of Cd-induced proximal tubule injury. Toxicol Appl Pharmacol. 2009; 238(3): 306-314.

[65] Royakkers AANM, van Sujilen JDE, Hofstra LS et al. Serum cystatin C-A useful endogenous marker of renal function in intensive care unit patients at risk for or with acute renal failure? Curr Med Chem. 2007; 14: 2314-2317.

[66] Royakkers A, Korevaar J, van Suijlen J et al. Serum and urine cystatin-áC are poor biomarkers for acute kidney injury and renal replacement therapy. Intensive Care Med. 2011; 37(3): 493-501.

[67] Schaub S, Wilkins J, Weiler T et al. Urine protein profiling with surface-enhanced laser-desorption/ionization time-of-flight mass spectrometry. Kidney Int. 2004; 65(1): 323-332.

[68] Shemin D and Dworkin LD. Neutrophil gelatinase-associated lipocalin (NGAL) as a biomarker for early acute kidney injury. Crit Care Clin. 2011; 27: 379-389.

[69] Shusterman N, Strom BL, Murray TG et al. Risk factors and outcome of hospital-acquired acute renal failure: Clinical Epidemiologic Study. Am J Med. 1987; 83(1): 65-71.

[70] Siew ED, Ware LB, Gebretsadik T et al. Urine neutrophil gelatinase-associated lipocalin moderately predicts acute kidney injury in critically ill adults. J Am Soc Nephrol. 2009; 20: 1823-1832.

[71] Siew ED, Ikizler TA, Gebretsadik T et al. Elevated Urinary IL-18 Levels at the Time of ICU Admission Predict Adverse Clinical Outcomes. Clin J Am Soc Nephrol. 2010; 5(8): 1497-1505.

[72] Singbartl K and Kellum JA. AKI in the ICU: definition, epidemiology, risk stratification, and outcomes. Kidney Int. 2011; Epub ahead of print.

[73] Sirota JC, Klawitter J and Edelstein CL. Biomarkers of acute kidney injury. J Toxicol. 2011; 2011: 328120.

[74] Soto K, Coelho S, Rodrigues B et al. Cystatin C as a marker of acute kidney injury in the emergency department. Clin J Am Soc Nephrol. 2010; 5(10): 1745-1754.

[75] Star RA. Treatment of acute renal failure. Kidney Int. 1998; 54: 1817-1831.

[76] Stevens LA, Lafayette RD, Perrone RD et al. Laboratory evaluation of kidney function. 2007; 8th Edition: 299-366.
[77] Theodorescu D, Wittke S, Ross MM et al. Discovery and validation of new protein biomarkers for urothelial cancer: a prospective analysis. Lancet Oncol. 2006; 7(3): 230-240.
[78] Trachtman H, Christen E, Cnaan A et al. Urinary neutrophil gelatinase-associated lipocalin (NGAL) in D+HUS: a novel marker of renal injury. Pediatr Nephrol. 2006; 21: 989-994.
[79] Tuladhar SM, Puntmann VO, Soni M et al. Rapid detection of acute kidney injury by plasma and urinary neutrophil gelatinase-associated lipocalin after cardiopulmonary bypass. J Cardiovasc Pharmacol. 2009; 53: 261-266.
[80] Uchino S, Kellum JA, Bellomo R et al. Acute renal failure in critically ill patients: a multinational, multicenter study. JAMA. 2005; 294: 813-818.
[81] Urbschat A, Obermüller N and Haferkamp A. Biomarkers of kidney injury. Biomarkers. 2011; 16(S1): S22-S30.
[82] van Timmeren MM, van den Heuvel MC, Bailly V et al. Tubular kidney injury molecule-1 (KIM-1) in human renal disease. J Pathol. 2007; 212(2): 209-217.
[83] Vecchi C, Montosi G, Zhang K et al. ER stress controls iron metabolism through induction of hepcidin. Science. 2009; 325(5942): 877-880.
[84] Vlahou A. Back to the future in bladder cancer research. Expert Rev Proteomics. 2011; 8(3): 295-297.
[85] Wagener G, Gubitosa G, Wang S et al. Urinary neutrophil gelatinase-associated lipocalin and acute kidney injury after cardiac surgery. Am J Kidney Dis. 2008; 52: 425-433.
[86] Wagener G, Minhaz M, Mattis FA et al. Urinary neutrophil gelatinase-associated lipocalin as a marker of acute kidney injury after orthotopic liver transplantation. Nephrol Dial Transplant. 2011; 26(5): 1717-1723.
[87] Waikar SS, Liu KD and Chertow GM. Diagnosis, Epidemiology and Outcomes of Acute Kidney Injury. Clin J Am Soc Nephrol. 2008; 3(3): 844-861.
[88] Wald R, Liangos O, Perianayagam MC et al. Plasma cystatin C and acute kidney injury after cardiopulmonary bypass. Clin J Am Soc Nephrol. 2010; 5(8): 1373-1379.
[89] Washburn KK, Zappitelli M, Arikan AA et al. Urinary interleukin-18 is an acute kidney injury biomarker in critically ill children. Nephrol Dial Transpl. 2008; 23(2): 566-572.
[90] Westenfelder C. Earlier diagnosis of acute kidney injury awaits effective therapy. Kidney Int. 2011; 79(11): 1159-1161.
[91] Wheeler DS, Devarajan P, Ma Q et al. Serum neutrophil gelatinase-associated lipocalin (NGAL) as a marker of acute kidney injury in critically ill children with septic shock. Crit Care Med. 2008;36:1297-1303.
[92] Wittke S, Fliser D, Haubitz M et al. Determination of peptides and proteins in human urine with capillary electrophoresis-mass spectrometry, a suitable tool for the establishment of new diagnostic markers. J Chromatogr A. 2003; 1013: 173-181.
[93] Xin C, Yulong X, Yu C et al. Urine Neutrophil Gelatinase-Associated Lipocalin and Interleukin-18 Predict Acute Kidney Injury after Cardiac Surgery*. Ren Fail. 2008; 30(9): 904-913.
[94] Xue JL, Daniels F, Star RA et al. Incidence and Mortality of Acute Renal Failure in Medicare Beneficiaries, 1992 to 2001. J Am Soc Nephrol. 2006; 17(4): 1135-1142.

[95] Yilmaz A, Sevketoglu E, Gedikbasi A et al. Early prediction of urinary tract infection with urinary neutrophil gelatinase associated lipocalin. Pediatr Nephrol. 2009; 24: 2387-2392.
[96] Ympa YP, Sakr Y, Reinhart K et al. Has mortality from acute renal failure decreased? A systematic review of the literature. Am J Med. 2005; 118(8): 827-832.
[97] Zappitelli M, Washburn KK, Arikan AA et al. Urine neutrophil gelatinase-associated lipocalin is an early marker of acute kidney injury in critically ill children: a prospective cohort study. Crit Care. 2007; 11(4): R84.
[98] Zhang PL, Rothblum LI, Han WK et al. Kidney injury molecule-1 expression in transplant biopsies is a sensitive measure of cell injury. Kidney Int. 2008; 73(5): 608-614.
[99] Zhang Z, Humphreys BD and Bonventre JV. Shedding of the Urinary Biomarker Kidney Injury Molecule-1 (KIM-1) Is Regulated by MAP Kinases and Juxtamembrane Region. J Am Soc Nephrol. 2007; 18(10): 2704-2714.
[100] Zhang Z, Lu B, Sheng X et al. Cystatin C in Prediction of Acute Kidney Injury: A Systemic Review and Meta-analysis. Am J Kidney Dis. 2011; 58(3): 356-365.

7

Sepsis and Dialysis Disequilibrium Syndrome

Nissar Shaikh
Dept Anesthesia/ICU, Hamad Medical Corporation, Doha Qatar

1. Introduction

Dialysis disequilibrium syndrome (DDS) is a central nervous system disorder, usually occurs in patients during hemodialysis (HD) or within 24 hours of HD. DDS was first described by Kennedy *et al.* in 1962. [11] If a critically ill patient on HD develops severe sepsis and septic shock with multiple organ failure (MOF), the adverse effect of HD on the brain is likely to be amplified, which may predispose to the DDS.

Severe sepsis and septic shock are the common indications for intensive care therapy admission. Sepsis/ severe sepsis are usually manifested by inadequate organ perfusion/function. Multiple organ dysfunction syndrome (MODS) is the presence of altered organ function, in an acutely ill septic patient whose homeostasis is maintained with the intervention.[4]

Mechanism (Fig1) for the occurrence of MODS is result of imbalance between the pro and anti-inflammatory response and the dominance of pro-inflammatory reaction. This leads to the systemic microvascular thrombosis, hypoxic hypoxia, immunosuppressant and apoptosis.[9] Which ultimately leads to organ dysfunction/failure in severe sepsis/ septic shock patients

Acute renal failure is one of the common complications of severe sepsis and septic shock. It occurs in 23% of severe sepsis and 51% of septic shock patients and requires hemodialysis. In case of renal failure due to sepsis, the renal vasoconstriction occurs due to the increased sympathetic tone; in contrast to the systemic vasodilatation. [16]

Twenty three percent of septic shock patients develop septic encephalopathy.[8] various anatomical abnormalities are found in these patients of severe sepsis and septic shock with brain involvement, these are collectively termed as the septic encephalopathy. These abnormalities includes proliferation of astrocytes, cerebral infarcts, multiple white matter hemorrhages, central pontine myelinolysis, multiple microabceses, reduction in cerebral blood flow , cerebral capillary leakage, and malfunctioning of the blood brain barrier.[10]

These septic encephalopathy changes can be amplified if patient is having traumatic brain injury, subarachnoid hemorrhage or on hemodialysis.

Critically ill patients frequently require renal replacement therapy and intermittent HD. DDS is an acute neurological manifestation due to cerebral edema that occurs during or after dialysis, these manifestations can be mild, such as nausea and vomiting, or severe, as seizures, coma, and death.[3] Walter *et al.* demonstrated by CT scan of the brain that about 2% of patients who underwent HD developed brain edema.[22] In all reported cases of DDS, the patients were conscious and undergoing HD for the first time. Hence DDS was easy to detect and treated promptly. Di-Fresco *et al.* successfully treated a case of DDS.[5]

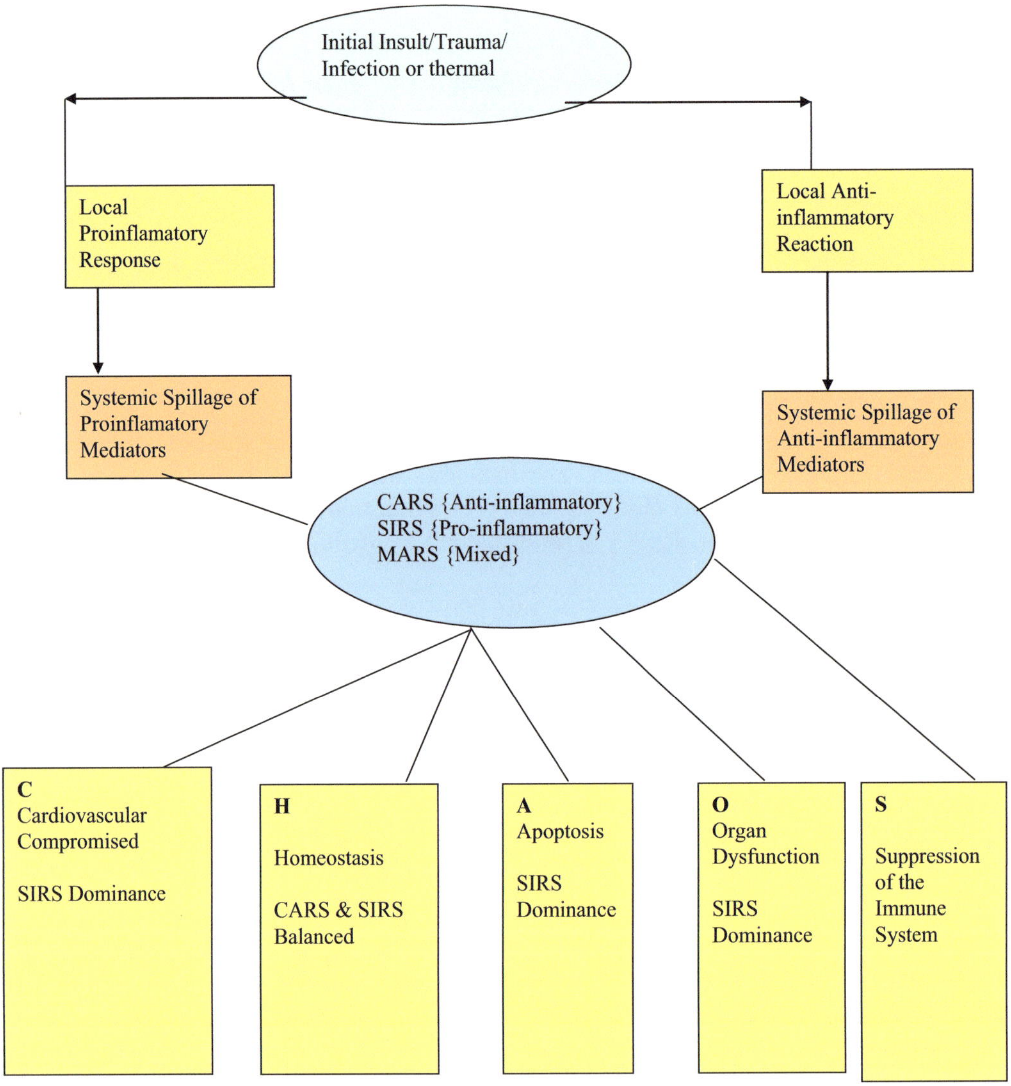

Fig. 1. Mechanism for MODS[8].

The risk factors for the development of DDS are rapid elevation of pCO_2,[14] head injury,[7] young age, metabolic acidosis,[1] and severe sepsis.[17] Patients requiring intensive care therapy are different from patients with end-stage renal failure or chronic renal failure, they usually have severe sepsis or septic shock, MOF; and are sedated. Bagshaw *et al.* reported a fatal case of DDS in a patient with sepsis, but this patient was awake and not in septic shock.

He underwent his first episode of aggressive HD resulting in severe and fatal DDS. [2] If patients are on slow HD for several consecutive days, develops septic shock; and they are supposed to have sepsis-induced changes in the brain.

Severe sepsis and septic shock with polymicrobial bacteremia causes a widespread of immune activation. This may alter the blood-brain permeability and may lead to DDS.[2]

Overall, there are 2 main theories for the development of DDS. The first theory, also called the reverse osmotic shift, relates to the acute removal of urea, which occurs comparatively slower across the blood-brain barrier than in plasma, thus generating a reverse osmotic gradient. This might promote the movement of water to the brain and cause brain edema. [20] This reverse osmotic shift in DDS has been demonstrated in experimental animals. Silver *et al.* demonstrated that rats undergoing rapid HD, urea nitrogen levels were lowered from 72 to 34 mmol in 90 min. This change was associated with a 6% increase in brain water. Surprisingly, neither undialysed nor dialysed rats with urea bath developed cerebral edema. [18] The second theory suggests that increased osmolarity of the extracellular fluid leads to adoptive accumulation of intracellular osmolytes in the brain. This decreases the cerebral cell dehydration and causes paradoxical reduction in the cerebral pH, resulting in brain edema during or after HD. [6] Recently, experimental studies helped in demonstrating the molecular basis for the development of DDS; the water and urea movement across the plasma membrane is facilitated by specific channels, called, aquaporins and urea transporters (UT), respectively. In the absence of these channels, water and urea diffusion through the cell membrane is slow. Also, because of the less number of UT, the urea exit from the astrocytes may be delayed, while rapid removal of extracellular urea during fast HD can lead to water entry into the cells, subsequently causing brain edema. [21] The aim of treatment of DDS is to reduce brain edema and to avoid its complication. Only one case of DDS has been reported in the literature, which was successfully treated using mannitol and hyperventilation. [5] Ideal management of DDS is prevention. The following methods have been tried to prevent DDS: Doorenbos *et al.* used urea to keep blood urea levels constant during HD and succeeded in avoiding DDS. [6] Another way is a gentle initiation of HD and gradual correction of biochemical abnormalities with slow and less efficient HD. [12] When aggressive HD is indicated, phenytoin may be used to prevent the development of DDS. [15]

If the patient has fluid overload, he can be shifted to hemofiltration and a short period of HD, or he can be started on peritoneal dialysis. So far, DDS is not reported with peritoneal dialysis. [1] To our knowledge, there are 2 reported cases of DDS occurring after more than 1 week of daily HD. Both these patients had septic shock, but were stable with inotropic and ventilatory support.[13] Their follow-up CT of brain and radiography of chest was without any major pathology. Both patients suffered neurologic deterioration during or 1 hour after the HD session and an emergency CT of brain showed severe brain edema with brain herniation (Fig2). Authors made the DDS diagnosis because the neurologic deterioration and herniation occurred during or within a few hours of the HD session, and after excluding other risk factors for hypotension and fatality as per advanced cardiac life support guidelines. [13] Severe sepsis and septic shock affects brain by reducing the blood flow to the brain and also causing capillary leakage and dysfunction of the blood-brain barrier. These effects are due to either toxic mediators or the indirect effect of hypoperfusion, hyperthermia, and increased intracranial pressure. [19] These effects will also be amplified if the patient is having a brain injury. [19] Patients on regular daily HD are likely to have brain edema, if they also develop septic shock, the effects on the brain may be amplified and leading to DDS.

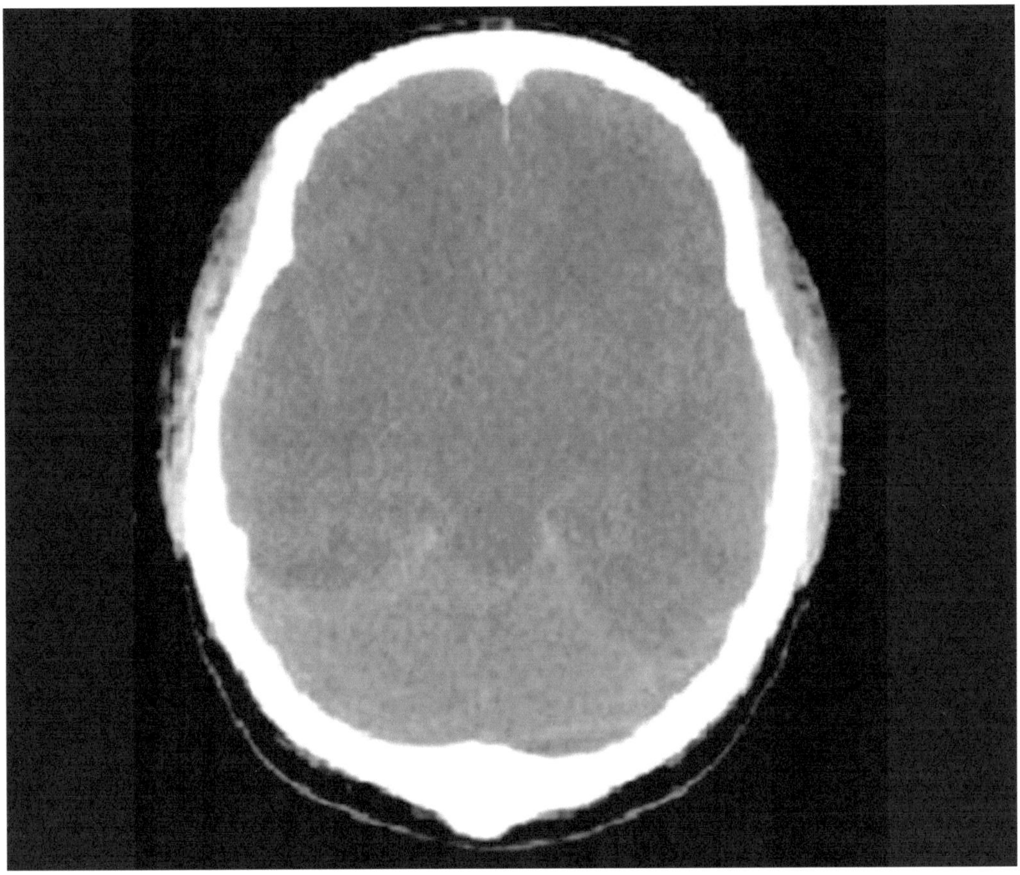

Fig. 2. Diffuse and severe brain edema in DDS

2. Conclusion

If a patient on HD develops severe sepsis or septic shock, DDS can occur even after repeated sessions of HD. DDS may contribute to the sudden deterioration and death in these septic patients. The acute care physicians, intensivists, and nephrologists should be aware of the risks of DDS and act accordingly.

3. References

[1] Arieff AI. Dialysis disequilibrium syndrome. Current concept on pathogenesis and prevention. Kidney Int 1994;45:629-35.

[2] Bagshaw SM, Peets AD, Hameed M, Boiteau PJ, Laupland KB, Doig CJ. Dialysis Disequilibrium syndrome: brain death following hemodialysis for metabolic acidosis and acute renal failure - a case report. BMC Nephrol 2004;5:9.

[3] Bergman H, Daugirdas JT, Ing TS. Complications during haemodialysis. In: Daugirdas JT, Blake PG, Ing TS, editors. Handbook of dialysis. 3 rd ed. Philadelphia: Lippincott, Williams and Wilkins; 2001. p. 148-68

[4] Bone RC, Balk RA, Cerra FB et al. Definition of sepsis, organ failure and guidelines for the use of innovative therapies. Chest 1992;101:1644-55

[5] DisFresco V, Landman M, White AC. Dialysis disequilibrium syndrome: An unusual cause of respiratory failure, in medical intensive care unit. Intensive Care Med 2000;26:628-30

[6] Doorenbos CJ, Bosma RJ, Lamberts PJN. Use of urea containing dialysate to avoid disequilibrium syndrome, enabling intensive dialysis, treatment of diabetic patient with renal failure and severe metformin induced lactic acidosis. Nephrol Dial Transplant 2001;16:1303-4.

[7] Grushkin CM, Korsch B, Fine RN. Haemodialysis in small children. JAMA 1972;221:869-73.

[8] Green R, Scott LK, Minagar A, Conrad s. Sepsis associated encephalopathy: a review. Frontiers in Bioscience 2004;9:1637-410

[9] Hotchkiss RS, Karl IE. The pathophysiology and treatment of sepsis. N Engl J Med 2003;348:138-50

[10] Jackson AC, Gilbert JJ, Young GB, Bolton CF. The encephalopathy of sepsis. Can J Neurol Sci 1985;12:303-7

[11] Kennedy AC, Linton AL, Eaton JC. Urea levels in cerebral fluid after haemodialysis. Lancet 1962;1:410-1.

[12] Krane NK. Intracranial pressure measurement in a patient undergoing hemodialysis and peritoneal dialysis. Am J Kidney Dis 1989;13:336-9.

[13] Nissar Shaikh, Andr'e Louon, Yolande Hanssens. Fatal dialysis disequilibrium syndrome: A tale of two patients. JETS 2010;3:300

[14] Oertel M, Kelly DF, Lee JH, McArthur DL, Glenn TC, Vespa P, *et al.* Efficacy of hyperventilation, blood pressure elevation and metabolic suppression therapy in controlling intracranial pressure after head injury. J Neurosurg 2002;97:1045-53.

[15] Owen WF, Lazarus JM. Dialytic management of acute renal failure: In: Lazarus JM, Brenner BM, editors. Acute renal failure. New York: Churchill Livingstone; 1993. p. 487-95.

[16] Schrier RW, Wang W. Acute renal failure and sepsis. N Engl J Med 2004;351:159-69

[17] Schilling L, Wahi M. Brain oedema: pathogenesis and therapy. Kidney Int 1997;59:S69-75.

[18] Silver SM, Stern RH, Halerpin ML. Brain swelling after dialysis: old urea or new osmoles? Am J Kidney Dis 1996;28:1-13.

[19] Stocchetti N. Brain and sepsis: functional impairment, structural damage and markers. Anesth Analg 2005;101:1463-4

[20] Trachtman H, Futterweit S, Tonidandel W, Gullans SR. The role of organic osmolytes in cerebral cell volume regulating response to acute and chronic renal failure. J Am Soc Nephrol 1993;3:1913-9.

[21] Trinh-Trang-Tan MM, Cartron JP, Bankir L. Molecular basis for dialysis disequilibrium syndrome: altered acuaporin and urea transporter expression in brain. Nephrol Dial Transplant 2005;20:1984-8.
[22] Walters RJ, Fox NC, Crum WR, Taube D, Thomas DJ. Haemodialysis and brain oedema. Nephron 2001;87:143-7.

8

Acute Kidney Injury Following Cardiac Surgery: Prevention, Diagnosis, and Management

Emmanuel Moss[1,3] and Yoan Lamarche[1,2,3]
[1]*Department of Cardiac Surgery, Montreal Heart Institute,*
[2]*Departments of Cardiac Surgery and Intensive Care, Hópital du Sacré-Coeur de Montréal,*
[3]*Université de Montréal,*
Montreal, Quebec
Canada

1. Introduction

Acute kidney injury (AKI) following cardiac surgery is associated with increased morbidity and mortality, longer hospital stays, and significantly increased health care costs. The physiological functions performed by the kidney, which include acid-base control, blood pressure regulation, water balance, and waste excretion, are crucial to the maintenance of homeostasis and can only partially be accomplished using renal replacement therapy (RRT). A number of risk factors have been identified that should be recognized in order to counsel patients appropriately and attempt to prevent AKI. Several pharmacologic and therapeutic modalities have been suggested, with varying levels of evidence, to aid in prevention of AKI and limit the extent of injury and morbidity once renal dysfunction has been recognized. The purpose of this chapter is to review the epidemiology, prevention, diagnosis, and treatment of acute kidney injury following cardiac surgery. These topics will be reviewed in detail in the discussion that follows.

2. Epidemiology

The incidence of AKI following cardiac surgery has historically been difficult to determine. Mild renal injury (creatinine rise <25%) may occur in as many as 50% of patients undergoing cardiac surgery. Moderate kidney injury has been reported in 8-15% of patients, while up to 5% of patients develop renal failure requiring dialysis following cardiac surgery. (Shaw, Swaminathan et al. 2008) Individual reports differ significantly as a result of inconsistent definitions, varied surgeries, and a heterogeneous patient population.(Bellomo, Ronco et al. 2004)

In many series, renal failure is defined as a 50% rise in serum creatinine, while others define it arbitrarily as a doubling of the creatinine, and yet others include only dialysis dependent patients in their analyses.(Bellomo, Kellum et al. 2004) The RIFLE and AKIN criteria were developed by panels of experts to provide a uniform definition of acute kidney injury and facilitate recommendations for patients suffering from renal failure.(Kellum, Mehta et al. 2002; Mehta, Kellum et al. 2007) (Figure 1) These definitions rely upon serum creatinine levels and urine output to define and categorize the severity of kidney injury. Regardless of the definition, once renal failure progresses and a patient becomes dialysis dependant, mortality rates rise considerably and are often reported to be above 50%.(Andersson, Ekroth et al. 1993; Chertow, Levy et al. 1998) Even with the progress of modern medicine and implementation of newer dialysis technology, the mortality associated with postoperative renal failure has not noticeably improved. (Ympa, Sakr et al. 2005) One may suggest that this is because renal failure in itself is often not the primary problem, but only a sign of significant low cardiac output and multi-organ failure, however, this is likely not the case. Other authors have proposed that the high mortality associated with renal failure is not related to RRT itself, rather it predisposes patients to other morbidities. A large study reviewing 16,000 patients with contrast induced nephropathy suggested that patient's whose hospitalisations were complicated by sepsis, coagulopathies, respiratory, or neurologic failure, were more likely to die during their hospitalisation, while it was rare for patients with uncomplicated renal failure not to survive. (Levy, Viscoli et al. 1996) Chertow et al, reporting on over 43,000 patients with AKI following cardiac surgery, found that these patients were more likely to suffer myocardial infarction, require reoperation for bleeding, and develop endocarditis or mediastinitis.(Chertow, Lazarus et al. 1997) Patients with renal failure also had an overall greater risk of death in the index hospitalization.

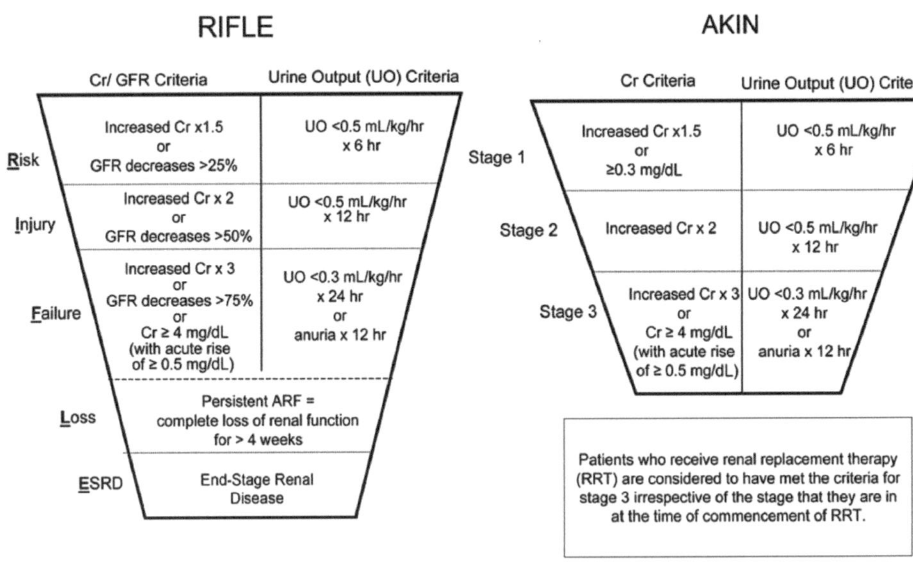

Fig. 1. RIFLE and AKIN criteria. Reproduced from Reproduced with permission from Biomed Central (Cruz, Ricci et al. 2009)

While patients with AKI requiring RRT demonstrate substantially elevated mortality rates, even patients with milder renal dysfunction not requiring RRT show decreased survival and worse outcomes compared to those without postoperative AKI.(1994; Conlon, Stafford-Smith et al. 1999) Although it may be intuitive that morbidity will increase with severe renal dysfunction, it is less obvious that a modest rise in creatinine can negatively affect quality of life and life expectancy.(Lassnigg, Schmidlin et al. 2004; Lassnigg, Schmid et al. 2008) In addition to increasing mortality, acute kidney injury prolongs ICU stay and increases the proportion of patients discharged to a nursing care facility. This data suggests that the ill-effects of acute kidney injury are not simply a sign of sicker patients with other comorbid conditions, rather AKI is an independent predictor of morbidity and mortality following cardiac surgery. As a result, all efforts must be made to identify patients at risk for AKI, focusing on prevention of renal dysfunction rather than simply treating it once the injury has occurred.

3. Pathophysiology of AKI following cardiac surgery

The pathophysiology and etiology of postoperative AKI in cardiac surgery is multifactorial, resulting from a combination vascular and tubular injury.(Mahon and Shorten 2006) A variety of events occur in the perioperative period that could individually and cumulatively result in renal dysfunction. During cardiopulmonary bypass (CPB), the kidneys are exposed to interruptions and alterations in blood flow due to changes in pump flow and the lack of pulsatility, which can lead to ischemia-reperfusion injury. Concurrently, the kidneys risk being affected by embolic materials originating from air entry into the circulation, platelet aggregates, lipids, and atheromatous plaques.(Sear 2005) Exposure to the CPB circuit initiates several cascades that can cause kidney injury, such as complement activation, free radical formation, and inflammatory cytokine production.(Mahon and Shorten 2006) Bellomo et al developed the following comprehensive list of pathophysiologic mechanisms behind AKI: (1) exogenous and endogenous toxins, (2) metabolic factors, (3) ischemia-reperfusion, (4) neurohormonal activation, (5) inflammation, and (6) oxidative stress.(Bellomo, Auriemma et al. 2008) The sum of these factors culminates in a significant and constant risk of renal tubular injury in patients undergoing cardiac surgery. While it is important to appreciate the pathophysiology of renal dysfunction, understanding and considering the differential diagnosis is clearly necessary to provide appropriate therapy. Figure 2 summarizes the differential diagnosis of acute renal failure.

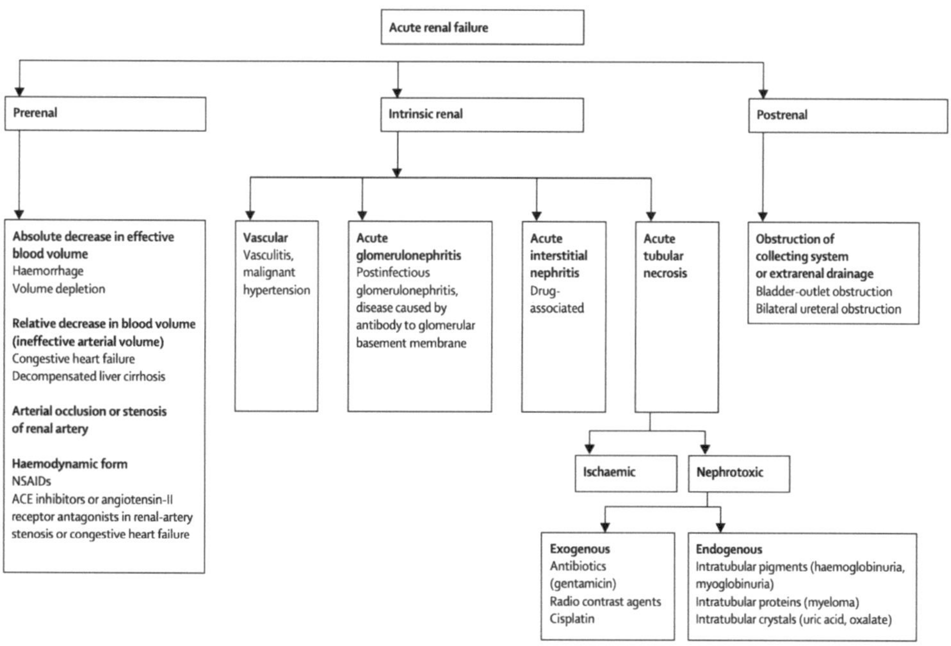

Fig. 2. Classification and major causes of acute renal failure. NSAIDs = non-steroidal anti-inflammatory agents; ACE = angiotensin-converting enzyme. Reproduced with permission from Elsevier (Lameire, Van Biesen et al. 2005)

4. Diagnosis of postoperative AKI

Although new concepts such as RIFLE and AKIN have helped standardize the definition of AKI, the criteria involved in making the diagnosis can take hours to days, leading to delayed recognition of renal dysfunction. This delay may be partly responsible for the limited progress that has been made in preventing and treating postoperative renal failure, and highlights the need for more immediate markers of AKI. The present and future tools available to diagnose AKI in cardiac surgery will be discussed below.

4.1 Creatinine

When comparing the progress in the diagnosic tools available for AKI to that of myocardial infarction, the state-of-the-art is lagging significantly. Fifty years ago creatinine kinase (CK) was the only available marker for cardiac injury, as was serum creatinine for renal injury. In current practice, cardiac injury is identified through several laboratory tests, such as levels CK-MB, Troponin-I, Troponin-T, Myoglobin, and BNP. However, creatinine is still the only biomarker routinely used to identify kidney injury. Creatinine and urine output together are relied upon to assess global kidney function. While creatinine is a relatively specific marker of renal injury, its sensitivity can be called into question and it bears some inherent limitations. Circulating levels vary with age, gender, muscle mass, vigorous exercise, and medications. In addition, levels rise only when GFR is reduced by more than 50% and it can take up to 24 hours before there is a sufficient increase to allow for the diagnosis of AKI.(Bagshaw and Gibney 2008) In light of these shortcomings, there is a clear need for newer, more sensitive, methods of diagnosing renal dysfunction.

4.2 Urine output

The most readily available surrogate marker of renal function is urine output. Compared to creatinine, it is more sensitive to changes in renal hemodynamics. Unfortunately, variations in urine output are considerably less specific, except when severely diminished or absent. Oliguria is defined as urine output of less than 0.5mg/kg/hour. The presence of an oliguric state gives physicians a sign that their patient's kidney function is at risk or already perturbed, however, the presence of normal urine output cannot provide assurance that renal function is unperturbed. In non-oliguric renal failure, the kidney's ability to produce urine is preserved but its ability to excrete water-soluble waste products is lost or markedly reduced. The reality is that even the combination of urine output and serum creatinine cannot reliably diagnose renal injury in a timely manner. This once again highlights the importance of uncovering and validating other methods to identify AKI.

4.3 Urinalysis

In patients with decreased urine output or suspected acute kidney injury, urinalysis is an important tool that can differentiate prerenal from renal failure. Consequently, it can be very useful in guiding treatment. Table 1 describes select variables and their association with the etiology of acute kidney injury.

	Prerenal	Renal
Urinalysis	Normal	Abnormal
Specific gravity	1.020	1.010
Osmolality (mmol/kg)	>500	>300
Sodium (mmol/L)	<20	>40
Fractional excretion of sodium (%)	<1	>2
Fractional excretion of urea (%)	<35	>35
Fractional excretion of uric acid (%)	<7	>35
Fractional excretion of lithium	<7	>15
Low-molecular weight proteins	Low	High
Brush border enzymes	Low	High

Table 1. Important variables in differentiating prerenal from renal acute renal failure. Adapted from Lameire et al (Lameire, Van Biesen et al. 2005)

4.4 Neutrophil gelatinase-associated lipocalin (NGAL)

NGAL is a protein, known to bind small iron-carrying molecules, that is significantly upregulated in response to acute renal injury. Its concentration rises within three hours in response to renal tubular injury and can precede the rise in creatinine by more than 24 hours.(Schmidt-Ott, Mori et al. 2006) The use of this protein to diagnose AKI has been most extensively studied in cardiac surgery. When evaluated in both adult and pediatric cardiac surgery patients, NGAL has shown good sensitivity and specificity for diagnosis of AKI, with a significantly earlier rise following injury when compared to creatinine. NGAL began to rise within two hours after renal insult, while creatinine rise occurred over a period of one to three days.(Mishra, Dent et al. 2005; Wagener, Jan et al. 2006; Dent, Ma et al. 2007; Bennett, Dent et al. 2008) NGAL levels have been shown predictive when measured both in the serum and the urine. The performance of NGAL in these and other clinical studies appears sufficient to recommend its inclusion in an early diagnostic panel for AKI, suggesting that we will likely see rapid expansion of its use in the coming years.

4.5 Cystatin C

Cystatin C is a cysteine protease inhibitor. Serum level of cystatin C is a reflection of GFR, making changes in serum and urine levels a reflection on changes in GFR. This is in contrast to NGAL, which is a reactive protein and a measure of tubular stress. Cystatin C levels are not significantly affected by age, race, gender, muscle mass, or infection, making it a better measure of GFR than serum creatinine.(Dharnidharka, Kwon et al. 2002) Due to these promising characteristics, cystatin C has been investigated in a variety of clinical settings, including cardiac surgery. With the exception of one inconclusive study, cystatin C has consistently been shown superior to serum creatinine in predicting AKI following cardiac surgery.(Koyner, Bennett et al. 2008; Haase-Fielitz, Bellomo et al. 2009; Heise, Waeschle et al. 2009) Cystatin C, like NGAL, also appears to offer prognostic value in this setting. When considering all available data, cystatin C appears to be a reliable marker of chronic renal dysfunction and both cystatin C and NGAL are dependable early predictors of AKI. However, NGAL may slightly outperform in cystatin C as an early predictor of injury.

4.6 Liver-type fatty acid binding protein (L-FABP)

L-FABP is a protein expressed in various organs, including the kidney, and plays a role in the cellular uptake of fatty acids. The molecule is filtered and reabsorbed by the kidney, resulting in elevated urine L-FABP levels in the presence of decreased GFR.(Negishi, Noiri et al. 2008; Portilla, Dent et al. 2008; Negishi, Noiri et al. 2009) Some clinical studies have demonstrated usefulness for L-FABP in identifying patients at risk for AKI.(Nakamura, Sugaya et al. 2006) It has also shown promise as a marker for postoperative AKI, although it appears to rise later than NGAL.(Portilla, Dent et al. 2008) The literature to date suggests that L-FABP may be a useful addition to preoperative risk assessment and postoperative diagnosis of AKI, with further investigation being warranted.

4.7 Interleukin-18 (IL-18)

IL-18 is a proinflammatory cytokine and a reliable signal for ischemia-induced AKI in animal models.(Melnikov, Ecder et al. 2001) Data from pediatric cardiac surgery, kidney transplantation, and acute respiratory distress syndrome have shown that urine IL-18 performs well as an early predictor of AKI.(Parikh, Abraham et al. 2005; Parikh, Jani et al. 2006; Parikh, Mishra et al. 2006) A recent prospective observational trial questioned the specificity of IL-18 as a marker of renal injury in cardiac surgery, suggesting that it may be a non-specific sign of post cardiopulmonary bypass inflammation.(Haase, Bellomo et al. 2008) As a consequence of these inconsistent results, IL-18 will require further investigation and validation before it can be considered for routine inclusion on urinary panels.

4.8 Kidney injury molecule-1 (KIM-1)

KIM-1 is a transmembrane glycoprotein that can be detected in the urine following AKI.(Zhang, Humphreys et al. 2007) Although it is not expressed in normal kidneys, KIM-1 is upregulated following nephrotoxic or ischemic injury.(Han, Bailly et al. 2002) Clinical studies have suggested that KIM-1 may be useful in improving early detection of AKI following cardiac surgery, particularly when measured in conjunction with other novel biomarkers.(Han, Wagener et al. 2009)

4.9 Summary of novel biomarkers of AKI in cardiac surgery

The cause of AKI in cardiac surgery is multifactorial, making it is unlikely that a single biomarker will prove sufficiently accurate and reliable to be trusted for risk stratification and diagnosis of AKI. Outlined above are the most promising biomarkers, which recognize damage in different pathways of renal injury. Table 2 is a summary of novel biomarkers and their key properties. In the future, combinations of these markers, used in parallel with clinical parameters, will likely emerge as practical tools to help predict and verify the onset of AKI in a variety of settings, including cardiac surgery.

Biomarker	Variable assessed	Time to detection (h)
Serum Cystatin	GFR	12-14
Serum NGAL	Proximal tubular injury	2-4
Urine NGAL	Proximal tubular injury	2-4
Urine L-FABP	Proximal tubular injury	4-6
Urine IL-18	Proximal tubular injury	4-6
Urine KIM-1	Proximal tubular injury	12-24

Table 2. Novel biomarkers for detection of acute kidney injury. GFR = glomerular filtration rate, NGAL = neutrophil gelatinase-associated lipocalin, L-FABP = Liver-type fatty acid binding protein IL = interleukin, KIM = kidney injury molecule.

5. Risk factors for acute kidney injury

5.1 Preoperative

Prevention postoperative renal failure begins by identifying patients at risk. Several risk factors have been for postoperative AKI have been identified, some more consistently than others. One of the largest studies addressing the topic was published by Chertow et al in 1997.(Chertow, Lazarus et al. 1997) This group developed a model for preoperative renal risk stratification by prospectively following 43,000 patients in 43 different centres over a seven-year period. The overall incidence of acute renal failure requiring dialysis was 1.1 %. Thirty-day mortality in patients requiring dialysis was 64%, compared to 4.3% for patients without renal failure. The authors identified ten clinical variables as independent predictors of dialysis dependant renal failure following cardiac surgery. (Table 3) These included preoperative renal dysfunction (OR 1.3-5.8, depending on creatinine clearance), valvular surgery (OR 1.98), intra-aortic balloon pump (OR 3.19), redo surgery (OR 1.93), NYHA class IV (OR 1.55), decreased left ventricular ejection fraction (OR 1.45), peripheral vascular disease (OR 1.51), chronic obstructive pulmonary disease (OR 1.26), pulmonary rales (OR 1.37), and the extremes of systolic blood pressure. Based on these factors, the authors developed a clinical algorithm to quantify risk and identify patients most in danger of requiring postoperative dialysis. Mangano et al studied a smaller population and identified other preoperative characteristics associated with postoperative dialysis.(Mangano, Diamondstone et al. 1998) Similar to Chertow, they identified congestive heart failure (RR 1.8), previous surgery (RR 1.8), and elevated creatinine (RR 2.3) as predisposing factors, and they also showed that age 70-79 years (RR 1.6) and 80-95 years (RR 3.5), type-1 diabetes (RR 1.8), and elevated preoperative serum glucose (exceeding 16.6 mmol/L, RR 3.7) significantly increased the risk of postoperative dialysis. These findings have been echoed by several other studies.(Abrahamov, Tamariz et al. 2001; Diaz, Moitra et al. 2008) Preoperative renal dysfunction has consistently been the most predictive of postoperative renal complications. A preoperative creatinine between 175 and 350mmol/L is associated with a 10-20% risk of postoperative dialysis, while patients with a creatinine greater than 350mmol/L may have a 25-28% risk of dialysis.(Frost, Pedersen et al. 1991; Chertow, Lazarus et al. 1997; Fortescue, Bates et al. 2000; Thakar, Liangos et al. 2003; Thakar, Liangos et al. 2003) Other authors have also found female gender, left main coronary disease, concomitant liver disease, and pre-existing sepsis to contribute to postoperative renal dysfunction.(Conlon, Stafford-Smith et al. 1999; Rosner and Okusa 2006; Rosner, Portilla et al. 2008) (Table 3)

Preoperative renal dysfunction
Valvular surgery
Intra-aortic balloon pump
Redo surgery
NYHA class IV
Decreased LVEF
Peripheral vascular disease
COPD
Pulmonary rales
Extremes of systolic blood pressure
Advanced age
Type-1 diabetes
Preoperative hyperglycemia

Table 3. Risk factors for dialysis dependant renal failure following cardiac surgery. LVEF = Left ventricular ejection fraction, COPD = chronic obstructive pulmonary disease

A significant modifiable risk factor that may play a role in postoperative AKI is the timing of surgery following contrast angiography. Medalion et al reviewed data on 365 patients who underwent CABG surgery.(Medalion, Cohen et al. 2010) Multivariate analysis identified several risk factors for postoperative AKI, including surgery within 24 hours of contrast administration and preoperative renal dysfunction (clearance < 60mL/min). Contrast dose greater than >1.4ml/kg was predictive of AKI if surgery was performed within five days of angiography. The authors suggest avoiding surgery within 24 hours of angiography whenever possible and delaying surgery for five days in patients having received a large contrast dose, particularly if the presence of chronic renal dysfunction.

It is unclear whether medications such as nonsteroidal anti-inflammatory drugs and angiotensin receptor blocker should be discontinued prior to surgery. Several authors have suggested that these medications increase the risk of postoperative AKI.(Rosner, Portilla et al. 2008). Finally, genetic predispositions to AKI have been reported more recently. A study from Duke University found that patient with the inherited apolipoprotein epsilon-4 allele were less likely to develop AKI compared to patients with other forms of the allele.(Chew, Newman et al. 2000)

It is essential to remember that preoperative renal dysfunction may not be obvious when looking at the creatinine alone. It is paramount to calculate the creatinine clearance for all patients, but particularly for those in extremes of age and body habitus, as this will permit a better identification of patients with increased risk of perioperative renal dysfunction.

5.2 Intraoperative risk factors

Many preoperative risk factors have become accepted by the community, as a large amount of data suggested their role in the development of postoperative renal dysfunction. Intraoperative risk factors, however, are notoriously difficult to control for and are sometimes challenged.

The maintenance of cardiovascular stability during CPB is dependant on many factors, including a proper functioning CPB circuit and patient factors, such as venous compliance, systemic vascular resistance, and autoregulatory systems. The goal of CPB is to maintain adequate end-organ perfusion at a level that allows optimal cellular functioning. Any deviation in perfusion pressure and flow rates can significantly affect the oxygen delivery to all organs and may result in periods of decreased flow or perfusion pressure, leading to renal injury.(Urzua, Troncoso et al. 1992; Fischer, Weissenberger et al. 2002)

Prolonged cardiopulmonary bypass and aortic cross-clamp times are relatively well-accepted as being linked to increased postoperative AKI, although this finding has not been present in all studies.(Fischer, Weissenberger et al. 2002; Tuttle, Worrall et al. 2003) Unfortunately, because of the heterogenous patient populations, no specific time frame has been established after which the risk of AKI increases. Additionally, although prolonged bypass times may play a role in postoperative AKI, it is likely a combination of all of the previously mentioned factors that will decide each individual patient's propensity for postoperative renal dysfunction. Other modifiable characteristics of CPB that may influence the incidence of AKI include pulsatile versus non-pulsatile flow during CPB, and normothermic versus hypothermic CPB. However, neither of these factors has been shown clinically to affect the incidence of postoperative AKI.(Urzua, Troncoso et al. 1992; Abramov, Tamariz et al. 2003; Provenchère, Plantefève et al. 2003)

Dilutional anemia during CPB has been associated with increased overall morbidity following cardiac surgery. Specifically, lowest on-pump hematocrit below 22-24% may put patients at risk for postoperative AKI.(Habib, Zacharias et al. 2003; Habib, Zacharias et al. 2005) Aprotinin is a serine protease inhibitor that, until recently, was commonly given perioperatively to decrease blood loss related to open-heart surgery.(van Oeveren, Jansen et al. 1987; Royston 1995) It has been suggested that aprotinin may cause vasoconstriction of the afferent arteriole, thus reducing glomerular perfusion pressure and occasioning renal dysfunction. A propensity based analysis of over 4000 patients receiving aprotinin and other fibrinolytic agents perioperatively concluded that the administration of aprotinin was associated with a doubling of the risk acute renal failure requiring RRT.(Mangano, Tudor et al. 2006) This finding has since been supported and opposed by similar large observational studies.(Furnary, Wu et al. 2007; Dietrich, Busley et al. 2008; Shaw, Stafford-Smith et al. 2008) More recently, an increased 30-day mortality in the aprotinin arm of the BART study (Blood Conservation Using Antifibrinolytics in a Randomized Trial) prompted the Food and Drug Administration to suspend marketing of the drug.(Fergusson, Hébert et al. 2008)

5.2.1 On vs Off pump CABG

One of the most debated topics on the subject of AKI prevention is the proposed renal protection offered by off-pump coronary artery bypass surgery (OPCAB) compared to

CABG with CPB. Advocates of off-pump surgery generally cite a reduced risk of AKI as a benefit of the OPCAB approach, however, there is little data to support this claim. Critics of OPCAB surgery suggest that instances of perioperative low cardiac output due to contortion of the heart may offset the detrimental effects of the CPB circuit. Niwekar et al. recently published a meta-analysis evaluating the results of on-pump vs off-pump surgery in twenty-two studies, including six randomized controlled trials (RCT) comprising over 27,000 patients.(Nigwekar, Kandula et al. 2009) In the pooled analysis there was a reduction in the overall incidence of AKI and in AKI requiring RRT. In a separate analysis of the RCTs only, overall incidence of AKI was reduced but there was no significant difference in the proportion of patients requiring renal replacement therapy. It is worth noting that one of the major limitations of this report is the lack of a uniform definition of AKI across the studies. The authors also report that the RCTs tended to enroll healthier patients with a lower risk of postoperative AKI. This bias, combined with smaller sample sizes, made the RCTs underpowered to study AKI.

In the absence of a randomized trial focusing on AKI after cardiac surgery, the best available evidence consists mostly of observational studies from which our conclusions must be drawn. Based on this data, it is reasonable to conclude that in patients at higher risk for AKI, an OPCAB approach, when appropriate, may reduce the likelihood of developing postoperative renal dysfunction. When interpreting this data, one must remember that renal protection is just one of the many important factors to consider when choosing an appropriate revascularisation method. The pros and cons of OPCAB versus CABG surgery with CPB must be analysed while considering each individual patient and each surgeon's preference and experience.

6. Prevention of postoperative AKI

A vast number of therapies have been proposed for limiting the incidence of perioperative renal dysfunction. These range from simple manoeuvres, such as maintaining hydration, to more advanced pharmacological interventions. The most well studied methods will be reviewed here.

6.1 Hydration

There is little argument that adequate hydration is a prerequisite to maintaining healthy kidney function. A randomized study evaluating contrast-induced nephropathy compared patients receiving an intravenous infusion of sodium chloride for twelve hours preceding their intervention to a control group of patients with unrestricted fluid ingestion. The authors found that intravenous fluid administration protected patients from AKI.(Trivedi, Moore et al. 2003) Other studies have echoed these results, particularly in patients with underlying renal dysfunction.(Solomon, Werner et al. 1994; Dussol, Morange et al. 2006) Another randomized trial compared a regimen of half-isotonic saline infusion to standard preoperative fluid restriction in patients with known renal dysfunction, defined as glomerular filtration rate <45mL/min.(Marathias, Vassili et al. 2006) Patients in the hydration group were significantly less likely to develop postoperative renal failure and no patients required RRT, compared to 27% of patients in the control group. While these may be arguments for preoperative fluid loading and avoiding perioperative hypovolemia, the ideal method of perioperative volume resuscitation remains a highly debated topic. Much effort has been put into identifying the ideal fluid, or ideal combination of fluids, to maintain perioperative circulating volume. This question has been investigated most thoroughly in the critical care literature, with several observational studies, randomized trials, and meta-analyses addressing the issue. Unfortunately, many studies have had conflicting results and little has been concluded on the subject.(Choi, Yip et al. 1999; Finfer, Bellomo et al. 2004; Roberts, Alderson et al. 2004; Rioux, Lessard et al. 2009; Bunn, Trivedi et al. 2011) Regarding renal failure specifically, a recent Cochrane review found that evidence was lacking to conclude that colloid use is associated with renal failure in a non-septic population.(Dart, Mutter et al. 2010) Data specific to cardiac surgery is also available but offers little help. A recent randomized pilot study by Magder et al compared the use of colloids to crystalloids in a postoperative cardiac surgery population.(Magder, Potter et al. 2010) The colloid based resuscitation protocol was associated with less catecholamine use, a lower incidence of pneumonia and mediastinal infection, and less need for cardiac pacing. A conflicting study found that there was indeed a dose-dependant relationship between pentastarch administration and AKI, with an optimal cutoff volume at 14mL/kg.(Rioux, Lessard et al. 2009) It is likely that either colloids or crystalloids are suitable solutions for fluid resuscitation and that a balanced resuscitation avoiding high doses of colloids or crystalloids alone would lead to optimal patient outcome.

6.2 Glycemic control

In 2001, van den Berghe published a seminal randomized trial establishing the benefit of intensive insulin therapy to maintain tight glycemic control in postoperative critically ill patients.(van den Berghe, Wouters et al. 2001) More than 60% of patients studied had undergone cardiac surgery. In addition to a significant mortality benefit, intensive insulin therapy was associated with a 41% reduction in patients requiring dialysis or hemofiltration. A subsequent large observational study found an even more prominent effect on prevention of AKI after instituting a similar protocol. (Krinsley 2004) Studies addressing diabetic patients specifically have also found increased postoperative AKI associated with poor perioperative glycemic control, however, it is unclear whether interventions to treat and prevent hyperglycemia can improve outcomes in this population.(Furnary, Gao et al. 2003; Ouattara, Lecomte et al. 2005) In fact, some groups have found that although tight glycemic control can prevent AKI, there may be a tradeoff for other complications, such as an increased incidence of death and stroke.(Gandhi, Nuttall et al. 2007; Investigators, Finfer et al. 2009)

6.3 Dopamine

Dopamine is an endogenous catecholamine with dose-dependent effects on dopaminergic, alpha- and beta1-adrenergic receptors. Experimentally, dopamine stimulates the renal dopaminergic receptors to result in increased renal blood flow and GFR, and acts as a diuretic and natriuretic. Based on promising studies in animals and healthy volunteers, the clinical use of low-dose dopamine (3 mg/kg/min) became popular and has been used routinely in some institutions.(MacGregor, Smith et al. 2000) Unfortunately, these results have not been reproduced in clinical reports, including several well-designed studies and meta-analyses.(Kellum 1997; Marik and Iglesias 1999; Bellomo, Chapman et al. 2000; Marik 2002) After reviewing the available data from 1966-2000, comprised of 2149 patients, Kellum at el concluded that "the use of low-dose dopamine for the treatment or prevention of acute renal failure cannot be justified on the basis of available evidence and should be eliminated from routine clinical use."(Kellum and M Decker 2001)

6.4 Other dopaminergic drugs

Fenoldopam is a synthetic derivative of dopamine with DA1 receptor selectivity that increases blood flow to the kidneys.(Mathur, Swan et al. 1999; Meco and Cirri 2010) Several small studies have reported favorable effects of fenoldopam on GFR and serum creatinine in cardiac surgery patients.(Halpenny, Lakshmi et al. 2001; Caimmi, Pagani et al. 2003; Garwood, Swamidoss et al. 2003) However, a number of well-designed trials have found no benefit with fenoldopam when compared to placebo, dopamine, or other treatments.(Bove, Landoni et al. 2005; Morelli, Ricci et al. 2005; Brienza, Malcangi et al. 2006) A 2007 meta-analysis published pooled results from 16 RCTs and concluded that fenoldopam reduces the need for renal replacement therapy and mortality in patients with AKI.(Landoni, Biondi-Zoccai et al. 2007) The results of this analysis may be questioned, however, due to the heterogeneity of the trials, including an inconsistant definition of AKI and no clear criteria for the commencement of renal replacement therapy. **Dopexamine** is a predominantly B2-agonist. This molecule has been less-thoroughly studied than the other dopamingeic drugs, but existing data is also inconsistent.(Hakim, Foulds et al. 1988; Stephan, Sonntag et al. 1990; MacGregor, Butterworth et al. 1994; Sherry, Tooley et al. 1997) As a result, dopexamine cannot be recommended as an effective way to reduce postoperative AKI.

Although none of the dopaminergic medications appear to be associated with prohibitive side effects, the evidence to date does not support their use in the context of preventing AKI following cardiac surgery. Further study may be warranted in the case of fenoldopam.

6.5 Loop diuretics

Furosemide is a loop diuretic that inhibits sodium absorption in the medullary portion of the loop of Henle. It has been suggested that by decreasing tubular cell workload, it may limit hypoxia within the nephron. Although this theoretical mechanism exists, there is little evidence supporting its use in preventing and treating AKI. Ho et al performed a meta-analysis of nine randomized controlled trials studying 849 patients with an increased risk of renal failure.(Ho and Sheridan 2006) A pooled analysis of the data failed to show improvements in mortality, requirement of RRT, or number of dialysis sessions. The review also found that high doses of furosemide put patients at risk for deafness and tinnitus. An earlier systematic review reported similar results. Not only has administration of loop diuretics failed to show a benefit when given in the perioperative setting, there is evidence that if may worsen renal dysfunction. Lassnigg et al randomized 126 low-risk patients to receive furosemide infusion, low-dose dopamine, or saline infusion during and after cardiac surgery.(Lassnigg, Donner et al. 2000) The maximum postoperative creatinine was doubled in the furosemide group compared to the other two groups. The mechanism of increased renal injury was not clearly elucidated but intravascular hypovolemia likely played a role.

In summary, there is no clear evidence to support the use of loop diuretics in decreasing the incidence or extent of renal injury following cardiac surgery. These medications should be prescribed when indicated for volume overload and other clinically appropriate scenarios.

6.6 Mannitol

Mannitol is an osmotic diuretic with several suggested benefits in the perioperative period. Theoretically, it increases intravascular volume, improving preload and cardiac output, increases blood to the kidneys through the release of atrial natriuretic peptide, and facilitates the flushing of debris from renal tubules by increasing urinary output.(Better, Rubinstein et al. 1997) Mannitol is known to have additional properties as a free radical scavenger, which may help attenuate the effects of reperfusion injury. Routine mannitol use became popular in cardiac surgery as a result of limited data published several decades ago.(BARRY and BERMAN 1961) More recent publications have consistently failed to show a benefit with mannitol therapy when given in the perioperative period.(Ip-Yam, Murphy et al. 1994; Better, Rubinstein et al. 1997; Poullis 1999; Carcoana, Mathew et al. 2003)

In light of these results, although it has become routine practice in many institutions to add mannitol to the pump prime solution, there is little evidence to support this therapy. It is also important to consider the possible detrimental effect of induced osmotic diuresis, which may include hypovolemia and hypernatremia. Unfortunately, until more robust data is available, individual cardiac surgery teams must base their decision to use mannitol on their own interpretation of the limited information available in the literature.

6.7 N-acetylcysteine

There is conflicting evidence supporting the use of the antioxidant n-acetylcysteine in the prevention of contrast-induced nephropathy.(Marenzi, Assanelli et al. 2006; Krämer and Hoffmann 2007) When studied in high-risk patients undergoing on-pump cardiac surgery, n-acetylcysteine failed to show a benefit compared to placebo in the prevention of postoperative renal failure.(Burns, Chu et al. 2005; El-Hamamsy, Stevens et al. 2007; Haase, Haase-Fielitz et al. 2007; Sisillo, Ceriani et al. 2008) Several meta-analyses reviewing this subject support the results of these individual trials.(Baker, Anglade et al. 2009; Nigwekar and Kandula 2009) The lack of benefit in cardiac surgery populations compared to contrast-induced nephropathy is likely related to the different mechanism of AKI, which is more clearly related to ischemia-reperfusion injury than nephrotoxicity.

6.8 Calcium channel blockers

Calcium channel blockers have been shown experimentally to promote renal vasodilatation, increase renal blood flow, and increase GFR. Studies in patients undergoing cardiac surgery have been contradictory.(Young, Diab et al. 1998; Piper, Kumle et al. 2003)

6.9 Natriuretic peptides

Natriuretic peptides are known to oppose the renin-angiotensin-aldosterone and arginine vasopressin systems through multiple mechanisms.(Nakao, Itoh et al. 1989) As a result they can induce natriuresis and vasodilatation to prevent hypervolemia and oppose the vasoconstrictive response induced by hypovolemia. Synthetic analogues of these proteins have been suggested as therapies to prevent renal failure following cardiac surgery.

Anaritide, the human recombinant form of atrial natriuretic peptide (ANP), is administered intravenously to induce arterial and venous dilatation, thus decreasing blood pressure. This drug failed to show a benefit in two randomized controlled trials of critically ill patients with acute tubular necrosis.(Allgren, Marbury et al. 1997; Lewis, Salem et al. 2000)

Nesiritide, a human recombinant form of Brain-type natriuretic peptide (BNP) is used in the treatment of decompensated heart failure. In a randomized controlled trial of heart failure patients, nesiritide improved diuresis and decreased pulmonary congestion and edema.(Mills, LeJemtel et al. 1999) Despite these benefits, a recent meta-analysis raised concerns about a possible detrimental effect on renal function.(Sackner-Bernstein, Skopicki et al. 2005) More recently, the NAPA investigators randomized 303 patients with left ventricular dysfunction undergoing cardiac surgery to receive nesiritide or placebo.(Mentzer, Oz et al. 2007) The primary outcomes were postoperative renal function, hemodynamics, and drug use. The authors found that nesiritide attenuated peak increase in creatinine, decreased hospital stay, and improved survival at 180 days. Two other randomized trials published in recent years showed favorable laboratory results in the nesiritide groups, however, they failed to show a significant clinical benefit.(Chen, Sundt et al. 2007; Ejaz, Martin et al. 2009) Although data regarding this drug has been conflicting, interesting results would suggest that further investigation is justified.

6.10 Sodium bicarbonate

Sodium bicarbonate is known to alkalinize urine and, when given intravenously, has been shown to attenuate renal dysfunction in the context of contrast infusion.(Merten, Burgess et al. 2004; Briguori, Airoldi et al. 2007; Recio-Mayoral, Chaparro et al. 2007) A recent randomized pilot study evaluated the effect of perioperative sodium bicarbonate infusion in a group of patients at increased risk of renal failure undergoing cardiac surgery.(Haase, Haase-Fielitz et al. 2009) Patients were randomized to receive a 24-hour infusion of sodium bicarbonate or sodium chloride, beginning just after the induction of anesthesia. A lower rate of renal dysfunction was found in the treatment group, evidenced by a lower incidence of increased creatinine and neutrophil gelatinase-associated lipocalin. Base on these results, the authors suggest that further trials are merited

6.11 Summary of results for preventive strategies

It is not surprising that no single molecule has been shown unequivocally to prevent or effectively treat renal failure following cardiac surgery. The mechanisms of renal injury are multifactorial and the incidence of significant renal failure requiring is RRT is relatively low. Additionally, most RCTs enroll low risk patients, making most studies underpowered to demonstrate any benefits that may exist. The two drugs that have shown the most promise and would benefit from further study are fenoldopam and nesiritide.

7. Principles of treatment and renal replacement therapy

7.1 General principles and supportive care

Once the diagnosis of AKI has been established, it is important to understand the clinical situation and initiate supportive care without delay. As with any patient in an acute care setting, vital signs and basic hemodynamics must be evaluated. Assessment of cardiac output and filling pressures will give clues as to whether cardiac tamponade should be suspected. Subsequently, any drugs with potentially adverse effects on the kidney should be identified and, if possible, withdrawn. Finally, it is important to complete the clinical picture, with the help of additional laboratory tests if necessary, and determine whether there is a renal or pre-renal cause of injury.

Serum values of BUN, creatinine, electrolytes and osmolality, as well as examination of urinary sediment, electrolytes and osmolality, will help determine whether there is a pre-renal cause correctable with fluid administration, or if an acute tubular injury is more likely. For example, a slight increase in creatinine with a large jump in BUN often suggests a pre-renal process, while a proportional rise in BUN and creatinine often signals AKI. Urine sodium >20 mEq/L and urine osmolality >500mOsm/kg are often seen in pre-renal disease. Calculation of the fractional excretion of sodium (FE_{Na}) can be useful in oliguric patients, with FE_{Na} <1% reflecting preserved renal function, consistent with a pre-renal disease state. FE_{Na} will usually be >2% in the context of AKI with impaired kidney function. (See Table 1)

Once the nature of kidney injury is understood, the practical management of patients with acute renal failure remains primarily supportive. If pre-renal oliguria is likely, it should be treated early and aggressively to prevent further tubular injury and loss of renal function. If AKI is established, only supportive care can be offered and efforts must be directed toward prevention of further kidney damage, hypervolemia, and treatment of metabolic and electrolyte issues as they arise. Frequent assessment of electrolytes, blood glucose, and acid-base balance is imperative to permit corrections if necessary.

When AKI is suspected or proven, optimization of hemodynamics should be prioritized to prevent further injury. Practically speaking, this includes optimizing preload and cardiac output. If oliguria persists despite these measures, symptomatic treatment can be instituted. This included managing the consequences of renal failure, which include hypervolemia, hyperkalemia, acidosis, and hyperphosphatemia.

As a result of earlier diagnosis and greater access to dialysis, mortality from hyperkalemia has decreased significantly. In patients with AKI, it is important to restrict daily potassium intake by withholding food and medications containing potassium. When potassium levels become high or ECG changes develop, emergency treatment may include intravenous infusion of calcium, sodium bicarbonate, or glucose and insulin, or an inhaled beta-agonist(Kim and Han 2002). These medications cause an intracellular potassium shift, thus decreasing serum levels. Since these medications do not actually remove potassium from the body, their effect is only temporary, and other interventions are necessary to eliminate it from the body. Administration of loop diuretics can be useful to eliminate potassium, however, varied responses to this medication render the effect unreliable. A sodium-potassium exchange resin, such as sodium polystyrene sulfonate (Kayexalate), can be effective in removing potassium, although the maximal effect occurs only after 4-6 hours. Kayexalate can be administered orally or intrarectally in doses of 15-60 grams, one to four times daily. The most significant complication of Kayexalate administration is gastrointestinal necrosis, which occurs very rarely but can be extremely morbid. Constipation is a more common side effect. While loop diuretics and Kayexalate are options in select patients, the most effective and rapid method of potassium elimination is hemodialysis.

Acidosis occurs frequently in acute renal failure, often complicating treatment in the critically ill patient due to altered homeostasis, decreased cardiac contractility, and attenuated responses to catecholamines. Management of metabolic acidosis should focus on correction of the cause and concomitant morbidity. If acidosis remains once treatment is optimized, hemodialysis is the most effective and proven method of correction. There is significant controversy regarding the use of bicarbonate in management of acidosis in the critically ill patient. Observational and randomized studies have failed to show a mortality or morbidity benefit when sodium bicarbonate is administered to correct acidosis.(Forsythe and Schmidt 2000; Kraut and Kurtz 2001; Kurtz, Kraut et al. 2008) The proposed rationale for the lack of benefit is that, while bicarbonate may increase extracellular pH, it exacerbates intracellular acidosis by the generation of carbon dioxide in the buffering process. Consequently, the practice of many critical care physicians is to administer sodium bicarbonate only in the presence of profound acidosis (pH <7.1) and associated hemodynamic instability. The goal of treatment should be a pH of approximately 7.2. Continuous infusion is favored over bolus injection in order to limit carbon dioxide production.(Kraut and Madias 2010)

As discussed above, loop diuretics have not been shown to prevent or attenuate renal failure. Despite a seemingly positive effect on urine output, the available literature suggests that routine furosemide administration may even have deleterious effects, particularly if given at high doses or if it results in an unwarranted delay in commencement of RRT.(Kellum, Leblanc et al. 2008) Furosemide may be useful when acute kidney injury is accompanied by hyperkalemia or hypervolemia. If none are present, furosemide is not indicated.

7.2 Renal replacement therapy

7.2.1 Indications

The primary roles of the kidney are to excrete toxins, maintain volemia, control electrolytes, and preserve acid-base homeostasis. Failure of the kidneys to perform any of these functions may precipitate an urgent indication for RRT. While there are no absolute guidelines mandating the initiation of RRT in the context of acute kidney injury, generally accepted indications for RRT in critically ill patients include electrolyte imbalances, hypervolemia with pulmonary edema, uremia, and metabolic acidosis. Specific suggested criteria are described in Table 4.

There is an ongoing debate regarding the ideal timing of initiation of RRT in the critically-ill patient, particularly following cardiac surgery. Several factors are responsible for the lack of a definitive answer, including the heterogeneous definition of AKI in the literature and a paucity of well-designed studies. Bouman et al analysed two RCTs and four retrospective studies addressing the question.(Bouman and Oudemans-Van Straaten 2007) Five of these studies, two of which focused uniquely on cardiac surgical patients, found a survival advantage with earlier initiation of RRT.(Gettings, Reynolds et al. 1999; Bouman, Oudemans-Van Straaten et al. 2002; Demirkiliç, Kuralay et al. 2004; Elahi, Lim et al. 2004; Jiang, Xue et al. 2005; Piccinni, Dan et al. 2006) Unfortunately the criteria for early and late initiation were different for each study and, due to the retrospective nature of several studies, they were fraught with confounding variables. In general, criteria for early initiation was dependent on oliguria, while late RRT was instituted based on serum biomarkers or clinical indications. The single randomized study in a surgical population found no difference in mortality between the early and late initiation groups.(Bouman, Oudemans-Van Straaten et al. 2002) However, it has been suggested that the severity of disease in this study was too low to demonstrate a significant difference between the two approaches, resulting in an underpowered trial.(John and Eckardt 2007) Conversely, there may have been a significant selection bias in the retrospective studies showing a benefit with early RRT. The question of early versus late initiation of RRT will remain until larger RCTs are available. In the interim, it may be reasonable to consider early hemodialysis in patients with other organ failure, persistent shock, or to avoid the contribution of acidosis and electrolyte abnormalities to an underlying shock state.

Indication	Description
Metabolic acidosis	• pH < 7.0
Electrolyte abnormalities	• Hyperkalemia (>6.5mmol/L) • Hyper/hyponatremia (Na >155 or <120 mmol/L)
Fluid overload	• Pulmonary edema • Oliguria (urine output <200mL/12 hours) • Anuria (urine output <50mL/12 hours)
Uremia	• Azotemia (Urea >30mmol/L) • Neuropathy, myopathy • Encephalopathy • Pericarditis

Table 4. Proposed indications for RRT in acute renal failure. Adapted from John et al, 2007 (John and Eckardt 2007)

7.2.2 Dosing and mode of RRT

A detailed discussion of the many dosing regimens and modes of RRT is beyond the scope of this chapter. Numerous retrospective and randomized trials have studied each of these topics, with a brief summary of the literature presented here.

The quantification of urea removal is usually referred to as the dose of dialysis. It is an important parameter when measuring the efficiency of RRT, with increased removal of urea being equivalent to a higher dialysis dose. While there is some evidence suggesting that a very low dialysis dose (0.5-0.6L/hr) is associated with worse outcomes, the results of several studies with regard to moderate (20mL/kg/hr) or high dosing (35mL/kg/hr) have been either neutral or in favour of high doses.(Storck, Hartl et al. 1991; Ronco, Bellomo et al. 2000; Bouman, Oudemans-Van Straaten et al. 2002) The VA/NIH Acute Renal Failure Trial Network study randomized 1124 patients undergoing either intermittent hemodialysis (hemodynamically stable) or continuous venovenous hemodiafiltration (hemodynamically unstable) to low intensity or high intensity regimens.(Network, Palevsky et al. 2008) At 60 days, there was no difference between the two groups in the rate of mortality, recovery of kidney function, or the rate of nonrenal organ failure. The authors suggest that other strategies will be necessary to decrease mortality in critically ill patients with acute kidney injury.

	Intermittent hemodialysis	Continuous renal replacement therapy
Advantages	• Lower risk of systemic bleeding • More time available for diagnostic and therapeutic interventions • More suitable for severe hyperkalemia • Lower cost	• Better hemodynamic stability • Fewer cardiac arrhythmias • Improved nutritional support • Better pulmonary gas exchange • Better fluid control • Better biochemical control Shorter stay in intensive-care unit
Disadvantages	• Availability of dialysis staff • More difficult hemodynamic control • Inadequate dialysis dose • Inadequate fluid control • Inadequate nutritional support • Not suitable for patients with intracranial hypertension • No removal of cytokines • Potential complement activation by non-biocompatible membranes	• Greater vascular access problems • Higher risk of systemic bleeding • Long-term immobilization of patient • More filter problems (ruptures, clotting) • Greater cost

Table 5. Advantages and disadvantages of intermittent versus continuous renal replacement therapy. Adapted from Lemaire et at, 2009(Lemaire, Jones et al. 2009)

The mode of RRT is a complex subject, primarily because such a wide variety of modes exist. The two principle categories of RRT are intermittent hemodialysis (IHD) and continuous renal replacement therapy (CRRT). Intermittent hemodialysis is performed over several hours at variable intervals, ranging from once daily to three times per week. Sustained, low-efficiency dialysis (SLED) and extended daily dialysis are subgroups of IHD and are useful in less stable patients that may not tolerate large fluid shifts.(Kihara, Ikeda et al. 1994) CRRT, which is performed continuously, uses much slower flow rates compared to IHD, thus affording better hemodynamic stability. The most common modes of CRRT are continuous venovenous hemofiltration, continuous venovenous hemodialysis, and continuous venovenous hemodiafiltration(Pannu, Klarenbach et al. 2008) One of the significant disadvantages of CRRT is the requirement for anticoagulation due to the slower flow through the system. In the postoperative setting with a patient at increased risk of bleeding, alternative strategies can be applied, such as regular saline flushes or citrate infusion.(Kutsogiannis, Gibney et al. 2005)

Pannu et al reviewed data from 9 RCTs and found no difference in survival between IHD and CRRT.(Pannu, Klarenbach et al. 2008) Despite these equivocal results, there may be distinct clinical advantages for individual patients that must be considered. For example, while IHD might be an obvious choice for patients who have passed the critical stage of their illness, a patient in severe shock on high doses of catecholamines would be more likely to tolerate CRRT. Cost is another important consideration, with IHD being considerably less costly. Table 5 summarizes the advantages and disadvantages of IHD and CRRT in the ICU setting.

8. Summary

Acute kidney injury is one of the most common complications following cardiac surgery, particularly in high-risk patients. Although our understanding of the pathophysiology of AKI has improved over time, we have been unable to significantly improve the prognosis of patients with this serious complication. Strategies for prevention, diagnosis and treatment are still in development, with significant effort being put into advancing our knowledge and progressing beyond our current limitations. While it is clear that further study is necessary to address the shortcomings in the variety of topics reviewed here, there is no substitute for astute clinical evaluation and adherence to basic principles of care in critically ill patients. Clinicians must be conscious of individual patient's risks and recognize early signs of AKI in order to optimize treatment and limit sequelae.

9. References

(1994). "Randomised trial of normothermic versus hypothermic coronary bypass surgery. The Warm Heart Investigators." *Lancet* 343(8897): 559-563.

Abrahamov, D., M. Tamariz, et al. (2001). "Renal dysfunction after cardiac surgery." *Can J Cardiol* 17(5): 565-570.

Abramov, D., M. Tamariz, et al. (2003). "The influence of cardiopulmonary bypass flow characteristics on the clinical outcome of 1820 coronary bypass patients." *Can J Cardiol* 19(3): 237-243.

Allgren, R. L., T. C. Marbury, et al. (1997). "Anaritide in acute tubular necrosis. Auriculin Anaritide Acute Renal Failure Study Group." *N Engl J Med* 336(12): 828-834.

Andersson, L. G., R. Ekroth, et al. (1993). "Acute renal failure after coronary surgery--a study of incidence and risk factors in 2009 consecutive patients." *Thorac Cardiovasc Surg 41(4): 237-241.*

Bagshaw, S. M. and R. T. N. Gibney (2008). "Conventional markers of kidney function." *Critical Care Medicine* 36(4 Suppl): S152-158.

Baker, W. L., M. W. Anglade, et al. (2009). "Use of N-acetylcysteine to reduce post-cardiothoracic surgery complications: a meta-analysis." *European journal of cardio-*

thoracic surgery : official journal of the European Association for Cardio-thoracic Surgery 35(3): 521-527.

Barry, K. G. and A. R. Berman (1961). "Mannitol infusion. III. The acute effect of the intravenous infusion of mannitol on blood and plasma volumes." *N Engl J Med* 264: 1085-1088.

Bellomo, R., S. Auriemma, et al. (2008). "The pathophysiology of cardiac surgery-associated acute kidney injury (CSA-AKI)." *Int J Artif Organs* 31(2): 166-178.

Bellomo, R., M. Chapman, et al. (2000). "Low-dose dopamine in patients with early renal dysfunction: a placebo-controlled randomised trial. Australian and New Zealand Intensive Care Society (ANZICS) Clinical Trials Group." *Lancet* 356(9248): 2139-2143.

Bellomo, R., J. A. Kellum, et al. (2004). "Defining acute renal failure: physiological principles." *Intensive Care Medicine* 30(1): 33-37.

Bellomo, R., C. Ronco, et al. (2004). "Acute renal failure - definition, outcome measures, animal models, fluid therapy and information technology needs: the Second International Consensus Conference of the Acute Dialysis Quality Initiative (ADQI) Group." *Crit Care* 8(4): R204-212.

Bennett, M., C. L. Dent, et al. (2008). "Urine NGAL predicts severity of acute kidney injury after cardiac surgery: a prospective study." *Clin J Am Soc Nephrol* 3(3): 665-673.

Better, O. S., I. Rubinstein, et al. (1997). "Mannitol therapy revisited (1940-1997)." *Kidney Int 52(4): 886-894.*

Bouman, C. S. C. and H. M. Oudemans-Van Straaten (2007). "Timing of renal replacement therapy in critically ill patients with acute kidney injury." *Curr Opin Crit Care* 13(6): 656-661.

Bouman, C. S. C., H. M. Oudemans-Van Straaten, et al. (2002). "Effects of early high-volume continuous venovenous hemofiltration on survival and recovery of renal function in intensive care patients with acute renal failure: a prospective, randomized trial." *Critical Care Medicine* 30(10): 2205-2211.

Bove, T., G. Landoni, et al. (2005). "Renoprotective action of fenoldopam in high-risk patients undergoing cardiac surgery: a prospective, double-blind, randomized clinical trial." *Circulation* 111(24): 3230-3235.

Brienza, N., V. Malcangi, et al. (2006). "A comparison between fenoldopam and low-dose dopamine in early renal dysfunction of critically ill patients." *Critical Care Medicine* 34(3): 707-714.

Briguori, C., F. Airoldi, et al. (2007). "Renal Insufficiency Following Contrast Media Administration Trial (REMEDIAL): a randomized comparison of 3 preventive strategies." *Circulation* 115(10): 1211-1217.

Bunn, F., D. Trivedi, et al. (2011). "Colloid solutions for fluid resuscitation." *Cochrane Database Syst Rev(*3): CD001319.

Burns, K. E. A., M. W. A. Chu, et al. (2005). "Perioperative N-acetylcysteine to prevent renal dysfunction in high-risk patients undergoing cabg surgery: a randomized controlled trial." *JAMA* 294(3): 342-350.

Caimmi, P.-P., L. Pagani, et al. (2003). "Fenoldopam for renal protection in patients undergoing cardiopulmonary bypass." *Journal of Cardiothoracic and Vascular Anesthesia* 17(4): 491-494.

Carcoana, O. V., J. P. Mathew, et al. (2003). "Mannitol and dopamine in patients undergoing cardiopulmonary bypass: a randomized clinical trial." *Anesth Analg* 97(5): 1222-1229.

Chen, H. H., T. M. Sundt, et al. (2007). "Low dose nesiritide and the preservation of renal function in patients with renal dysfunction undergoing cardiopulmonary-bypass surgery: a double-blind placebo-controlled pilot study." *Circulation* 116(11 Suppl): I134-138.

Chertow, G. M., J. M. Lazarus, et al. (1997). "Preoperative renal risk stratification." *Circulation* 95(4): 878-884.

Chertow, G. M., E. M. Levy, et al. (1998). "Independent association between acute renal failure and mortality following cardiac surgery." *Am J Med* 104(4): 343-348.

Chew, S. T., M. F. Newman, et al. (2000). "Preliminary report on the association of apolipoprotein E polymorphisms, with postoperative peak serum creatinine concentrations in cardiac surgical patients." *Anesthesiology* 93(2): 325-331.

Choi, P. T., G. Yip, et al. (1999). "Crystalloids vs. colloids in fluid resuscitation: a systematic review." *Critical Care Medicine* 27(1): 200-210.

Conlon, P. J., M. Stafford-Smith, et al. (1999). "Acute renal failure following cardiac surgery." *Nephrol Dial Transplant* 14(5): 1158-1162.

Cruz, D. N., Z. Ricci, et al. (2009). "Clinical review: RIFLE and AKIN--time for reappraisal." *Critical Care* 13(3): 211.

Dart, A. B., T. C. Mutter, et al. (2010). "Hydroxyethyl starch (HES) versus other fluid therapies: effects on kidney function." *Cochrane Database Syst Rev*(1): CD007594.

Demirkiliç, U., E. Kuralay, et al. (2004). "Timing of replacement therapy for acute renal failure after cardiac surgery." *J Card Surg* 19(1): 17-20.

Dent, C. L., Q. Ma, et al. (2007). "Plasma neutrophil gelatinase-associated lipocalin predicts acute kidney injury, morbidity and mortality after pediatric cardiac surgery: a prospective uncontrolled cohort study." *Crit Care* 11(6): R127.

Dharnidharka, V. R., C. Kwon, et al. (2002). "Serum cystatin C is superior to serum creatinine as a marker of kidney function: a meta-analysis." *Am J Kidney Dis* 40(2): 221-226.

Diaz, G. C., V. Moitra, et al. (2008). "Hepatic and renal protection during cardiac surgery." *Anesthesiol Clin* 26(3): 565-590.

Dietrich, W., R. Busley, et al. (2008). "Effects of aprotinin dosage on renal function: an analysis of 8,548 cardiac surgical patients treated with different dosages of aprotinin." *Anesthesiology* 108(2): 189-198.

Dussol, B., S. Morange, et al. (2006). "A randomized trial of saline hydration to prevent contrast nephropathy in chronic renal failure patients." *Nephrol Dial Transplant* 21(8): 2120-2126.

Ejaz, A. A., T. D. Martin, et al. (2009). "Prophylactic nesiritide does not prevent dialysis or all-cause mortality in patients undergoing high-risk cardiac surgery." *The Journal of Thoracic and Cardiovascular Surgery* 138(4): 959-964.

El-Hamamsy, I., L.-M. Stevens, et al. (2007). "Effect of intravenous N-acetylcysteine on outcomes after coronary artery bypass surgery: a randomized, double-blind, placebo-controlled clinical trial." *The Journal of Thoracic and Cardiovascular Surgery* 133(1): 7-12.

Elahi, M. M., M. Y. Lim, et al. (2004). "Early hemofiltration improves survival in post-cardiotomy patients with acute renal failure." *European journal of cardio-thoracic surgery : official journal of the European Association for Cardio-thoracic Surgery* 26(5): 1027-1031.

Fergusson, D. A., P. C. Hébert, et al. (2008). "A comparison of aprotinin and lysine analogues in high-risk cardiac surgery." *N Engl J Med* 358(22): 2319-2331.

Finfer, S., R. Bellomo, et al. (2004). "A comparison of albumin and saline for fluid resuscitation in the intensive care unit." *N Engl J Med* 350(22): 2247-2256.

Fischer, U. M., W. K. Weissenberger, et al. (2002). "Impact of cardiopulmonary bypass management on postcardiac surgery renal function." *Perfusion* 17(6): 401-406.

Forsythe, S. M. and G. A. Schmidt (2000). "Sodium bicarbonate for the treatment of lactic acidosis." *Chest* 117(1): 260-267.

Fortescue, E. B., D. W. Bates, et al. (2000). "Predicting acute renal failure after coronary bypass surgery: cross-validation of two risk-stratification algorithms." *Kidney Int 57(6): 2594-2602.*

Frost, L., R. S. Pedersen, et al. (1991). "Prognosis and risk factors in acute, dialysis-requiring renal failure after open-heart surgery." *Scand J Thorac Cardiovasc Surg* 25(3): 161-166.

Furnary, A. P., G. Gao, et al. (2003). "Continuous insulin infusion reduces mortality in patients with diabetes undergoing coronary artery bypass grafting." *The Journal of Thoracic and Cardiovascular Surgery* 125(5): 1007-1021.

Furnary, A. P., Y. Wu, et al. (2007). "Aprotinin does not increase the risk of renal failure in cardiac surgery patients." *Circulation* 116(11 Suppl): I127-133.

Gandhi, G. Y., G. A. Nuttall, et al. (2007). "Intensive intraoperative insulin therapy versus conventional glucose management during cardiac surgery: a randomized trial." *Ann Intern Med* 146(4): 233-243.

Garwood, S., C. P. Swamidoss, et al. (2003). "A case series of low-dose fenoldopam in seventy cardiac surgical patients at increased risk of renal dysfunction." *Journal of Cardiothoracic and Vascular Anesthesia* 17(1): 17-21.

Gettings, L. G., H. N. Reynolds, et al. (1999). "Outcome in post-traumatic acute renal failure when continuous renal replacement therapy is applied early vs. late." *Intensive Care Med* 25(8): 805-813.

Haase, M., R. Bellomo, et al. (2008). "Urinary interleukin-18 does not predict acute kidney injury after adult cardiac surgery: a prospective observational cohort study." *Crit Care* 12(4): R96.

Haase, M., A. Haase-Fielitz, et al. (2007). "Phase II, randomized, controlled trial of high-dose N-acetylcysteine in high-risk cardiac surgery patients." *Critical Care Medicine* 35(5): 1324-1331.

Haase, M., A. Haase-Fielitz, et al. (2009). "Sodium bicarbonate to prevent increases in serum creatinine after cardiac surgery: a pilot double-blind, randomized controlled trial." *Critical Care Medicine* 37(1): 39-47.

Haase-Fielitz, A., R. Bellomo, et al. (2009). "Novel and conventional serum biomarkers predicting acute kidney injury in adult cardiac surgery--a prospective cohort study." *Critical Care Medicine* 37(2): 553-560.

Habib, R. H., A. Zacharias, et al. (2003). "Adverse effects of low hematocrit during cardiopulmonary bypass in the adult: should current practice be changed?" *J Thorac Cardiovasc Surg* 125(6): 1438-1450.

Habib, R. H., A. Zacharias, et al. (2005). "Role of hemodilutional anemia and transfusion during cardiopulmonary bypass in renal injury after coronary revascularization: implications on operative outcome." *Crit Care Med* 33(8): 1749-1756.

Hakim, M., R. Foulds, et al. (1988). "Dopexamine hydrochloride, a beta 2 adrenergic and dopaminergic agonist; haemodynamic effects following cardiac surgery." *Eur Heart J* 9(8): 853-858.

Halpenny, M., S. Lakshmi, et al. (2001). "Fenoldopam: renal and splanchnic effects in patients undergoing coronary artery bypass grafting." *Anaesthesia* 56(10): 953-960.

Han, W. K., V. Bailly, et al. (2002). "Kidney Injury Molecule-1 (KIM-1): a novel biomarker for human renal proximal tubule injury." *Kidney Int* 62(1): 237-244.

Han, W. K., G. Wagener, et al. (2009). "Urinary biomarkers in the early detection of acute kidney injury after cardiac surgery." *Clin J Am Soc Nephrol* 4(5): 873-882.

Heise, D., R. M. Waeschle, et al. (2009). "Utility of cystatin C for assessment of renal function after cardiac surgery." *Nephron Clin Pract* 112(2): c107-114.

Ho, K. M. and D. J. Sheridan (2006). "Meta-analysis of frusemide to prevent or treat acute renal failure." *BMJ* 333(7565): 420.

Investigators, N.-S. S., S. Finfer, et al. (2009). "Intensive versus conventional glucose control in critically ill patients." *N Engl J Med* 360(13): 1283-1297.

Ip-Yam, P. C., S. Murphy, et al. (1994). "Renal function and proteinuria after cardiopulmonary bypass: the effects of temperature and mannitol." *Anesth Analg* 78(5): 842-847.

Jiang, H.-L., W.-J. Xue, et al. (2005). "Influence of continuous veno-venous hemofiltration on the course of acute pancreatitis." *World J Gastroenterol* 11(31): 4815-4821.

John, S. and K.-U. Eckardt (2007). "Renal replacement strategies in the ICU." *Chest* 132(4): 1379-1388.

Kellum, J. (1997). "The use of diuretics and dopamine in acute renal failure: a systematic review of the evidence." *Crit Care* 1(2): 53-59.

Kellum, J. A., M. Leblanc, et al. (2008). "Acute renal failure." *Clin Evid (Online)* 2008.

Kellum, J. A. and J. M Decker (2001). "Use of dopamine in acute renal failure: a meta-analysis." *Critical Care Medicine* 29(8): 1526-1531.

Kellum, J. A., R. L. Mehta, et al. (2002). "The first international consensus conference on continuous renal replacement therapy." *Kidney Int* 62(5): 1855-1863.

Kihara, M., Y. Ikeda, et al. (1994). "Slow hemodialysis performed during the day in managing renal failure in critically ill patients." *Nephron* 67(1): 36-41.

Kim, H.-J. and S.-W. Han (2002). "Therapeutic approach to hyperkalemia." *Nephron* 92 Suppl 1: 33-40.

Koyner, J. L., M. R. Bennett, et al. (2008). "Urinary cystatin C as an early biomarker of acute kidney injury following adult cardiothoracic surgery." *Kidney Int* 74(8): 1059-1069.

Krämer, B. K. and U. Hoffmann (2007). "Benefit of acetylcysteine for prevention of contrast-induced nephropathy after primary angioplasty." *Nat Clin Pract Nephrol* 3(1): 10-11.

Kraut, J. A. and I. Kurtz (2001). "Use of base in the treatment of severe acidemic states." Am J *Kidney Dis* 38(4): 703-727.

Kraut, J. A. and N. E. Madias (2010). "Metabolic acidosis: pathophysiology, diagnosis and management." *Nat Rev Nephrol* 6(5): 274-285.

Krinsley, J. S. (2004). "Effect of an intensive glucose management protocol on the mortality of critically ill adult patients." *Mayo Clin Proc* 79(8): 992-1000.

Kurtz, I., J. Kraut, et al. (2008). "Acid-base analysis: a critique of the Stewart and bicarbonate-centered approaches." *Am J Physiol Renal Physiol* 294(5): F1009-1031.

Kutsogiannis, D. J., R. T. N. Gibney, et al. (2005). "Regional citrate versus systemic heparin anticoagulation for continuous renal replacement in critically ill patients." *Kidney Int* 67(6): 2361-2367.

Lameire, N., W. Van Biesen, et al. (2005). "Acute renal failure." *Lancet* 365(9457): 417-430.

Landoni, G., G. G. L. Biondi-Zoccai, et al. (2007). "Beneficial impact of fenoldopam in critically ill patients with or at risk for acute renal failure: a meta-analysis of randomized clinical trials." *Am J Kidney Dis* 49(1): 56-68.

Lassnigg, A., E. Donner, et al. (2000). "Lack of renoprotective effects of dopamine and furosemide during cardiac surgery." *J Am Soc Nephrol* 11(1): 97-104.

Lassnigg, A., E. R. Schmid, et al. (2008). "Impact of minimal increases in serum creatinine on outcome in patients after cardiothoracic surgery: do we have to revise current definitions of acute renal failure?" *Critical Care Medicine* 36(4): 1129-1137.

Lassnigg, A., D. Schmidlin, et al. (2004). "Minimal changes of serum creatinine predict prognosis in patients after cardiothoracic surgery: a prospective cohort study." *J Am Soc Nephrol* 15(6): 1597-1605.

Lemaire, S. A., M. M. Jones, et al. (2009). "Randomized comparison of cold blood and cold crystalloid renal perfusion for renal protection during thoracoabdominal aortic aneurysm repair." *Journal of Vascular Surgery* 49(1): 11-19.

Levy, E. M., C. M. Viscoli, et al. (1996). "The effect of acute renal failure on mortality. A cohort analysis." *JAMA* 275(19): 1489-1494.

Lewis, J., M. M. Salem, et al. (2000). "Atrial natriuretic factor in oliguric acute renal failure. Anaritide Acute Renal Failure Study Group." *Am J Kidney Dis* 36(4): 767-774.

MacGregor, D. A., J. F. Butterworth, et al. (1994). "Hemodynamic and renal effects of dopexamine and dobutamine in patients with reduced cardiac output following coronary artery bypass grafting." *Chest* 106(3): 835-841.

MacGregor, D. A., T. E. Smith, et al. (2000). "Pharmacokinetics of dopamine in healthy male subjects." *Anesthesiology* 92(2): 338-346.

Magder, S., B. J. Potter, et al. (2010). "Fluids after cardiac surgery: a pilot study of the use of colloids versus crystalloids." *Critical Care Medicine* 38(11): 2117-2124.

Mahon, P. and G. Shorten (2006). "Perioperative acute renal failure." *Current Opinion in Anaesthesiology* 19(3): 332-338.

Mangano, C. M., L. S. Diamondstone, et al. (1998). "Renal dysfunction after myocardial revascularization: risk factors, adverse outcomes, and hospital resource utilization. The Multicenter Study of Perioperative Ischemia Research Group." *Ann Intern Med* 128(3): 194-203.

Mangano, D. T., I. C. Tudor, et al. (2006). "The risk associated with aprotinin in cardiac surgery." *N Engl J Med* 354(4): 353-365.

Marathias, K. P., M. Vassili, et al. (2006). "Preoperative intravenous hydration confers renoprotection in patients with chronic kidney disease undergoing cardiac surgery." *Artif Organs* 30(8): 615-621.

Marenzi, G., E. Assanelli, et al. (2006). "N-acetylcysteine and contrast-induced nephropathy in primary angioplasty." *N Engl J Med* 354(26): 2773-2782.

Marik, P. E. (2002). "Low-dose dopamine: a systematic review." *Intensive Care Medicine* 28(7): 877-883.

Marik, P. E. and J. Iglesias (1999). "Low-dose dopamine does not prevent acute renal failure in patients with septic shock and oliguria. NORASEPT II Study Investigators." *Am J Med* 107(4): 387-390.

Mathur, V. S., S. K. Swan, et al. (1999). "The effects of fenoldopam, a selective dopamine receptor agonist, on systemic and renal hemodynamics in normotensive subjects." *Critical Care Medicine* 27(9): 1832-1837.

Meco, M. and S. Cirri (2010). "The effect of various fenoldopam doses on renal perfusion in patients undergoing cardiac surgery." *The Annals of Thoracic Surgery* 89(2): 497-503.

Medalion, B., H. Cohen, et al. (2010). "The effect of cardiac angiography timing, contrast media dose, and preoperative renal function on acute renal failure after coronary artery bypass grafting." *J Thorac Cardiovasc Surg* 139(6): 1539-1544.

Mehta, R. L., J. A. Kellum, et al. (2007). "Acute Kidney Injury Network: report of an initiative to improve outcomes in acute kidney injury." *Crit Care* 11(2): R31.

Melnikov, V. Y., T. Ecder, et al. (2001). "Impaired IL-18 processing protects caspase-1-deficient mice from ischemic acute renal failure." *J Clin Invest* 107(9): 1145-1152.

Mentzer, R. M., M. C. Oz, et al. (2007). "Effects of perioperative nesiritide in patients with left ventricular dysfunction undergoing cardiac surgery:the NAPA Trial." *Journal of the American College of Cardiology* 49(6): 716-726.

Merten, G. J., W. P. Burgess, et al. (2004). "Prevention of contrast-induced nephropathy with sodium bicarbonate: a randomized controlled trial." *JAMA* 291(19): 2328-2334.

Mills, R. M., T. H. LeJemtel, et al. (1999). "Sustained hemodynamic effects of an infusion of nesiritide (human b-type natriuretic peptide) in heart failure: a randomized, double-blind, placebo-controlled clinical trial. Natrecor Study Group." *Journal of the American College of Cardiology* 34(1): 155-162.

Mishra, J., C. Dent, et al. (2005). "Neutrophil gelatinase-associated lipocalin (NGAL) as a biomarker for acute renal injury after cardiac surgery." *Lancet* 365(9466): 1231-1238.

Morelli, A., Z. Ricci, et al. (2005). "Prophylactic fenoldopam for renal protection in sepsis: a randomized, double-blind, placebo-controlled pilot trial." *Critical Care Medicine* 33(11): 2451-2456.

Nakamura, T., T. Sugaya, et al. (2006). "Urinary excretion of liver-type fatty acid-binding protein in contrast medium-induced nephropathy." *Am J Kidney Dis* 47(3): 439-444.

Nakao, K., H. Itoh, et al. (1989). "[A family of natriuretic peptides (ANP.BNP)]." *Nippon Rinsho* 47(9): 1987-1995.

Negishi, K., E. Noiri, et al. (2009). "Monitoring of urinary L-type fatty acid-binding protein predicts histological severity of acute kidney injury." *Am J Pathol* 174(4): 1154-1159.

Negishi, K., E. Noiri, et al. (2008). "Renal L-type fatty acid-binding protein mediates the bezafibrate reduction of cisplatin-induced acute kidney injury." *Kidney Int* 73(12): 1374-1384.

Network, V. N. A. R. F. T., P. M. Palevsky, et al. (2008). "Intensity of renal support in critically ill patients with acute kidney injury." *N Engl J Med* 359(1): 7-20.

Nigwekar, S. U. and P. Kandula (2009). "N-acetylcysteine in cardiovascular-surgery-associated renal failure: a meta-analysis." *The Annals of Thoracic Surgery* 87(1): 139-147.

Nigwekar, S. U., P. Kandula, et al. (2009). "Off-pump coronary artery bypass surgery and acute kidney injury: a meta-analysis of randomized and observational studies." *Am J Kidney Dis* 54(3): 413-423.

Ouattara, A., P. Lecomte, et al. (2005). "Poor intraoperative blood glucose control is associated with a worsened hospital outcome after cardiac surgery in diabetic patients." *Anesthesiology* 103(4): 687-694.

Pannu, N., S. Klarenbach, et al. (2008). "Renal Replacement Therapy in Patients With Acute Renal Failure: A Systematic Review." *JAMA: The Journal of the American Medical Association* 299(7): 793-805.

Parikh, C. R., E. Abraham, et al. (2005). "Urine IL-18 is an early diagnostic marker for acute kidney injury and predicts mortality in the intensive care unit." *J Am Soc Nephrol* 16(10): 3046-3052.

Parikh, C. R., A. Jani, et al. (2006). "Urine NGAL and IL-18 are predictive biomarkers for delayed graft function following kidney transplantation." *Am J Transplant* 6(7): 1639-1645.

Parikh, C. R., J. Mishra, et al. (2006). "Urinary IL-18 is an early predictive biomarker of acute kidney injury after cardiac surgery." *Kidney Int* 70(1): 199-203.

Piccinni, P., M. Dan, et al. (2006). "Early isovolaemic haemofiltration in oliguric patients with septic shock." *Intensive Care Med* 32(1): 80-86.

Piper, S. N., B. Kumle, et al. (2003). "Diltiazem may preserve renal tubular integrity after cardiac surgery." *Can J Anaesth* 50(3): 285-292.

Portilla, D., C. Dent, et al. (2008). "Liver fatty acid-binding protein as a biomarker of acute kidney injury after cardiac surgery." *Kidney Int* 73(4): 465-472.

Poullis, M. (1999). "Mannitol and cardiac surgery." *Thorac Cardiovasc Surg* 47(1): 58-62.

Provenchère, S., G. Plantefève, et al. (2003). "Renal dysfunction after cardiac surgery with normothermic cardiopulmonary bypass: incidence, risk factors, and effect on clinical outcome." *Anesth Analg* 96(5): 1258-1264, table of contents.

Recio-Mayoral, A., M. Chaparro, et al. (2007). "The reno-protective effect of hydration with sodium bicarbonate plus N-acetylcysteine in patients undergoing emergency percutaneous coronary intervention: the RENO Study." *Journal of the American College of Cardiology* 49(12): 1283-1288.

Rioux, J.-P., M. Lessard, et al. (2009). "Pentastarch 10% (250 kDa/0.45) is an independent risk factor of acute kidney injury following cardiac surgery." *Critical Care Medicine* 37(4): 1293-1298.

Roberts, I., P. Alderson, et al. (2004). "Colloids versus crystalloids for fluid resuscitation in critically ill patients." *Cochrane Database Syst Rev*(4): CD000567.

Ronco, C., R. Bellomo, et al. (2000). "Effects of different doses in continuous veno-venous haemofiltration on outcomes of acute renal failure: a prospective randomised trial." *Lancet* 356(9223): 26-30.

Rosner, M. H. and M. D. Okusa (2006). "Acute kidney injury associated with cardiac surgery." *Clin J Am Soc Nephrol* 1(1): 19-32.

Rosner, M. H., D. Portilla, et al. (2008). "Cardiac surgery as a cause of acute kidney injury: pathogenesis and potential therapies." *J Intensive Care Med* 23(1): 3-18.

Royston, D. (1995). "Blood-sparing drugs: aprotinin, tranexamic acid, and epsilon-aminocaproic acid." *Int Anesthesiol Clin* 33(1): 155-179.

Sackner-Bernstein, J. D., H. A. Skopicki, et al. (2005). "Risk of worsening renal function with nesiritide in patients with acutely decompensated heart failure." *Circulation* 111(12): 1487-1491.

Schmidt-Ott, K. M., K. Mori, et al. (2006). "Neutrophil gelatinase-associated lipocalin-mediated iron traffic in kidney epithelia." *Curr Opin Nephrol Hypertens* 15(4): 442-449.

Sear, J. W. (2005). "Kidney dysfunction in the postoperative period." *Br J Anaesth* 95(1): 20-32.

Shaw, A., M. Swaminathan, et al. (2008). "Cardiac surgery-associated acute kidney injury: putting together the pieces of the puzzle." *Nephron Physiol* 109(4): p55-60.

Shaw, A. D., M. Stafford-Smith, et al. (2008). "The effect of aprotinin on outcome after coronary-artery bypass grafting." *N Engl J Med* 358(8): 784-793.

Sherry, E., M. A. Tooley, et al. (1997). "Effect of dopexamine hydrochloride on renal vascular resistance index and haemodynamic responses following coronary artery bypass graft surgery." *Eur J Anaesthesiol* 14(2): 184-189.

Sisillo, E., R. Ceriani, et al. (2008). "N-acetylcysteine for prevention of acute renal failure in patients with chronic renal insufficiency undergoing cardiac surgery: a prospective, randomized, clinical trial." *Critical Care Medicine* 36(1): 81-86.

Solomon, R., C. Werner, et al. (1994). "Effects of saline, mannitol, and furosemide to prevent acute decreases in renal function induced by radiocontrast agents." *N Engl J Med* 331(21): 1416-1420.

Stephan, H., H. Sonntag, et al. (1990). "Cardiovascular and renal haemodynamic effects of dopexamine: comparison with dopamine." *Br J Anaesth* 65(3): 380-387.

Storck, M., W. H. Hartl, et al. (1991). "Comparison of pump-driven and spontaneous continuous haemofiltration in postoperative acute renal failure." *Lancet* 337(8739): 452-455.

Thakar, C. V., O. Liangos, et al. (2003). "ARF after open-heart surgery: Influence of gender and race." *Am J Kidney Dis* 41(4): 742-751.

Thakar, C. V., O. Liangos, et al. (2003). "Predicting acute renal failure after cardiac surgery: validation and re-definition of a risk-stratification algorithm." *Hemodial Int* 7(2): 143-147.

Trivedi, H. S., H. Moore, et al. (2003). "A randomized prospective trial to assess the role of saline hydration on the development of contrast nephrotoxicity." *Nephron Clin Pract* 93(1): C29-34.

Tuttle, K. R., N. K. Worrall, et al. (2003). "Predictors of ARF after cardiac surgical procedures." *Am J Kidney Dis* 41(1): 76-83.

Urzua, J., S. Troncoso, et al. (1992). "Renal function and cardiopulmonary bypass: effect of perfusion pressure." *Journal of Cardiothoracic and Vascular Anesthesia* 6(3): 299-303.

van den Berghe, G., P. Wouters, et al. (2001). "Intensive insulin therapy in the critically ill patients." *N Engl J Med* 345(19): 1359-1367.

van Oeveren, W., N. J. Jansen, et al. (1987). "Effects of aprotinin on hemostatic mechanisms during cardiopulmonary bypass." *The Annals of Thoracic Surgery* 44(6): 640-645.

Wagener, G., M. Jan, et al. (2006). "Association between increases in urinary neutrophil gelatinase-associated lipocalin and acute renal dysfunction after adult cardiac surgery." *Anesthesiology* 105(3): 485-491.

Ympa, Y. P., Y. Sakr, et al. (2005). "Has mortality from acute renal failure decreased? A systematic review of the literature." *Am J Med* 118(8): 827-832.

Young, E. W., A. Diab, et al. (1998). "Intravenous diltiazem and acute renal failure after cardiac operations." *The Annals of Thoracic Surgery* 65(5): 1316-1319.

Zhang, Z., B. D. Humphreys, et al. (2007). "Shedding of the urinary biomarker kidney injury molecule-1 (KIM-1) is regulated by MAP kinases and juxtamembrane region." *J Am Soc Nephrol* 18(10): 2704-2714.

9

Acute Kidney Injury Induced by Snake and Arthropod Venoms

Markus Berger[1], Maria Aparecida Ribeiro Vieira[2] and Jorge Almeida Guimarães[1]
[1]*Center of Biotechnology, Departament of Molecular Biology and Biotechnology, Federal University of Rio Grande do Sul (UFRGS), Porto Alegre,*
[2]*Institute of Biological Sciences, Department of Fisiology and Biology, Federal University of Minas Gerais (UFMG)*
Brazil

1. Introduction

Snakebites and accidents caused by venomous arthropods (mainly spiders, scorpions, bees, wasps and caterpillars) are important public health problem. Despite of this, public health authorities, nationally and internationally, have given little attention to this problem worldwide (Warrell, 2010; Williams et al., 2010). As a consequence, the morbidity and mortality associated with snake and arthropod envenoming produce a great impact on the population and on the health-care systems. One of the most important and lethal effect of these animal venoms is nephrotoxicity (Sitprija, 2006). Specifically in South America and Brazil, the main snakes responsible for cases of acute kidney injury (AKI) are those from *Bothrops* and *Crotalus* genus. Among venomous arthropods, AKI has been reported after accidents with bees, spiders of the genus *Loxosceles* and caterpillars of the genus *Lonomia*.

Taking in account the importance of accidents with these venomous animals, in this chapter we reviewed the main mechanisms that play a role in AKI induced by the most common snakes and arthropods found in South America. The following key aspects are addressed: Epidemiology, clinical renal manifestations, renal pathophysiology, diagnosis, clinical management of AKI and the currently experimental models used to study the venom-induced AKI.

2. Epidemiology and prevalence of venomous snakes and arthropods in South America

Given the wide distribution of venomous animals, particularly in tropical and subtropical regions, the extensive number of accidents and the complexity of the clinical conditions it causes, the distint types of envenomation can be considered a global problem because they assume great public health importance, especially in the poorest areas of the world (World Health Organization [WHO], 2007). This environmental and occupational disease affects mainly agricultural workers and their children in some of the most impoverished rural communities of developing countries in Africa, Asia, Latin America and Oceania. Populations in these regions experience high morbidity and mortality because of the poor access to health services, which are often suboptimal, and, in some instances, a scarcity of antivenom, which is the only specific treatment so far tecnically possible to be available. A large number of victims survive with permanent physical and psychological sequelae (Gutiérrez et al., 2010; Kasturiratne et al., 2008; Warrell, 2010).

A group of venomous animals is responsible for medically important accidents: snakes, scorpions, spiders, caterpillars, bees and wasps. Global epidemiological data on accidents with these different types of animals are scarce and often depend on the existence of country-specific estimates based on hospital admissions data and community-based population surveys. Unfortunately, in the low-income countries, where most accidents occur, there is not such a well organized health systems in order to correctly report the envenomation cases (Kasturiratne et al., 2008; Williams et al., 2010). Nevertheless, after the incorporation of snakebite envenomations on the World Health Organization list of neglected tropical diseases in 2009 (www.who.int/neglected_diseases/diseases/snakebites/en/), more attention has been given to the lack of information on the true epidemiological impact of accidents, especially in the cases of snakebites. Current data indicate that 5.4 to 5.5 million people are bitten by snakes each year, resulting in near 400,000 amputations, and between 20,000 to 125,000 deaths (Chippaux, 1998, Kasturiratne et al., 2008; Williams et al., 2010). The highest burden of snakebite was identified in South and Southeast Asia, sub-Saharan Africa and Central and South America. Annually, Asia and Africa have incidence rates of 1.2 million and 1 million bites with 60,000 and 20,000 deaths, respectively. In Central and South America, epidemiological data indicate the occurrence of 300,000 snakebites per year which result in 4,000 deaths and approximately 12,000 cases of physical sequelae (Chippaux, 2011; Gutiérrez et al., 2010).

Specifically in Brazil, data from the System of Health Surveillance of the Ministry of Health indicate the ocorrence of 107,364 accidents with venomous animals in the year of 2009 (including cases of snake, scorpion, spider, caterpillar and bee envenomations) which resulted in 290 deaths. When compared to the 2008 year there were an increase of 12 % and 16 % in the total number of accidents and deaths, respectively (Boletim eletrônico epidemiológico, 2010). The majority of reported cases was caused by snakes and scorpions, which were also responsible for the highest rates of lethality (Table 1). Most snakebite (53 %) occurred from January to May, which reflect the influence of seasonal factors, such as an increase in temperature and humidity associated with the rainy season in some regions of Brazil. Human agricultural activities were also associated with envenomations, since 78 % of accidents occurred in rural areas. Snakes of *Bothrops* genus (Lance-headed pit vipers) were responsible for 90.5 % of the accidents while snakes of *Crotalus* genus (South American rattlesnakes) accounted for 7.7 % of total cases, showing however, a much higher lethality index (1.25 %) than that for *Bothrops* snakes (0.35 %) (Ministério da Saúde, 2001). Analysing the different regions of Brazil, the highest proportion of snakebites in relation to the population is localized in the North Region (Amazon Forest) with 53.9 accidents/100,000 inhabitants, probably due to the difficulty of patients to access health services and/or to the delay in the administration of antivenom (Table 1). Among all venomous animals, the scorpion stands out for its high and growing number of accidents in Brazil. Compared to the 2008 year, there was an increase of 7,050 cases in 2009 (45,721 *versus* 38,671 cases in 2008).

According to Chippaux and Goyffon (2008), scorpions are responsible annually for 1.2 million accidents and for about 3,250 deaths in the world. In Brazil, the increased number of scorpion accidents has been attributed to its adaptation to urban and domiciliar areas (Ministério da Saúde, 2001). In this case, the highest incidence was registred in the Northeast Region (Table 1). In contrast, accidents with spiders, caterpillars and bees are a growing problem in states of Southern Brazil. Specifically in the state of Paraná the brown spider (*Loxosceles* genus) is the most important venomous animal responsible for the high incidence of spider envenomation in the whole South Region (da Silva et al., 2004). In contrast, in the states of Rio Grande do Sul and Santa Catarina the caterpillar *Lonomia obliqua*, also called *taturana* (from the American-Indian Tupi-Guarani *tatá*, which means fire, and *raná*, similar to), has been associated with severe cases of hemorrhagic syndrome (Veiga et al., 2009). In this case, although accidents may occur throughout the year, 80 % of cases were reported during summer, when the animal is in the larval stage of its life cycle. Between 1997 and 2005 there were 984 accidents only in the state of Rio Grande do Sul, resulting in a mortality rate of 0.5 % (Abella et al., 2006). Currently, the therapeutic use of specific antivenom (antilonomic serum) has decreased the number of deaths (Table 1). Among bee accidents, the most dangerous are caused by *Apis mellifera* (Africanized bees). In these cases the high number of deaths (30 in 2009) has been associated mainly with the absence of a specific antivenom and the occurence of allergic reactions (Boletim eletrônico epidemiológico, 2010).

ACCIDENTS WITH VENOMOUS ANIMALS IN BRAZIL. REPORTED DATA: YEAR 2009 *.					
	Snakes	**Spiders**	**Scorpions**	**Caterpillars**	**Bees**
Total number of accidents	27,655	23,515	45,721	4,028	6,445
Incidence per 100,000 inhabitants	14.4	12.3	24	2.1	3.4
Number of deaths	125	26	104	5	30
Lethality (%)	0.45	0.11	0.23	0.13	0.05
Brazilian Regions	**Incidence per 100,000 inhabitants**				
North	53.9	3.6	16.2	1.7	1.9
Northeast	14.6	1.3	39.6	0.4	2.5
Midwest	20	2.6	13.3	0.7	2.2
Southeast	7.4	7.1	23.7	1.7	3.2
South	10.1	58.5	3.5	7.3	7

* Data from Brazilian Ministry of Health, 2010 (Boletim Eletrônico Epidemiológico, April 2010).

Table 1. Epidemiological data of accidents with venomous animals in Brazil.

3. Clinical renal manifestations due to snake and arthropod envenomation

A broad clinical spectrum of renal function impairment has been reported in snake and arthropod envenomations (Sitprija, 2006). As the kidneys are highly vascularized organs and have the ability to concentrate substances into the urine they are particularly susceptible to venom toxins. The most common clinical renal manifestations seen in human patients is acute tubular necrosis, but all renal structures may be involved. Thus, the occurrence of acute tubulointerstitial nephritis, renal cortical necrosis, mesangiolysis, vasculitis, glomerulonephritis, proteinuria, haematuria and myoglobinuria have also been described (Sitprija, 2006).

In this subsection, we reviewed the clinical characteristics of human accidents with snakes and arthropods that cause AKI which are highly prevalent in Brazil and other regions of Latin America. Envenomations by the following animals were analysed: *Bothrops* and *Crotalus* snakes, the brown spider *Loxosceles*, africanized bees, wasps and the caterpillars of genus *Lonomia*. Despite the significant number of accidents with scorpions (Table 1), cases of AKI have not been associated to them. In fact, it is known that the main target of scorpion venom is the nervous and cardiac systems (Cologna et al., 2009).

3.1 Snakebite envenomation

Envenomation by snakebite, indenpendently of the species responsible for the bite, enforces medical emergencies since different organs and tissues can be affected at the same time. In Brazil, most severe cases result from bites by snakes of the family Viperidae (pit vipers and true vipers). Within this family are the *Bothrops* and *Crotalus* snakes. Specifically in the *Bothrops* genus there are more than 30 species distributed from southern Mexico to Argentina, including Brazil. The most important species are *Bothrops asper, B. jararaca, B. atrox, B. moojeni, B. jararacussu* and *B. alternatus*. *Bothrops* snakes preferentially inhabit rural areas and moist forest environments. But these snakes also invade cultivated areas and ambients with rodents' proliferation. *Bothrops* snakes have nocturnal habits and an aggressive defensive behavior and its venom present proteolytic, coagulant and hemorrhagic active principles that are directly or indirectly implicated in the local and systemic effects observed upon envenoming acidents (Warrel, 2010). Local effects due to the envenoming by these snakes are characterized by bleeding, swelling, pain and sometimes blisters, and can be frenquently complicated by the development of local abscesses and necrosis. Occasionally, compartmental syndrome may develop, which results in functional or anatomic loss of the bitten limb (Gutiérrez et al., 2006). Signs of systemic envenoming include gingival hemorrhage, microscopic hematuria, ecchymosis and consumption coagulopathy and, more rarely, epistaxis, hemoptosis, menorrhagia and hematemesis (Gutiérrez et al., 2006; Otero et al., 2002). Disturbances of hemostasis also include severe afibrinogenemia, thrombocytopenia and platelet aggregation dysfunction (Santoro and Sano-Martins, 2004). Deaths are usually attributed to renal injury, shock, severe bleeding, and complicating sepsis.

Renal dysfunction can occur early in the human bothropic envenomation which often induces oliguria and is accompanied by an increase in the plasma creatinine concentration. The need for dialysis ranges from 33 % to 75 % of cases (Pinho et al., 2008). AKI is mainly due to acute tubular necrosis and acute cortical necrosis and occasionally glomerulonephritis (Table 2) (Rodrigues-Sgrignolli et al., 2011). These renal pathological alterations have been attributed mainly to hemodynamic changes in response to envenomation, hemoglobinuria, intravascular clot formation and direct venom nephrotoxicity.

By analyzing a series of retrospective studies, Pinho et al. (2008) reported that the prevalence of AKI after *Bothrops* envenomation ranges from 1.6 % to 38.5 %. In most of these reports AKI diagnosis was based on the increase in the plasma creatinine and/or blood nitrogen urea being, the creatinine *clearance* barely estimated. The main reported factors influencing AKI prevalence upon such envenomation are: the patient's age (children under 10 year of age have been shown to be more susceptible to develop AKI); the snake's age (venom composition can vary even within the same species, according to the snake's age); bite site and amount of inoculated venom; and the time elapsed until antivenom treatment. Moreover, pre-existing diseases such as hypertension, diabetes or previous nephropathies may become patients more vulnerable to the effects of venom (Rodrigues-Sgrignolli et al., 2011; Zelanis et al., 2010). Taking in consideration all the above factors, the mortality rate of *Bothrops* venom-induced AKI range from 13 % to 19 %.

Other snakes well known for their nephrotoxicity are the South American rattlesnakes (*Crotalus* snakes). In Brazil, the *Crotalus* genus is represented by a single specie, *Crotalus durissus*, that is composed of six subspecies: *Crotalus durissus terrificus, C. d.collilineatus, C.d. cascavella, C.d. ruruima, C.d. marajoensis* and *C.d. trigonicus*. Besides sharing some common characteristics with other venomous snakes, the *Crotalus* genus presents a rattle at the end of its tail, which is a particular characteristic of these snakes making easier their identification. In general the *Crotalus* snakes are found in rocky and drier regions. They are rarely found in humid forests and feed mainly of small rodents. They are robust (may reach 1 meter in length) and are less agressive than *Bothrops* snakes (Ministério da Saúde, 2001).

Among the six different subspecies, *C.d. terrificus* is the most frequently implicated in envenomation cases registered in Brazil. The venom has neurotoxic, myotoxic, and nephrotoxic activities (Table 2). In neuromuscular junctions, the venom leads to a powerful presynaptic inhibition of acetylcholine release, which is responsible for the neuromuscular blockade and progressive flaccid paralysis of variable degrees. Eyelid ptosis, blurred and/or double vision, ophthalmoplegia and facial muscle paralysis are common manifestations of venom neurotoxicity. The myotoxic activity of the venom also produces severe skeletal muscle injury leading to myalgia and rhabdomyolysis with the subsequent release of myoglobin from damaged skeletal muscle into serum and urine (Azevedo-Marques et al., 1987). Indeed, the serum creatine kinase (CK) levels are significantly higher (260-folds that of normal values) in patients who develop AKI after a *Crotalus* bite. Other markers of rhabdomyolysis, such as aspartate aminotransferase (AST), alanine aminotransferase (ALT) and lactate dehydrogenase (LDH) are also increased in patients with AKI (Pinho et al., 2005). High serum and urine levels of myoglobin are potentially nephrotoxic, leading to acute tubular necrosis, which is the primary and most serious complication of human crotalid envenomation. Tissue damage at the site of the bite has been reported to be minimal or absent, a feature that differentiates the South American rattlesnake from other species of *Crotalus* and from *Bothrops* envenomations. Spontaneous bleeding has only been rarely observed in human patients, despite the presence of blood incoagulability in some cases (Jorge & Ribeiro, 1992). AKI is the main cause of death among patients surviving to the early effects of *Crotalus* snakebites.

In a study of 100 cases of *Crotalus* bites, Pinho et al. (2005) showed that AKI develops within the first 24 to 48 hours after envenomation. Envenomed patients presented a significant reduction in glomerular filtration rate (estimated by the creatinine *clearance*). AKI patients also presented dark-brown urine and a fractional excretion of sodium significantly higher than the normal (Pinho et al., 2005). The major kidney pathological alteration is acute tubular necrosis, although interstitial nephritis has also been observed (Amaral et al., 1986; Azevedo-Marques et al., 1985) (Table 2). In this type of envenomation the occurrence of severe rhabdomyolysis is one of the more accepted explanations for the acute tubular necrosis. Other factors potentially associated with venom-induced AKI such as shock, hypotension and hemolysis are present in some cases, but have not been confirmed in *Crotalus* envenomation (Azevedo-Marques et al., 1987; Pinho et al., 2008). Despite of *in vitro* hemolytic activity of *Crotalus* venom, it was confirmed that *in vivo C.d. terrificus* envenomation causes myolysis rather than intravascular hemolysis (Azevedo-Marques et al., 1987).

The prevalence of AKI associated with Crotalid envenomation ranges from 10 to 29 % and 68 to 77 % of AKI patients require dialysis treatment. The mortality rate of *Crotalus* venom-induced AKI ranges from 8 to 17 % (Amaral et al., 1986; Pinho et al., 2008; Silveira & Nishioka, 1992). Although most risk factors for AKI are very similar to those described for bothropic envenomation it was reported that early after *Crotalus* snakebite the plasma levels of CK (higher than 2,000 U/L) were associated with a 12-fold increase in the risk of developing AKI (Pinho et al., 2005).

3.2 Brown spider envenomation

Among arthropods, spider and scorpion bites are the most frequent and of medical care importance. Although the number of accidents with scorpions often overcome those with spiders, reports of AKI after human envenomation with scorpion are scarce (Abdulkader et al., 2008). One species of spider that can cause severe renal injury is the brown spider (*Loxosceles* genus). Spiders of the genus *Loxosceles* have a worldwide distribution, since they can live under variable conditions such as temperature ranging from 8 to 43°C and that they can stay long time intervals living without food or water (Hogan et al., 2004; Swanson and Vetter, 2006). In Brazil, seven species have been described, but some of them are the most frequently implicated in bites in humans, namely *Loxosceles intermedia, L. gaucho* and *L. laeta*. These spiders are commonly found inside the residences both in rural and urban areas. They are small, measuring between 8 and 15 mm of body length while their legs measure 8-30 mm. Their colour varies from a pale brown (*L. laeta*) to a dark brown (*L. gaucho*). *Loxosceles* spiders are not aggressive and the bites usually occur when they are pressed against the body, mainly while the victim is sleeping or dressing (da Silva et al., 2004).

The venom has proteolytic, dermonecrotic, hemolytic and nephrotoxic activities (Isbister & Fan, 2011) (Table 2). The accident may have local and systemic manifestations that are exhibited in two different clinical forms: cutaneous and viscerocutaneous loxoscelism (da Silva et al., 2004). Most patients have only the local manifestation or cutaneous loxoscelism. In these cases, the accident may cause mild cutaneous inflammatory reaction or a local injury characterized by pain, edema and erithrema, later developing to dermonecrosis with gravitational spreading. In the minority of cases loxoscelism can cause a systemic injury or the viscerocutaneous loxoscelism. This form occurs predominantly in children, and patients can develop AKI, which is considered the main cause of death after brown spider envenomation. Viscerocutaneous loxoscelism is characterized by fever, malaise, weakness, nausea and vomiting, hemolysis, hematuria, jaundice, thrombocytopenia and disseminated intravascular coagulation. This severe multisystemic clinical picture can occur as early as 24 hours after the bite (Abdulkader et al., 2008; da Silva et al., 2004; Isbister & Fan, 2011).

Analysis of 267 loxoscelism cases reported in Brazil showed that the viscerocutaneous form was diagnosed in 13.1 % of the cases, where *L laeta* was the main specie implicated in the accidents. The investigators reported jaundice in 68.6 %, oliguria in 45.7 %, anuria in 8.6 %, dark urine in 28.6 %, hemorrhage in 25.7 %, and shock in 2.9 % of the patients. AKI occurred in 6.4 % of the patients, and most of them were diagnosed more than 24 hours after the bite. Four patients died (1.5 %), all of them were children under 14 years old (Sezerino et al., 1998). The main factors likely associated with AKI development are hemolysis, hypotension/shock, and direct venom nephrotoxicity (Table 2). Pigment-induced acute tubular necrosis was reported in human necropsies of viscerocutaneous loxoscelism (Zambrano et al., 2005). Thus, it was suggested that the pathological effect of the venom on the kidney may reflect hematological disturbances, such as intravascular hemolysis and disseminated intravascular coagulation (Abdulkader et al., 2008). Although only low myotoxic activity has been reported in *Loxosceles* venom, rhabdomyolysis can also occur after envenomation. In this cases, high levels of serum CK and deposits of myoglobin in tubular cells have been observed (França et al., 2002; Lucato-Junior et al., 2011).

3.3 Bee and wasp envenomation

Stings of insects from the order Hymenoptera, which includes several species of bees, hornets, wasps and yellow jacks, have also been implicated in cases of human envenomation (Vetter et al., 1999).

In general the victims present only local allergic reactions after one or a few stings. However, after a massive attack with hundreds or thousands of stings, a systemic envenomation may occur (Abdulkader et al., 2008). The majority of envenomation cases with medical importance is caused by the so-called Africanized bees (*Apis* genus). These bees are hybrids between bees of European origin (*Apis mellifera mellifera* and *Apis mellifera ligustica*) and African bees (*Apis mellifera scutellata*) which were originated by the introduction of different species in Brazil since 1957. Currently, due to the migratory behavior and a high reproductive rate they are found throughout South America, Central America and parts of North America. Because of their aggressive behavior and the number of accidents associated with them, the Africanized bees are also known as "killer bees" (Abdulkader et al., 2008; França et al., 1994).

The main venom activities are hemolytic, myotoxic, cardiotoxic and nephrotoxic (Table 2). Clinical manifestations can be divided into allergic and systemic reactions. Allergic reactions usually are observed in patients with a history of previous bee stings or asthma or other hypersensitivity disease. These reactions occur immediately after a single sting and can lead to anaphylaxis and death by laryngeal edema. Systemic reactions usually occur after multiple stings and are characterized by pain, erythema, urticaria, release of histamine, nausea, vomiting, respiratory failure, hypotension and shock (Abdulkader et al., 2008). Rhabdomyolysis and hemolysis can be detected a few hours after the accident (Chao et al., 2004). Fatalities are typically the result of renal damage or from cardiac arrest due to complications of the venom toxicity (Vetter et al., 1999).

AKI has been observed in cases of massive attacks with 150 stings to more than 1,500 stings. Envenomed patients commonly have anuria or oliguria, high levels of serum creatinine (10-30 mg/dL) and CK (>2,000 U/L), hypotension, tachycardia, myocardial damage and anemia (Daher et al., 2003; Gabriel et al., 2004; França et al., 1994; Xuan et al., 2010). Acute tubular necrosis is the main histologic finding in human beings, domestic dogs, and in experimental animals after bee and wasp envenomations. Allergic interstitial nephritis with concurrent pigment tubulopathy resulting from both hemoglobin and myoglobin has also been described after wasp stings (Chao et al., 2004; Zhang et al., 2001) (Table 2). A direct nephrotoxicity of the venom and/or hypotension caused by anaphylactic reaction are also mechanisms implicated in AKI induced by bees of *Apis* genus (Grisotto et al., 2006). By analyzing five cases of severe envenomation by Africanized bees, França et al. (1994) found high venom concentrations in serum and urine which remain for more than 50 h after the stings in two fatal cases; in one of them the total circulating unbound whole venom components was estimated at 27 mg, one hour after the attack. Despite the treatment with dialysis, antihistamines, corticosteroids, bronchodilators, vasodilators, bicarbonate, mannitol and mechanical ventilation, three out four patients died between 22 and 71 h after the attacks. However, in the majority of cases, the renal damage is usually reversible responding well to the dialysis. Complete recovery may require 3-6 weeks (Vetter et al., 1999).

3.4 Caterpillar envenomation

The accidental contact with some lepidopteran caterpillars can also cause human envenomation cases that vary from simple skin irritation and local allergic reactions to a systemic disease characterized by renal damage and hemorrhagic disturbances (Pinto et al., 2010; Veiga et al., 2009). From the medically important Saturniidae family, *Lonomia* genus has been attributed to cause human envenomations since late 1960's in Venezuela (Arocha-Piñango et al., 2000). In Southern Brazil, *Lonomia obliqua* caterpillar is becoming the most important venomous animal responsible for severe injuries, hemorrhagic disorders and often fatal outcome since the 1980's (Duarte et al., 1990). For instance, in the State of Rio Grande do Sul, located in this Brazilian region, more than a thousand accidents have been registered in the period from 1997 to 2005 (Abella et al., 2006). In fact, based on data from the year 2009, the Brazilian Ministry of Health registered an incidence of 7.3 lepidopteran envenomations per 100,000 inhabitants in Southern Brazil (Boletim eletrônico epidemiológico, 2010) (Table 1). Actually, these numbers are greatly underestimated due to the fact that most accidents are occurring in distant rural areas, where the cases are poorly reported. *Lonomia*'s accidents usually occur when the victim, leaning against tree trunks containing dozens or hundreds of caterpillars, comes into contact with their bristles. These structures are hard and spiny evaginations of the cuticle, underneath which the toxins are stored. Often, the whole animal is smashed in the accident, the insect's chitinous bristles get broken and the venomous secretions, including hemolymph, penetrate the human skin and enter the circulation (Veiga et al., 2001**a**).

The venom presents procoagulant, fibrinogenolytic, proteolytic and hemolytic activities (Table 2). Clinical symptoms of *Lonomia* envenomation include local pain (burning sensation) and inflammatory reaction, which starts immediately after contact; systemic reactions such as headache, fever, vomiting and asthenia, which appear a few hours after exposure; and bleeding diathesis characterized by hematomas and ecchymosis, gross hematuria, hematemesis, melena, pulmonary and intracerebral hemorrhage and AKI (Pinto et al., 2010). Intravascular hemolysis has also been described in human envenomation and experimental studies (Malaque et al., 2006; Seibert et al., 2004). The activation of blood coagulation, fibrinolysis and the systemic inhibition of platelet function are mechanisms that seem to contribute to the hemorrhagic syndrome commonly observed in *Lonomia* envenomation (Berger et al., 2010**a**). In human patients, this hemorrhagic syndrome manifests as a consumptive coagulopathy without thrombocytopenia (Berger et al., 2010**a;** Zannin et al., 2003).

The incidence of AKI varies from 2 to 5 % of envenomation cases reported in the literature (Duarte et al., 1990; Gamborgi et al., 2006). Of the 2,067 patients evaluated in southern Brazil (period from 1989 to 2003), 39 (1.9 %) developed AKI (serum creatinine levels > 1.5 mg/dL). Eleven (32 %) of these patients were treated with dialysis and four (10.3 %) developed chronic renal injury (CRI). All victims with AKI presented concomitantly coagulation disturbances and hematuria and/or hemoglobinuria. Seven deaths (4%) occurred during the period (Gamborgi et al., 2006). The impossibility of conducting early renal biopsies, due the coagulation disturbances inherent to the envenomation, has made it difficult to analyze the acute anatomopathological alterations. The few reports existing in the literature describe thickening of the Bowman's capsule, focal tubular atrophy and acute tubular necrosis (Burdmann et al., 1996; Fan et al., 1998) (Table 2). Similarly, the contribution of other factors possibly associated with AKI, such as hypotension or glomerular fibrin deposition, remains still obscure in *Lonomia* envenomation.

4. Toxins of snake and arthropod venoms and their role in the pathophysiology of acute kidney injury

Animal venoms are mixtures of biologically active proteins and peptides, and also non-protein toxins, carbohydrates, lipids, amines, and other small molecules. The clinical features of envenomation reflect the effects of these different venom components and thus, the contribution of the venom toxins to the pathophysiology of renal injury is complex and multifactorial (Sitprija, 2006).

Based on the current knowledge, the hypothesis for pathogenesis of venom-induced AKI include both a direct cytotoxic action of the venom on different renal structures, and a secondary response of the whole organism resulting from systemic envenomation. The secondary response is usually triggered by inflammation, release of cytokines and vasoactive substances that leads to changes in renal function and hemodynamics (Fig. 1). In fact, there is an increase in plasma concentration of different cytokines and vasoactive substances such as TNF-α, interleukins, nitric oxide, histamine, bradykinin and eicosanoids following several types of envenomations (Petricevich et al., 2000). The elevation of cytokines are mainly due to accumulation of pro-inflammatory cells and immune system response. Together, all these mediators can impair renal function ultimately contributing to a decrease in renal perfusion pressure, renal blood flow and glomerular filtration rate. As a result in association with the systemic hypotension (Table 2), there will be an inadequate tissue and cellular oxygen delivery which can generate an ischemic process. Since the intermediary metabolism and energy production have an absolute dependence on oxygen, and oxygen cannot be stored intracellularly, the inadequate oxygen availability rapidly leads to cellular dysfunction, injury, and cell death by necrosis (Deitch, 1992). Important contribution to venom-induced renal ischemia is also derived from the process of hemolysis, rhabdomyolysis and/or intravascular deposition of platelets and fibrin in the microcirculation (Table 2). The presence of hemoglobin and myoglobin also have a direct cytotoxic effect on renal tubules (Fig.1) (Khan, 2009; Zager, 1996). Thus, it seems that different, but interrelated processes may contribute to the nephrotoxicity and even to other pathological features observed in envenomed patients.

Venomous animals	**Main venom activities**	**General clinical manifestations**	**Characteristics of AKI and renal pathology**
Bothrops snakes	Hemorrhagic, Procoagulant, Proteolytic and Nephrotoxic	Local abscesses and necrosis, Spontaneous bleeding, DIC, Hypotension	Oliguria/anuria, Hemoglobinuria, Hematuria, ATN, AIN, RCN, GFD
Crotalus snakes	Neurotoxic, Myotoxic and Nephrotoxic	Flaccid paralysis, Myalgia, Rhabdomyolysis	Decrease in GFR, Myoglobinuria, ATN, AIN
Brown spiders (*Loxsosceles*)	Dermonecrotic, Proteolytic, Hemolytic and Nephrotoxic	Local abscesses and necrosis, Hemolysis, Rhabdomyolysis, DIC, Hypotension	Hematuria, Hemoglobinuria, Myoglobinuria, ATN
Africanized Bees (*Apis mellifera*)	Hemolytic, Myotoxic, Cardiotoxic and Nephrotoxic	Allergic reaction (anaphylaxis), Hypotension, Hemolysis, Rhabdomyolysis	Oliguria/anuria,ATN, AIN, Hemoglobinuria, Myoglobinuria
Lonomia caterpillars	Procoagulant, Fibrinogenolytic, Proteolytic and Hemolytic	Ecchymosis, Spontaneous bleeding, DIC, Hemolysis	Hematuria, Hemoglobinuria, ATN

DIC - Disseminated Intravascular Coagulation; ATN - Acute tubular necrosis, AIN - Allergic interstitial nephritis, RCN - Renal Cortical Necrosis, GFD - Glomerular Fibrin Deposition, GFR - Glomerular Filtration Rate.

Table 2. Clinical aspects of venom-induced Acute Kidney Injury (AKI).

Recently, advances in molecular biology, proteomics and transcriptomics, facilitated the isolation of toxins and contributed significantly to the study of their mechanisms of action on renal tissue. In this subsection, we reviewed the renal physiopathological effects of snake and arthropod venoms and their main isolated toxins. Special emphasis was given to experimental studies with venomous animals highly prevalent in Brazil and other regions of Latin America. As in the previous subsection the following animals were included: *Bothrops* and *Crotalus* snakes, the brown spider *Loxosceles*, africanized bees, wasps and the caterpillars of genus *Lonomia*.

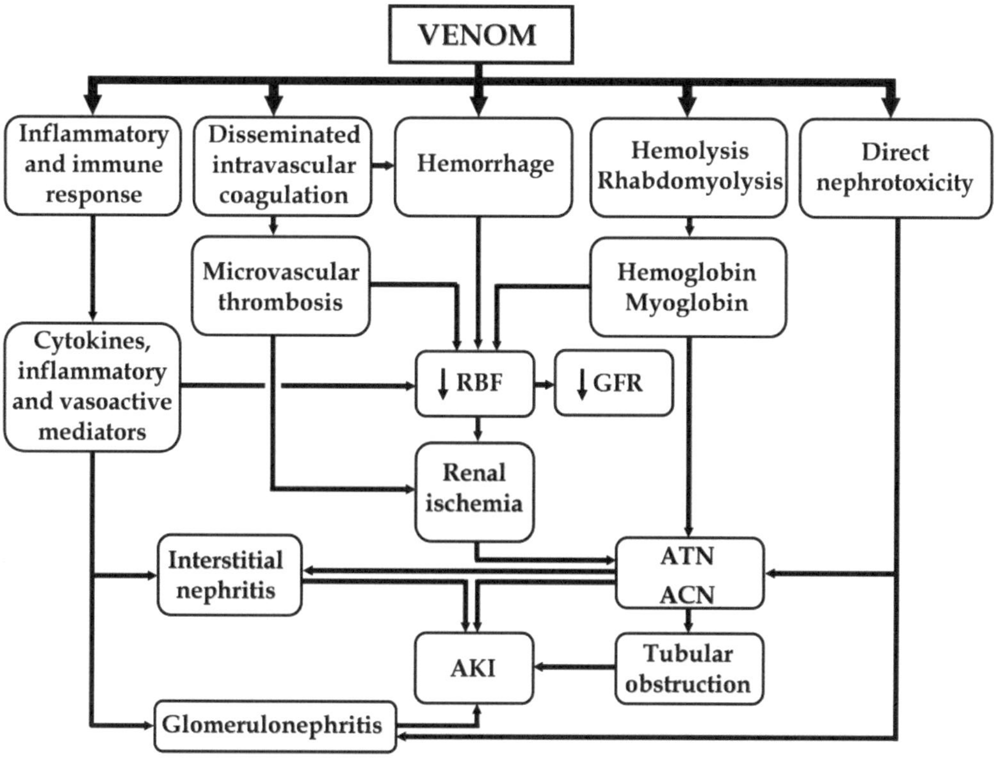

Fig. 1. Schematic summary of pathophysiological phenomena involved in the venom-induced acute kidney injury (AKI). RBF - Renal Blood Flow; GFR - Glomerular Filtratiton Rate; ATN - Acute Tubular Necrosis; ACN - Acute Cortical Necrosis.

4.1 Snake venoms

4.1.1 *Bothrops* venom

The venom of *bothrops* snakes can cause prominent local tissue damage usually characterized by swelling, blistering, hemorrhage and necrosis of skeletal muscle. Such local pathology is mostly due to the venom proteolytic action (Gutiérrez et al., 2006). Snake venom metalloproteinases (SVMPs), phospholipases A_2, , serine proteinases, esterases, L-amino acid oxidases, hyaluronidases, C-type lectins-like and bradykinin-potentiating peptides (BPPs) are the main venom components that acts inducing cellular injury or releasing inflammatory and vasoactive mediators (Warrell, 2010). Transcriptomic and proteomic studies have showed that SVMPs and serine proteinases are the major toxins in the venom, which explained the high local damage and hemorrhage seen in envenomed patients (Table 2) (Cidade et al., 2006; Zelanis et al., 2010). *Bothrops* toxins are also known for their multiple effects on hemostasis. In fact, the venom have thrombin-like enzymes, factor

X and prothrombin activators that are able to directly convert fibrinogen into fibrin (Berger et al., 2008; White, 2005). These actions produce intravascular coagulation and may lead to blood incoagulability by consumption coagulopathy. Systemic inhibition of platelet aggregation and thrombocytopenia are common (Rucavado et al., 2005; Santoro & Sano-Martins, 2004). Moreover, anti-hemostatic principles, such as thrombin and platelet aggregation inhibitors, are also found in *bothrops* venoms (Kamiguti , 2005; Zingali et al., 2005).

Regarding renal function, Boer-Lima et al. (1999) observed that the intravenous injection of *B. moojeni* venom in rats, produced renal tubular disturbances including an increase in proximal and post-proximal fractional excretion of sodium associated with acute tubular necrosis. The glomerular filtration rate decreased significantly, despite the absence of systemic hypotension. Severe morphologic disturbances in the renal glomeruli also occurred. The changes included mesangiolysis, glomerular microaneurysms, and glomerular basement membrane abnormalities. In addition, there was a reduction in the number and width of podocyte pedicels, which caused a reduction in the number of filtration slits. The morphophysiological changes observed in experimental animals also correlated with the levels of proteinuria (Boer-Lima et al., 2002). Similar renal functional alterations were observed after intravenous injection of *B. jararaca* venom into rats. In these animals, differently of human envenomation, *B. jararaca* venom was not able to induce systemic hypotension but significantly reduced the renal plasma flow and increased renal vascular resistance (Burdmann et al., 1993). There was no increase in CK, indicating that rhabdomyolysis is not an important consequence of *B. jararaca* envenomation. However, the venom caused marked fibrinogen consumption and intravascular hemolysis. Indeed, kidney of rats and rabbits envenomed with *B. jararaca* showed an extensive intraglomerular deposition of fibrin and platelets (Burdmann et al., 1993; Santoro & Sano-Martins, 2004). Contrarily to the findings with *B. jararaca* venom, Boer-Lima et al. (1999) did not observed any glomerular fibrin deposition in the *B. moojeni* envenomation. They suggested that the glomerular injury is more likely to be related to structural disorganization of the glomerular capillary tuft, consequent to a direct action of the venom on the mesangial matrix, glomerular basement membrane and podocytes rather than to fibrin deposition in the capillaries.

Studying the kinetic of renal distribution of injected *B. alternatus* venom in rats, Mello et al. (2010) detected the highest venom concentration in renal tissue 30 min post-venom injection. After this time, venom concentration decreased progressively. Venom components were also detected into urine 3, 6 and 24 h post-venom injection. By immunohistochemistry, venom proteins were detected in glomeruli, proximal and distal tubules, and vascular and perivascular tissue, suggesting that toxins bind to kidney structures where they probably exert a direct nephrotoxic action. In accordance to this observation, it was showed that *B. alternatus* venom is cytotoxic to canine renal epithelial cells (MDCK) in culture and causes extensive cytoskeletal alterations inducing impairment of the cell-matrix interaction (Nascimento et al., 2007). Additionally, it was described that *B. jararaca* venom also causes *in vitro* injury of isolated renal proximal tubules and that the *B. moojeni* venom increases cell release of lactate dehydrogenase and decreased cellular uptake of the vital neutral red in MDCK cells (de Castro et al., 2004; Collares-Buzato et al., 2002). Functionally, *B. alternatus* venom induced oliguria, urine acidification, decreased in glomerular filtration rate and hematuria. Morphologically, the venom caused lobulation of the capillary tufts, dilation of Bowman's capsular space, disruption of renal tubule brush border, and fibrosis around glomeruli and proximal tubules that persisted 7 days after envenomation (Linardi et al., 2011; Mello et al., 2010).

Some purified *Bothrops* toxins are able to reproduce the renal effects obtained with whole venom. Studies on the isolated perfused rat kidney have shown that L-amino acid oxidase (Braga et al., 2008), C-type lectins (Braga et al., 2006), phospholipase A2 myotoxins (Barbosa et al., 2005; Evangelista et al., 2010) and thrombin-like enzyme (Braga et al., 2007) from *Bothrops* venoms can alter renal function. The isolated perfused kidney technique also confirmed the direct acute tubular nephrotoxicity of *Bothrops* venoms and showed that platelet activating factor might play a role in some renal functional disturbances such as the decreased in glomerular filtration rate (Monteiro and Fonteles, 1999). However, the systemic injection of baltergin, a purified metalloproteinase from *B. alternatus* venom, only mildly affected the kidney structure. At high doses, baltergin causes congestion, subcapsular hemorrhage and inflammatory infiltrate (Gay et al., 2009). There was no detection of tubular necrosis indicating that different toxins act synergistically to produce the AKI observed in animals treated with whole venom.

4.1.2 *Crotalus* venom

The venom of *Crotalus* rattlesnakes is a complex combination of different enzymes and toxic peptides that mainly display neurotoxic and myotoxic activities (Boldrini-França et al., 2010). Toxins affecting hemostasis, such as thrombin-like enzymes and platelet activators are also found. The main protein families identified by proteomics included phospholipases A_2, serine proteinases, cysteine-rich secretory proteins (CRISP), vascular endothelial growth factor-like molecules (VEGF), L-amino acid oxidases, C-type lectins-like, and snake venom metalloproteinases (SVMP). Crotoxin, a neurotoxic phospholipase A_2, represents more than 60 % of the proteins in the whole venom and is the major component responsible for its neurotoxic and myotoxic effects (Boldrini-França et al., 2010). Additionally, crotoxin also exhibits cardiotoxic and direct nephrotoxic activities. Structurally, crotoxin is a heterodimeric β-neurotoxin that consists of a toxic basic phospholipase A_2 and a nonenzymatic, non-toxic acidic component (crotapotin). Crotapotin potentiates the activity of crotoxin, since it prevents the basic phospholipase subunit binding to non-specific sites (Sampaio et al., 2010; Soares et al., 2001). Crotoxin targets neuromuscular junctions and inhibits the release of acetylcholine, which leads to neuromuscular blockade and muscular and respiratory paralysis. In the muscle tissue, crotoxin causes selective injury of skeletal muscle groups composed of type I and IIa fibers, which are extremely vascularized and rich in myoglobin (Sampaio et al., 2010). Other important toxins are crotamine, convulxin and gyroxin. Crotamine is a toxic peptide with myonecrotic activity (Martins et al., 2002). Convulxin is a C-type lectin-like glycoprotein with high affinity to specific receptors in rabbit and human platelets. Convulxin binds to the putative collagen receptor glycoprotein VI (GPVI) and mediates platelet adhesion, aggregation and intracellular calcium mobilization (Francischetti et al., 1997). Gyroxin is a serine proteinase that displays several activities including the induction of blood coagulation (thrombin-like activity), vasodilation and neurotoxicity (Alves da Silva et al., 2011).

Intraperitoneal injection of *C.d. terrificus* venom in mice increased plasma creatinine and uric acid and caused urinary hypoosmolality. When compared to control groups injected with saline, the incidence of hypercreatinemia and hyperuricemia (plasma values higher than 1.8 mg/dL) occurred in 60 % and 100 % of the experimental animals, respectively (Yamasaki et al., 2008). *Crotalus* experimental envenomation was also associated with significant renal blood flow and glomerular filtration rate decreases and ischemia with consequent acute tubular necrosis. In isolated perfused rat kidneys treated with crude venom or crotoxin, a large amount of protein material was observed in the glomeruli, probably due to a direct toxic effect of the venom on the glomeruli and tubules and/or to an increase in vascular permeability (Monteiro et al., 2001). Prostaglandins and TNF-α release seems to be important since the treatment with indomethacin and pentoxifylline (inhibitors of cyclooxygenase and TNF-α synthesis, respectively) were able to blockade the renal effects induced by supernatant of macrophages activated with *Crotalus* venom (Martins et al., 2003; Martins et al., 2004). Among the main venom components, crotoxin was able to induce significant changes in glomerular filtration rate and electrolyte transport in isolated kidney. Gyroxin caused only mild alteration in renal parameters and convulxin had no effects (Martins et al., 2002).

Rhabdomyolysis is a well-known cause of AKI and is commonly observed in envenomed patients and envenomed experimental animals. Myoglobin toxicity has been related to renal vasoconstriction, intraluminal cast formation and direct heme-protein cytotoxicity. Myoglobin can contribute to renal vasoconstriction by directly binding to nitric oxide (NO). Thus, acting as NO scavenging molecules, heme-proteins (including myoglobin or hemoglobin) lead to renal hypoperfusion, reductions in the storage of ATP, ischemia and tissue injury (Zager, 1996). Intraluminal casts are formed due to the precipitation of myoglobin inside the renal tubules, forming obstructive casts. Precipitated myoglobin also can be degraded resulting in the release of free iron and heme. Once released, free iron and heme contribute to renal injury by generate reactive oxygen species (ROS) and lipid peroxidation (Khan, 2009; Zager, 1996). Indeed, Yamasaki et al. (2008), showed an increase of oxidized glutathione/reduced glutathione ratio (GSSG/GSH) in renal tissue during *Crotalus* envenomation. This data indicates a rise in the ROS generation by consumption of reduced glutathione (GSH) and production of oxidized glutathione (GSSH) which are the main antioxidant and oxido-reducing agents, respectively. Confirming the participation of ROS in *Crotalus* induced renal injury, envenomed animals treated with lipoic acid (an antioxidant molecule) had their GSSG/GSH ratios normalized when compared to control groups (Alegre et al., 2010). In addition to deleterious effects of obstructive myoglobin casts formation, the high levels of uric acid found in envenomed animals also contribute to tubular obstruction (Yamasaki et al., 2008). Marked hyperuricemia is known to cause AKI by supersaturation, crystallisation and deposition of crystals inside renal tubules (acute urate nephropathy). Moreover, experimental hyperuricemia causes renal vasoconstriction and soluble uric acid has been shown to inhibit endothelial NO bioavailability (Ejaz et al., 2007). Recently, it was observed that systemic inhibition of uric acid synthesis, by allopurinol treatment, significantly reduced lethality rate, normalized GSSG/GSH ratio and ameliorate the renal histopathological changes. Thus, uric acid also seems to have an important role in renal pathophysiology of *Crotalus* envenomation (Frezzatti & Silveira, 2011).

4.2 *Loxosceles* venom

The bites of brown spiders (*Loxosceles* genus) led to several clinical manifestations such as necrotic skin degeneration and gravitational spread at the bite site, renal injury and hematological disturbances. Several studies concerning the structural and biological roles of various venom components have shown the complex nature of these venomous secretions. Likewise, the venom of *Loxosceles* spiders is a complex mixture of protein-based toxins with a molecular mass profile ranging from 5 to 40 kDa. The main components belong to the classes of phospholipases D (or dermonecrotic toxins), serine proteinases, venom allergens, hyaluronidases, astacin-like metalloproteinases and insecticidal peptides (Gremski et al., 2010). Dermonecrotic toxins and astacin-like metalloproteinases are considered the major components responsible for the clinical profile observed in envenomed victims (Table 2) (da Silva et al., 2004). In fact, a transcriptomic study indicated that phospholipases D and astacin-like metalloproteinases represent 20.2 % and 22.6 % of total toxin-encoding transcripts, respectively. Other toxins also important to envenomation, such as serine proteinases, venom allergens and hyaluronidases represent the minority of encoding transcripts (Gremski et al., 2010).

Among all the toxins found in *Loxosceles* spider venom, dermonecrotic toxin is undoubtedly the component most investigated and characterized. This toxin is able to reproduce the major biological effects induced by whole venom. It is involved with the development of dermonecrotic lesions and can trigger neutrophil migration, complement system activation, cytokine and chemokine release, platelet aggregation, lysis of red blood cells, among other effects (Abdulkader et al., 2008; da Silva et al., 2004). Dermonecrotic toxin comprises a family of toxins with different related isoforms that have biological, amino acid and immunological similarities which are found in several *Loxosceles* species. Only in *L. intermedia* venom, many isoforms were described being 9 out of them already expressed as recombinant proteins (Gremski et al., 2010). *Loxosceles* dermonecrotic toxins belong to phospholipases D (30–35 kDa) class of enzymes which was primarily designated as sphingomyelinases D due to their ability to convert sphingomyelin to choline and ceramide 1-phosphate (N-acylsphingosine1-phosphate). As some *Loxosceles* sphingomyelinases D have broad substrate specificity, being able to hydrolyze not only sphingophospholipids but also lysoglycerophospholipids, they are now classified as phospholipases D (Lee and Lynch, 2005). Due to sequence, structural and biochemical differences these toxins are grouped in two classes and their structures and substrate specificities have been recently elucidated (de Giuseppe et al., 2011; Murakami et al., 2005). Other important components of *Loxosceles* venom are the metalloproteinases. The enzymes have molecular weights ranging from 20 to 35 kDa displaying gelatinolytic, fibronectinolytic and fibrinogenolytic activities. They are zinc endopeptidases homologous to the astacin family of metalloproteinases from the crayfish, *Astacus astacus*. The *Loxosceles* astacin-like metalloproteinases possess a digestive function used to initiate the degradation of prey molecules, facilitating the posterior ingestion process (Trevizan-Silva et al., 2010). Furthermore, these enzymes have an important role in the pathogenesis observed in envenomation, particularly inducing hemorrhage into the dermis, injury of blood vessels, imperfect platelet adhesion, and the defective wound healing observed in some cases. Likewise, these metalloproteases can also render tissue structures more permeable, facilitating other noxious toxins to spread throughout the body of victims (Veiga et al., 2000; Veiga et al., 2001**b**).

The nephrotoxic effect of the *L. intermidia* spider venom was demonstrated experimentally in mice exposed to the whole venom (Luciano et al., 2004). Histhopathological analysis showed morphological renal alterations including hyalinization of proximal and distal tubules, erythrocytes in Bowman's space, glomerular collapse, tubule epithelial cell blebs and vacuoles, interstitial edema, and deposition of a protein-rich material inside the Bowman's space and tubule lumen. Morphometric analysis showed that 75–80 % of the kidney area was affected by the venom and no glomerular or tubule leukocyte infiltration was described, suggesting that the involvement of inflammatory process is not important to renal injury in this type of envenomation. Despite the presence of erythrocytes and protein deposits in glomerular and tubular structures, no signs of intravascular hemolysis or hemoglobin were detected in envenomed animals. Supporting the evidence that *L. intermidia* venom has toxins with direct nephrotoxicity, confocal microscopy studies with antibodies against venom proteins were able to show direct binding of toxins to renal structures. Venom proteins were detected in glomerular and tubular epithelial cells and in renal basement membranes. Toxins with molecular weights of 30 kDa were also identified in renal tissue extracts by immunoblotting (Luciano et al., 2004). One of these venom proteins that can bind to the kidney tissue is the dermonecrotic toxin. Chaim et al. (2006), injecting the recombinant dermonecrotic toxin in mice, found glomerular edema and tubular necrosis without signs of inflammatory response. Additionally, the dermonecrotic toxin was detected in kidney tissue and induced changes in renal function such as urine alkalinization, hematuria and elevation of blood urea nitrogen levels. The treatment of renal epithelial cells (MDCK) with recombinant dermonecrotic toxin also caused morphological alterations and reduced the cell viability, confirming its direct citotoxicity (Chaim et al., 2006). Both effects upon renal structures *in vivo* and renal cells *in vitro* were dependent of the phospholipase D catalytic activity, since a mutated toxin without phospholipase activity showed no nephrotoxic effect (Kusma et al., 2008). Another mechanism involved in AKI induced by *Loxosceles* venom is the renal vasoconstriction and rhabdomyolysis. Recently, it was reported that *L. gaucho* caused a sharp and significant drop in glomerular filtration rate, renal blood flow and urinary output and increased renal vascular resistance in rats (Lucato-Júnior et al., 2011). In this model, the authors also found deposits of myoglobin in tubular cells and degenerative lesions indicative of an ischemic process (Lucato-Júnior et al., 2011).

4.3 Bee and wasp venoms

Bee and wasp venoms are composed of a mixture of proteins, peptides, and small molecules, which are related to different mechanisms of envenomation. In the Africanized bee (*Apis mellifera*) venom the most important components are melittin and phospholipase A2. Melittin is a highly toxic peptide and the most abundant component of bee venom comprising about 50 % of its dry weight. This peptide is able to disrupt biological membranes, producing many effects on living cells (Fletcher et al., 1993). Melittin has antibacterial activity, induces voltage-gated channel formation and can also produce micellization of phospholipids bilayers due to its membrane-interacting effect. This peptide is responsible for the direct hemolytic effect of *Apis* venom (Dempsey, 1990; Terra et al., 2007). The enzyme phospholipase A2 represents approximately 11 % of whole venom and acts synergically with melittin. Once melittin has disrupted the membrane, phospholipase

A2 cleaves bonds in the fatty acid portion of the bilipid membrane layer (Vetter et al., 1999; Lee et al., 2001). In association, melittin and phospholipase A2, can act on erythrocytes, myocytes, hepatocytes, fibroblasts, mast cells, and leukocytes (Abdulkader et al., 2008; Fletcher et al., 1993; Habermann, 1972). Additionally, bee venom also has hyaluronidase (an enzyme that disrupts the hyaluronic acid in connective-tissue matrix), apamin (a neurotoxin), mast cell degranulating peptide (a peptide that releases histamine from mast cells) and other small molecules such as histamine, dopamine, and noradrenaline. Among all *Apis mellifera* venom components the main allergens are melittin, phospholipase A2 and hyaluronidase (Vetter et al., 1999). In wasp venoms the components are active amines (serotonin, histamine, tyramine, catecholamines); wasp kinins (similar in composition to bradykinin), which are mostly responsible for pain; and histamine-releasing peptides, which are responsible for the inflammatory response. The major allergens identified in wasp venoms are phospholipase A1, a hyaluronidase and a serine-protease (Pantera et al., 2003; Vetter et al., 1999).

Despite the current knowledge on the composition of wasp venoms, little is known about the participation of its components, and even the whole venom, on the AKI observed in envenomed patients. On the other hand, the mechanisms of bee venom-induced AKI have been more explored in experimental models *in vivo* and *in vitro*. In the case of bee envenomation, the experimental injection of venom in rats caused a significant and early reduction in glomerular filtration rate and diuresis and an increase in plasma creatinine levels (dos Reis et al., 1997; Grisotto et al., 2006). Tubular alterations such as increased fractional sodium and potassium excretions and a reduced water transport through collecting tubules, were also described (dos Reis et al., 1997). The early glomerular filtration rate reduction was concomitant with marked cortical and medullary renal blood flow decrease (Grisotto et al., 2006). Neither hypertension and hypotension nor intravascular hemolysis were detected in experimental models. Despite of the absence of hemolysis, rhabdomyolysis was present with massive myoglobin deposition in the lumen of the tubules as well as into the tubular cells (dos Reis et al., 1997; Grisotto et al., 2006). The injection of purified melittin or phospholipase A2 also induced rhabdomyolysis, due to their capacity to disrupt the membranes of myocytes (Ownby et al., 1997). Additionally, *in vitro* studies have been demonstrated that bee venom is citotoxic to cultured isolated proximal tubule cells (Grisotto et al., 2006). Histological analysis showed acute tubular necrosis mainly in cortex and outer medulla, and cast formation in the distal and collecting tubules (dos Reis et al., 1998). These degenerative lesions observed in AKI induced by the bee venom have been associated with the ischemic process induced by melittin, phospholipase A2 and histamine (Abdulkader et al., 2008; Grisotto et al., 2006). Indeed, melittin and phospholipase A2 may be related to impaired renal blood flow by causing direct vasoconstriction, smooth muscle cell contraction, increased renal renin secretion and release of vasoconstrictor eicosanoids and catecholamines. Histamine and the mast cell degranulating peptides present in the venom also play a role in renal blood flow decrease, since histamine can directly induce vascular changes (Cerne et al., 2010; Churchill et al., 1990).

4.4 *Lonomia* venom

Caterpillars of the species *L. obliqua* are well known in Southern Brazil by causing a severe hemorrhagic syndrome characterized by coagulation disorders, AKI and generalized hemorrhage. The venom is composed of several active principles, including procoagulant and fibrinolytic activities (Pinto et al., 2010). Even though many studies have been performed with toxic secretions from *L. obliqua* aiming a better elucidation of the hemorrhagic syndrome resulting from this envenomation, few active principles have been purified from the venom and fully characterized so far. Thus, most of the molecules identified in this caterpillar have been characterized as putative enzymes and other proteins based solely on cDNA and amino acid sequences obtained by transcriptomic and proteomic methods (Ricci-Silva et al., 2008; Veiga et al., 2005). Through these techniques, the major protein found in *Lonomia* is a biliverdin-binding protein of the lipocalin family, which is mainly concentrated in the bristles and plays an important role in the caterpillar's camouflage behavior. Along with the lipocalin and other housekeeping proteins, *L. obliqua*'s integument, hemolymph and bristles produce and store a variety of active principles. Among these proteins, the most abundant ones are serine proteases and their inhibitors (serpins) in the integument, and serine proteases, kininogen and lectins in the bristles. Besides these molecules, cysteine proteinases, phospholipase A2, cystatins, Kazal-type inhibitors and other protease inhibitors are also found. Serine proteases are the most relevant protein family when considering their potential of interfering with blood coagulation. Moreover, serine proteases are an expressive group, representing 16.7 % and 25 % of the clusters derived from tegument and bristle transcriptome, respectively (Veiga et al., 2005). This protein group presents coagulation factors-like activities, so it is expected that these enzymes participate in the generation of thrombin, by activation of factor X and prothrombin (Berger et al., 2010**a;** Veiga et al., 2003), and in the activation of the fibrinolytic system, contributing directly and indirectly to fibrinogen degradation (Pinto et al., 2006) and resulting in the hemorrhagic disorder. In fact, proteases with fibrinogenolytic, prothrombin and factor X activating activities have been purified and characterized in this venom (Alvarez-Flores et al., 2006; Pinto et al., 2004; Reis et al., 2006). The phospholipase A2 enzyme also has a function in envenomation. This enzyme was isolated and characterized as the major component responsible to the *in vitro* and *in vivo* hemolytic activity of *L. obliqua* venom (Seibert et al., 2004; Seibert et al., 2006). Additionally, the phospholipase A2 seems to be involved in platelet aggregation inducing activity present in the venom (Berger et al., 2010**b**). Lectins, particularly c-type lectins, are a relatively well-studied group of proteins in snake venoms that may exert an additional function in hemostasis modulation by interacting with coagulations factors and/or platelet receptors. Three lectin clusters were found in the bristle cDNA library with homology to many snake venom lectins being then another important candidate contributing to the hemorrhagic disorder (Veiga et al., 2005).

Although AKI is the leading cause of death in *L. obliqua* envenomation, the mechanisms involved in kidney disorders are poorly understood. In contrast to hemostatic disturbances, to date, there is no experimental studies describing the renal effects of *L. obliqua* venom. Current knowledge is based only on a few case reports in which hematuria, high levels of serum creatinine and acute tubular necrosis are described as the main features of *L. obliqua* induced AKI. Due to this lack of knowledge, nowadays we are focused on the investigation of the effects of *L. obliqua* venom on renal function in rats. Preliminary results, indicate that subcutaneous injection of *L. obliqua* bristle extract caused severe hematuria with the presence of intact erythrocytes and leukocytes in urinary sediment (Berger et al., unpublished data). Envenomed animals also show proteinuria and significant changes in glomerular filtration rate and tubular electrolytic transport (Berger et al., unpublished data). Currently, the contribution of intravascular coagulation, deposits of hemoglobin in renal tubules and hemodynamic changes are under investigation.

5. Diagnosis and management of acute kidney injury in snake and arthropod envenomation

The early intravenous administration of animal-derived antivenoms is the only specific treatment against snake and arthropod envenomations. Antivenoms are concentrated of immunoglobulins (usually pepsin-refined F(ab')2 fragment of whole IgG) purified from the plasma of a horse or sheep that has been immunized with the venoms of one or more species of venomous animal (WHO, 2010**a**). The preparation of antivenoms is expensive and technically demanding. Around the world different manufacturers, which include public and private laboratories of diverse sizes and strengths, are able to produce the antivenoms (Gutiérrez et al., 2010; Williams et al., 2010). Some of them are small facilities, mostly located in public institutions, which manufacture for the needs of specific countries. Others are larger laboratories that manufacture and distribute antivenoms throughout various countries or regions. Although some countries or regions manufacture enough antivenom for their national and regional needs, as in Europe, USA, Brazil, Central America, Mexico, Australia, Thailand and Japan, in other parts of the world, specially in some regions of Africa, there are very few antivenom producers (Gutiérrez et al., 2010). In Brazil, three main Institutions are responsible for production of antivenoms: Instituto Butantan, Fundação Ezequiel Dias and Hospital Vital Brasil. The manufacture is government-subsidized and the antivenom is usually provided free to the patients. However, failures in the distribution of antivenoms to places where they are needed still contribute to the maintenance of high mortality rates (Table 1). In some instances, antivenoms are held in the main cities, where envenomations are rare, instead of being distributed to peripheral health clinics in rural areas where the accidents are frequent. This reflects defective distribution planning which is associated with a lack of coordination between those who understand the epidemiological pattern of the disease and those responsible for the antivenom distribution. Also, inadequate storage and transportation of antivenoms may result in physical destruction of vials and ampoules (e.g. by freezing of liquid antivenom) (WHO, 2010**a**). Besides the inadequate supply, distribution and accessibility to safe and effective antivenoms, another major issue is the lack of trained of health workers on how to use these products and how to conduct appropriate clinical management of medical emergencies. In fact, it is estimated that in Brazil in 2009, 37% of accidents with scorpions and 9% of accidents with spiders received inadequate treatment with antivenom, mainly because the health authorities are uninformed of the treatment protocols (Boletim eletrônico epidemiológico, 2010).

The treatment with antivenom is indicated in moderate and severe cases when systemic signs of envenomation are observed. In general, patients with hemostatic abnormalities, neurotoxic signs, cardiovascular abnormalities, AKI, hemoglobinuria and myoglobinuria should receive antivenom therapy (WHO, 2010**a**). In these cases the time elapsed between the occurrence of the accident and administration of a correct dose of antivenom is decisive for a sucessful therapy. It was demonstrated that the time interval between the accident and administration of the antivenom of more than 2 hours was associated with the development of AKI, as well as with the risk of death or permanent injuries after *Bothrops* and *Crotalus* envenomations (Otero et al., 2002; Pinho et al., 2005). Although the correct use of antivenom is an effective form of treatment, the sorotherapy is also associated with the occurrence of severe adverse effects. The most serious adverse effect is anaphylactic reactions. Clinical features such as urticaria, itching, fever, tachycardia, vomiting, abdominal colic, headache, bronchospasm, hypotension and angioedema have been described after antivenom treatment (Fan et al., 1999; Ministério da Saúde, 2001). The incidence of adverse effects depends on the quality, dose and speed of intravenous injection or infusion. With antivenoms of good quality profile, there is a low incidence (less than 10%) of generally mild adverse reactions, mostly urticaria and itching. However, for products containing contaminant proteins, the incidence of such reactions may be as high as 85 %, including potentially life-threatening systemic disturbances such as hypotension and bronchospasm (WHO, 2007). Thus the adverse effects are directly associated with lack of good manufacturing practices adopted by laboratories that manufacture antivenoms. Recently, in an attempt to improve the quality of antivenom production the WHO established the guidelines for production, control and regulation of snake antivenom immunoglobulins. These guidelines provide detailed information on the recommended steps for antivenom manufacture and control (WHO, 2010**b**).

A number of additional interventions besides antivenom may be necessary to restore renal function in patients who developed AKI. Special attention should be given to hypotension, shock, electrolyte balance and maintenance of an adequate state of hydration. An urinary flow of 30 to 40 mL/h/kg is recommended for adults and 1 to 3 mL/h/kg for children to prevent AKI after snake envenomations (Ministério da Saúde, 2001; Pinho et al., 2008). Patients presenting oliguria or anuria, despite of fluid administration, are usually treated with intravenous furosemide or mannitol (WHO, 2010**a**). In these cases, a higher urinary flow may decrease the expousure of tubular cells to venom components and myoglobin or hemoglobin, which result in injury attenuation and prevention of tubular lumen obstruction (Zager, 1996). Cases that are unresponsive to fluid intake and diuretics are referred to renal units for dialysis (Pinho et al., 2008). Early alkalinization of urine by sodium bicarbonate in patients with myoglobinuria or hemoglobinuria is also recommended, because in the presence of acidic urine, myoglobin and uric acid precipitate and form obstructive cast (Khan, 2009).

6. Conclusion

Envenomation by different venomous snakes and arthropods is a neglected disease that afflicts the most impoverished inhabitants of rural areas in tropical developing countries. In this chapter, we reviewed some important aspects related to epidemiology, prevalence, clinical manifestations, pathophysiology and treatment of venom-induced AKI, which is one of the most significant and lethal effect of animal venoms. Despite of actual knowledge discussed here, several aspects involving the renal manifestations remain still unclear. Thus, further research are needed to cover the following key points: (i) biochemical composition of different animal venoms and their individual contribution to renal injury; (ii) renal pathological mechanisms induced by some specific venoms that are still unexplored; (iii) discovery of new and more specific therapeutic alternatives to treat envenomation cases and (iv) improvement in the production, distribution and availability of the antivenoms currently used.

7. Acknowledgments

The authors are grateful to Coordenação de Aperfeiçoamento de Pessoal de Nível Superior, Ministério da Educação, Brasil (CAPES-MEC) and Conselho Nacional de Desenvolvimento Científico e Tecnológico, Ministério da Ciência e Tecnologia, Brasil (CNPq-MCT) for funding and fellowships.

8. References

Abella, H.B; Marques, M.G.B.; Silva, K.R.L.M.; Rossoni, M.G. & Torres, J.B. (2006). Acidentes com lagartas do gênero Lonomia registrados no Centro de Informação Toxicológica do Rio Grande do Sul no período de 1997 a 2005, In: Nicolella, A. (Ed.), *Toxicovogilância - toxicologia clínica: dados e indicadores selecionados*. Secretaria da Saúde. Fundação Estadual de Produção e Pesquisa em Saúde. Centro de Informação Toxicológica, Porto Alegre, pp. 29-34.

Abdulkader, R.C.; Barbaro, K.C.; Barros, E.J. & Burdmann, E.A. (2008). Nephrotoxicity of insect and spider venoms in Latin America. *Seminars in Nephrology*. Vol.28, No.4, pp. 373-82.

Alegre, V.S.; Barone, J.M.; Yamasaki, S.C.; Zambotti-Villela, L. & Silveira, P.F. (2010). Lipoic acid effects on renal function, aminopeptidase activities and oxidative stress in *Crotalus durissus terrificus* envenomation in mice. *Toxicon*. Vol.56, No.3, pp.402-10.

Alvarez-Flores, M.P.; Fritzen, M.; Reis, C.V. & Chudzinski-Tavassi, A.M. (2006). Losac, a factor X activator from *Lonomia obliqua* bristle extract: its role in the pathophysiological mechanisms and cell survival. *Biochemical and Biophysical Research Communications*. Vol. 343, No. 4, pp. 1216-23.

Alves da Silva, J.A.; Oliveira, K.C. & Camillo, M.A. (2011). Gyroxin increases blood-brain barrier permeability to Evans blue dye in mice. *Toxicon*. Vol.57, No.1, pp.162-7.

Amaral, C.F.; de Rezende, N.A.; da Silva, O.A.; Ribeiro, M.M.; Magalhães, R.A.; dos Reis, R.J.; Carneiro, J.G. & Castro, J.R. (1986). Acute kidney failure secondary to ophidian bothropic and crotalid accidents. Analysis of 63 cases. *Revista do Instituto de Medicina Tropical de Sao Paulo*. Vol.28, No.4, pp. 220-7.

Arocha-Piñango, C.L.; Marval, E. & Guerrero, B. (2000). *Lonomia* genus caterpillar toxins: biochemical aspects. *Biochimie*. Vol.82, No.9-10, pp.937-42.

Azevedo-Marques, M.M.; Cupo, P.; Coimbra, T.M.; Hering, S.E.; Rossi, M.A. & Laure, C.J. (1985). Myonecrosis, myoglobinuria and acute renal failure induced by South American rattlesnake (*Crotalus durissus terrificus*) envenomation in Brazil. *Toxicon*. Vol.23, No.4, pp. 631-6.

Azevedo-Marques, M.M.; Hering, S.E. & Cupo, P. (1987). Evidence that *Crotalus durissus terrificus* (South American rattlesnake) envenomation in humans causes myolysis rather than hemolysis. *Toxicon*. Vol.25, No.11, pp. 1163-8.

Barbosa, P.S.; Martins, A.M.; Havt, A.; Toyama, D.O.; Evangelista, J.S.; Ferreira, D.P.; Joazeiro, P.P.; Beriam, L.O.; Toyama, M.H.; Fonteles, M.C. & Monteiro, H.S. (2005).

Renal and antibacterial effects induced by myotoxin I and II isolated from *Bothrops jararacussu* venom. *Toxicon*. Vol.15, No.4, pp 376-86.

Berger, M.; Pinto, A.F. & Guimarães, J.A. (2008). Purification and functional characterization of bothrojaractivase, a prothrombin-activating metalloproteinase isolated from *Bothrops jararaca* snake venom. *Toxicon*. Vol.51, No.4, pp. 488-501.

Berger, M.; Reck-Jr, J.; Terra, R.M.; Pinto, A.F.; Termignoni, C. & Guimarães, J.A. (2010a) *Lonomia obliqua* caterpillar envenomation causes platelet hypoaggregation and blood incoagulability in rats. *Toxicon*. Vol.55, No.1, pp. 33-44.

Berger, M.; Reck-Jr, J.; Terra, R.M.; Beys da Silva, W.O; Santi, L.; Pinto, A.F.; Vainstein, M.H.; Termignoni, C. & Guimarães, J.A. (2010b). *Lonomia obliqua* venomous secretion induces human platelet adhesion and aggregation. *Journal of Thrombosis and Thrombolysis*. Vol.30, No.3, pp. 300-10.

Boer-Lima, P.A.; Gontijo, J.A. & da Cruz-Höfling, M.A. (1999). Histologic and functional renal alterations caused by *Bothrops moojeni* snake venom in rats. *American Journal of Tropical Medicine and Hygiene*. Vol.61, No.5, pp. 698-706.

Boer-Lima, P.A.; Gontijo, J.A. & Cruz-Höfling, M.A. (2002). *Bothrops moojeni* snake venom-induced renal glomeruli changes in rat. *American Journal of Tropical Medicine and Hygiene*. Vol.67, No.2, pp. 217-22.

Boldrini-França, J.; Corrêa-Netto, C.; Silva, M.M.; Rodrigues, R.S.; De La Torre, P.; Pérez, A.; Soares, A.M.; Zingali, R.B.; Nogueira, R.A.; Rodrigues, V.M.; Sanz, L. & Calvete, J.J. (2010). Snake venomics and antivenomics of *Crotalus durissus* subspecies from Brazil: assessment of geographic variation and its implication on snakebite management. *Journal of Proteomics*. Vol.73, No.9, pp. 1758-76.

Boletim eletrônico epidemiológico, 2010. Secretaria de Vigilância em Saúde/Ministério da Saúde (SVS/MS), Brasil. Available from: www.portal.saude.gov.br/portal/arquivos/pdf/ano10_n02_sit_epidemiol_zoonoses_br.pdf

Braga, M.D.; Martins, A.M.; Amora, D.N.; de Menezes, D.B.; Toyama, M.H.; Toyama, D.O.; Marangoni, S.; Barbosa, P.S.; de Sousa Alves, R.; Fonteles, M.C. & Monteiro, H.S. (2006) Purification and biological effects of C-type lectin isolated from *Bothrops insularis* venom. *Toxicon*. Vol.47, No.8, pp. 859-67.

Braga, M.D.; Martins, A.M.; de Menezes, D.B.; Barbosa, P.S.; Evangelista, J.S.; Toyama, M.H.; Toyama, D.O.; Fonteles, M.C. & Monteiro, H.S. (2007). Purification and biological activity of the thrombin-like substance isolated from *Bothrops insularis* venom. *Toxicon*. Vol.49, No.3, pp. 329-38.

Braga, M.D.; Martins, A.M.; Amora, D.N.; de Menezes, D.B.; Toyama, M.H.; Toyama, D.O.; Marangoni, S.; Alves, C.D.; Barbosa, P.S.; de Sousa Alves, R.; Fonteles, M.C. & Monteiro HS. (2008). Purification and biological effects of L-amino acid oxidase isolated from *Bothrops insularis* venom. *Toxicon*. Vol.51, No.2, pp. 199-207.

Burdmann, E.A.; Woronik, V.; Prado, E.B.; Abdulkader, R.C.; Saldanha, L.B.; Barreto, O.C. & Marcondes, M. (1993). Snakebite-induced acute renal failure: an experimental model. *American Journal of Tropical Medicine and Hygiene*. Vol.48, No.1, pp. 82-8.

Burdmann, E.A.; Antunes, I.; Saldanha, L.B. & Abdulkader, R.C. (1996). Severe acute renal failure induced by the venom of *Lonomia* caterpillars. *Clinical Nephrololgy*. Vol.46, No.5, pp. 337-9.

Cerne, K.; Kristan, K.C.; Budihna, M.V. & Stanovnik, L. (2010). Mechanisms of changes in coronary arterial tone induced by bee venom toxins. *Toxicon*. Vol.56, No.3, pp. 305-12.

Chaim, O.M.; Sade, Y.B.; da Silveira, R.B.; Toma, L.; Kalapothakis, E.; Chávez-Olórtegui, C.; Mangili, O.C.; Gremski, W.; von Dietrich, C.P.; Nader, H.B. & Veiga S.S. (2006). Brown spider dermonecrotic toxin directly induces nephrotoxicity. *Toxicology and Applied Pharmacology*. Vol.211, No.1, pp. 64-77.

Chao, Y.W.; Yang, A.H.; Ng, Y.Y. & Yang, W.C. (2004). Acute interstitial nephritis and pigmented tubulopathy in a patient after wasp stings. *American Journal of Kidney Diseases*. Vol.43, No.2, pp. 15-19.

Chippaux, J.P. (1998). Snake-bites: appraisal of the global situation. *Bulletin of the World Health Organization*. Vol.76, No.5, pp. 515-24.

Chippaux, J.P. & Goyffon, M. (2008). Epidemiology of scorpionism: a global appraisal. *Acta Tropica*. Vol.107, No.2, pp. 71-9.

Chippaux, J.P. (2011). Estimate of the burden of snakebites in sub-Saharan Africa: a meta-analytic approach. *Toxicon*. Vol.57, No.4, pp. 586-99.

Churchill, P.C.; Rossi, N.F.; Churchill, M.C. & Ellis, V.R. (1990). Effect of melittin or renin and prostaglandin E2 release from rat renal cortical slices. *Journal of Physiolology*. Vol.428, pp. 233–241.

Cidade, D.A.; Simão, T.A.; Dávila, A.M.; Wagner, G.; Junqueira-de-Azevedo, I.L.; Ho, P.L.; Bon, C.; Zingali, R.B. & Albano, R.M. (2006). *Bothrops jararaca* venom gland transcriptome: analysis of the gene expression pattern. *Toxicon*. Vol.48, No.4, pp. 437-61.

Collares-Buzato, C.B.; de Paula Le Sueur, L. & da Cruz-Höfling, M.A. (2002). Impairment of the cell-to-matrix adhesion and cytotoxicity induced by *Bothrops moojeni* snake venom in cultured renal tubular epithelia. *Toxicology and Applied Pharmacolology*. Vol.181, No.2, pp. 124-32.

Cologna, C.T.; Marcussi, S.; Giglio, J.R.; Soares, A.M. & Arantes, E.C. (2009). *Tityus serrulatus* scorpion venom and toxins: an overview. *Protein and Peptide Letters*. Vol.16, No.8, pp. 920-32.

Daher, E.F.; Silva-Junior, G.B.; Bezerra, G.P.; Pontes, L.B.; Martins, A.M.C. & Guimarães, J.A. (2003). Acute renal failure after massive honeybee stings. *Revista do Instituto de Medicina Tropical de Sao Paulo*. Vol.45, No.1, pp. 45-50.

da Silva, P.H.; da Silveira, R.B.; Appel, M.H.; Mangili, O.C.; Gremski, W. & Veiga, S.S. (2004). Brown spiders and loxoscelism. *Toxicon*. Vol.44, No.7, pp. 693-709.

de Castro, I.; Burdmann, E.A.; Seguro, A.C. & Yu, L. (2004). *Bothrops* venom induces direct renal tubular injury: role for lipid peroxidation and prevention by antivenom. *Toxicon*. Vol.43, No.7, pp. 833-9.

de Giuseppe, P.O.; Ullah, A.; Silva, D.T.; Gremski, L.H.; Wille, A.C.; Chaves-Moreira, D.; Ribeiro, A.S.; Chaim, O.M.; Murakami, M.T.; Veiga, S.S. & Arni, R.K. (2011). Structure of a novel class II phospholipase D: catalytic cleft is modified by a disulphide bridge. *Biochemical and Biophysical Research Communications*. Vol. 409, No.4, pp. 622-7.

Deitch, E.A. (1992). Multiple organ failure. Pathophysiology and potential future therapy. *Annals of Surgery*. Vol. 216, No. 2, pp. 117-34.

Dempsey, C.E. (1990). The actions of melittin on membranes. *Biochimica et Biophysica Acta*. Vol.1031, No.2, pp. 143-61.

dos Reis, M.A.; Costa, R.S.; Coimbra, T.M.; Dantas, M. & Gomes, U.A. (1997). Renal changes induced by envenomation with Africanized bee venom in female Wistar rats. *Kidney and Blood Pressure Research*. Vol. 20, No. 4, pp. 271-7.

dos Reis MA.; Costa, R.S.; Coimbra, T.M.; Teixeira, V.P. (1998). Acute renal failure in experimental envenomation with Africanized bee venom. *Renal Failure*. Vol.20, No.1, pp. 39-51.

Duarte, A.C.; Caovilla, J.J.; Lorini, J.D.; Mantovani, G.; Sumida, J.; Manfre, P.C.; Silveira, R.C. & de Moura, S.P. (1990). Insuficiência renal aguda por acidentes com lagartas. *Jornal Brasileiro de Nefrologia*. Vol.12, pp. 184-7.

Ejaz, A.A.; Mu, W.; Kang, D.H.; Roncal, C.; Sautin, Y.Y.; Henderson, G.; Tabah-Fisch, I.; Keller, B.; Beaver, T.M.; Nakagawa, T. & Johnson, R.J. (2007). Could uric acid have a role in acute renal failure. *Clinical Journal of the American Society of Nephrology*. Vol.2, No.1, pp. 16-21.

Evangelista, I.L.; Martins, A.M.; Nascimento, N.R.; Havt, A.; Evangelista, J.S.; de Norões, T.B.; Toyama, M.H.; Diz-Filho, E.B.; Toyama, O.; Fonteles, M.C. & Monteiro, H.S. (2010) Renal and cardiovascular effects of *Bothrops marajoensis* venom and phospholipase A2. *Toxicon*. Vol. 55, No. 6, pp. 1061-70.

Fan, H.W.; Marcopito, L.F.; Cardoso, J.L.; França, F.O.; Malaque, C.M.; Ferrari, R.A.; Theakston, R.D. & Warrell, D.A. (1999). Sequential randomised and double blind trial of promethazine prophylaxis against early anaphylactic reactions to antivenom for *Bothrops* snakebites. *British Medical Journal (BMJ)*. Vol. 318, pp. 1451–1453.

Fan, H.W.; Cardoso, J.L.; Olmos, R.D.; Almeida, F.J.; Viana, R.P. & Martinez, A.P. (1998). Hemorrhagic syndrome and acute renal failure in a pregnant woman after contact with *Lonomia* caterpillars: a case report. *Revista do Instituto de Medicina Tropical de São Paulo*. Vol. 40, No. 2, pp. 119-20.

Fletcher, J.E. & Jiang, M.S. (1993). Possible mechanisms of action of cobra snake venom cardiotoxins and bee venom melittin. *Toxicon*. Vol. 31, No. 6, pp. 669-95.

França, F.O.; Benvenuti, L.A.; Fan, H.W.; dos Santos, D.R.; Hain, S.H.; Picchi-Martins, F.R.; Cardoso, J.L.; Kamiguti, A.S.; Theakston, R.D. & Warrell, D.A. (1994). Severe and fatal mass attacks by 'killer' bees (Africanized honey bees-*Apis mellifera scutellata*) in Brazil: clinicopathological studies with measurement of serum venom concentrations. *The Quarterly Journal of Medicine (Q J Med)*. Vol. 87, No. 5, pp. 269-82.

França, F.O.; Barbaro, K.C. & Abdulkader, R.C. (2002). Rhabdomyolysis in presumed viscero-cutaneous loxoscelism: report of two cases. *Transactions of the Royal Society of Tropical Medicine and Hygiene*. Vol. 96, No. 3, pp. 287-90.

Francischetti, I.M.; Saliou, B.; Leduc, M.; Carlini, C.R.; Hatmi, M.; Randon, J.; Faili, A. & Bon, C. (1997). Convulxin, a potent platelet-aggregating protein from *Crotalus durissus terrificus* venom, specifically binds to platelets. *Toxicon*. Vol. 35, No. 8, pp. 1217-28.

Frezzatti, R. & Silveira, P.F. (2011). Allopurinol Reduces the Lethality Associated with Acute Renal Failure Induced by *Crotalus durissus terrificus* Snake Venom: Comparison with Probenecid. *PLoS Neglected Tropical Diseases*. Vol. 5, No. 9, pp. e1312.

Gabriel, D.P.; Rodrigues, A.G.; Barsante, R.C.; dos Santos-Silva, V.; Caramori, J.T.; Martim, L.C.; Barretti, P. & Balbi, A.L. (2004). Severe acute renal failure after massive attack of Africanized bees. *Nephrology, Dialysis, Transplantation*. Vol. 19, No. 10, pp. 2680.

Gamborgi, G.P.; Metcalf, E.B. & Barros, E.J. (2006). Acute renal failure provoked by toxin from caterpillars of the species *Lonomia obliqua*. *Toxicon*. Vol. 47, No. 1, pp. 68-74.

Gay, C.C.; Marunak, S.L.; Teibler, P.; Ruiz, R.; Acosta de Pérez, O.C. & Leiva, L.C. (2009). Systemic alterations induced by a *Bothrops alternatus* hemorrhagic metalloproteinase (baltergin) in mice. *Toxicon*. Vol. 53, No. 1, pp. 53-9.

Gremski, L.H.; da Silveira, R.B.; Chaim, O.M.; Probst, C.M.; Ferrer, V.P.; Nowatzki, J.; Weinschutz, H.C.; Madeira, H.M.; Gremski, W.; Nader, H.B.; Senff-Ribeiro, A. & Veiga, S.S. (2010). A novel expression profile of the *Loxosceles intermedia* spider venomous gland revealed by transcriptome analysis. *Molecular Biosystems*. Vol. 6, No. 12, pp. 2403-16.

Grisotto, L.S.; Mendes, G.E.; Castro, I.; Baptista, M.A.; Alves, V.A.; Yu, L. & Burdmann, E.A. (2006). Mechanisms of bee venom-induced acute renal failure. *Toxicon*. Vol. 48, No. 1, pp. 44-54.

Gutiérrez, J.M.; Theakston, R.D. & Warrell, D.A. (2006). Confronting the neglected problem of snake bite envenoming: the need for a global partnership. *PLoS Medicine*. Vol. 3, No. 6, pp. e150.

Gutiérrez, J.M.; Williams, D.; Fan, H.W. & Warrell, D.A. (2010). Snakebite envenoming from a global perspective: Towards an integrated approach. *Toxicon*. Vol. 56, No 7, pp. 1223-35.

Habermann, E. (1972). Bee and wasp venoms. *Science*. Vol. 177, No. 46, pp. 314-22.

Hogan, C.J.; Barbaro, K.C. & Winkel, K. (2004). Loxoscelism: old obstacles, new directions. *Annals of Emergency Medicine*. Vol. 44, pp. 608-622.

Isbister, G.K. & Fan, H.W. (2011). Spider bite. *Lancet*. (*in press*)

Jorge, M.T. & Ribeiro, L.A. (1992). The epidemiology and clinical picture of an accidental bite by the South American rattlesnake (*Crotalus durissus*). *Revista do Instituto de Medicina Tropical de São Paulo*. Vol. 34, No. 4, pp. 347-54.

Kamiguti, A.S. (2005). Platelets as targets of snake venom metalloproteinases. *Toxicon*. Vol. 45, No. 8, pp. 1041-9.

Kasturiratne, A.; Wickremasinghe, A.R.; de Silva, N.; Gunawardena, N.K.; Pathmeswaran, A.; Premaratna, R.; Savioli, L.; Lalloo, D.G. & de Silva, H.J. (2008). The global burden of snakebite: a literature analysis and modelling based on regional estimates of envenoming and deaths. *PLoS Medicine*. Vol. 5, No. 11, pp. e218.

Khan, FY. (2009). Rhabdomyolysis: a review of the literature. *Netherland Journal of Medicine*. Vol. 67, No. 9, pp. 272-83.

Kusma, J.; Chaim, O.M.; Wille, A.C.; Ferrer, V.P.; Sade, Y.B.; Donatti, L.; Gremski, W.; Mangili, O.C. & Veiga, S.S. (2008). Nephrotoxicity caused by brown spider venom phospholipase-D (dermonecrotic toxin) depends on catalytic activity. *Biochimie*. Vol. 90, No. 11-12, pp. 1722-36.

Lee, S. & Lynch, K.R. (2005). Brown recluse spider (*Loxosceles reclusa*) venom phospholipase D (PLD) generates lysophosphatidic acid (LPA). *Biochemical Journal*. Vol. 391, No. 2, pp. 317-23.

Lee, S.Y.; Park, H.S.; Lee, S.J. & Choi, M. (2001). Melittin exerts multiple effects on the release of free fatty acids from L1210 cells: lack of selective activation of phospholipase A2 by melittin. *Archives of Biochemistry and Biophysics*. Vol. 389, pp. 57-67.

Linardi, A.; Rocha e Silva, T.A.; Miyabara, E.H.; Franco-Penteado, C.F.; Cardoso, K.C.; Boer, P.A.; Moriscot, A.S.; Gontijo, J.A.; Joazeiro, P.P.; Collares-Buzato, C.B. & Hyslop, S. (2011). Histological and functional renal alterations caused by *Bothrops alternatus* snake venom: expression and activity of Na+/K+-ATPase. *Biochimica et Biophysica Acta*. Vol. 1810, No. 9, pp. 895-906.

Lucato-Junior, R.V.; Abdulkader, R.C.; Barbaro, K.C.; Mendes, G.E.; Castro, I.; Baptista, M.A.; Cury, P.M.; Malheiros, D.M.; Schor, N.; Yu, L. & Burdmann, E.A. (2011). *Loxosceles gaucho* venom-induced acute kidney injury - *in vivo* and *in vitro* studies. *PLoS Neglected Tropical Diseases*. Vol. 5, No. 5, pp. e1182.

Luciano, M.N.; da Silva, P.H.; Chaim, O.M.; dos Santos, V.L.; Franco, C.R.; Soares, M.F.; Zanata, S.M.; Mangili, O.C.; Gremski, W. & Veiga, S.S. (2004). Experimental evidence for a direct cytotoxicity of *Loxosceles intermedia* (brown spider) venom in renal tissue. *Journal of Histochemistry and Cytochemistry*. Vol. 52, No. 4, pp. 455-67.

Malaque, C.M.; Andrade, L.; Madalosso, G.; Tomy, S.; Tavares, F.L. & Seguro, A.C. (2006). Short report: A case of hemolysis resulting from contact with a *Lonomia* caterpillar in southern Brazil. *American Journal of Tropical Medicine and Hygiene*. Vol. 74, No. 5, pp. 807-9.

Martins, A.M.; Toyama, M.H.; Havt, A.; Novello, J.C.; Marangoni, S.; Fonteles, M.C. & Monteiro, H.S. (2002). Determination of *Crotalus durissus cascavella* venom components that induce renal toxicity in isolated rat kidneys. *Toxicon*. Vol. 40, No. 8, pp. 1165-171.

Martins, A.M.; Lima, A.A.; Toyama, M.H.; Marangoni, S.; Fonteles, M.C. & Monteiro, H.S. (2003). Renal effects of supernatant from macrophages activated by *Crotalus durissus cascavella* venom: the role of phospholipase A2 and cyclooxygenase. *Pharmacology & Toxicology*. Vol. 92, No. 1, pp. 14-20.

Martins, A.M.; Nobre, A.C.; Almeida, A.C.; Bezerra, G.; Lima, A.A.; Fonteles, M.C. & Monteiro, H.S. (2004). Thalidomide and pentoxifylline block the renal effects of supernatants of macrophages activated with *Crotalus durissus cascavella* venom. *Brazilian Journal of Medical and Biological Research*. Vol. 37, No. 10, pp. 1525-30.

Mello, S.M.; Linardi, A.; Rennó, A.L.; Tarsitano, C.A.; Pereira, E.M. & Hyslop, S. (2010). Renal kinetics of *Bothrops alternatus* (Urutu) snake venom in rats. *Toxicon*. Vol. 55, No. 2-3, pp. 470-80.

Ministério da Saúde (2001). Manual de Diagnóstico e Tratamento por Animais Peçonhentos. Fundação Nacional da Saúde, Brasil. Available from: http://portal.saude.gov.br/portal/saude/visualizar_texto.cfm?idtxt=21182.

Monteiro, H.S. & Fonteles, M.C. (1999). The effect of *Bothrops jararaca* venom on rat kidney after short-term exposure: preliminary results. *Pharmacology & Toxicology*. Vol. 85, No. 4, pp. 198-200.

Monteiro, H.S.; da Silva, I.M.; Martins, A.M. & Fonteles, M.C. (2001). Actions of *Crotalus durissus terrificus* venom and crotoxin on the isolated rat kidney. *Brazilian Journal of Medical and Biological Research*. Vol. 34, No. 10, pp. 1347-52.

Murakami, M.T.; Fernandes-Pedrosa, M.F.; Tambourgi, D.V. & Arni, R.K. (2005). Structural basis for metal ion coordination and the catalytic mechanism of sphingomyelinases D. *Journal of Biological Chemistry*. Vol. 280, No. 14, pp. 13658-64.

Nascimento, J.M.; Franchi, G.C.; Nowill, A.E.; Collares-Buzato, C.B. & Hyslop, S. (2007). Cytoskeletal rearrangement and cell death induced by *Bothrops alternatus* snake venom in cultured Madin-Darby canine kidney cells. *Biochemistry and Cell Biology*. Vol. 85, No. 5, pp. 591-605.

Ownby, C.L.; Powell, J.R.; Jiang, M.S. & Fletcher, J.E. (1997). Melittin and phospholipase A2 from bee (*Apis mellifera*) venom cause necrosis of murine skeletal muscle *in vivo*. *Toxicon*. Vol. 35, pp. 67-80.

Otero, R.; Gutiérrez, J.; Beatriz-Mesa, M.; Duque, E.; Rodríguez, O.; Luis-Arango, J.; Gómez, F.; Toro, A.; Cano, F.; María-Rodríguez, L.; Caro, E.; Martínez, J.; Cornejo, W.; Mariano-Gómez, L.; Luis-Uribe, F.; Cárdenas, S.; Núñez, V. & Díaz, A. (2002). Complications of *Bothrops*, *Porthidium*, and *Bothriechis* snakebites in Colombia. A clinical and epidemiological study of 39 cases attended in a university hospital. *Toxicon*. Vol. 40, No. 8, pp. 1107-114.

Pantera, B.; Hoffman, D.R.; Carresi, L.; Cappugi, G.; Turillazzi, S.; Manao, G.; Severino, M.; Spadolini, I.; Orsomando, G.; Moneti, G. & Pazzagli, L. (2003). Characterization of the major allergens purified from the venom of the paper wasp *Polistes gallicus*. *Biochimica et Biophysica Acta*. Vol. 1623, No. 2-3, pp. 72-81.

Petricevich, V.L.; Teixeira, C.F.P.; Tambourgi, D.V. & Gutiérrez, J.M. (2000). Increments in serum cytokine and nitric oxide levels in mice injected with *Bothrops asper* and *Bothrops jararaca* snake venoms. *Toxicon*. Vol. 38, No. 9, pp. 1253–66.

Pinho, F.M.; Zanetta, D.M. & Burdmann, E.A. (2005). Acute renal failure after *Crotalus durissus* snakebite: a prospective survey on 100 patients. *Kidney International*. Vol. 67, No. 2, pp. 659-67.

Pinho, F.M.; Yu, L. & Burdmann EA. (2008). Snakebite-induced acute kidney injury in Latin America. *Seminars in Nephrology*. Vol. 28, No. 4, pp. 354-62.

Pinto, A.F.; Dobrovolski, R.; Veiga, A.B. & Guimarães, J.A. (2004). Lonofibrase, a novel alpha-fibrinogenase from *Lonomia obliqua* caterpillars. *Thrombosis Research*. Vol.113, No. 2, pp. 147-54.

Pinto, A.F.; Silva, K.R. & Guimarães, J.A. (2006). Proteases from *Lonomia obliqua* venomous secretions: comparison of procoagulant, fibrin(ogen)olytic and amidolytic activities. *Toxicon*. Vol. 47, No. 1, pp.113-21.

Pinto, A.F.; Berger, M.; Reck-Jr, J.; Terra, R.M. & Guimarães, J.A. (2010). *Lonomia obliqua* venom: *In vivo* effects and molecular aspects associated with the hemorrhagic syndrome. *Toxicon*. Vol. 56, No. 7, pp. 1103-12.

Reis, C.V.; Andrade, S.A.; Ramos, O.H.; Ramos, C.R.; Ho, P.L.; Batista, I.F. & Chudzinski-Tavassi, A.M. (2006). Lopap, a prothrombin activator from Lonomia obliqua belonging to the lipocalin family: recombinant production, biochemical characterization and structure-function insights. *Biochemical Journal*. Vol. 398, No. 2, pp. 295-302.

Ricci-Silva, M.E.; Valente, R.H.; León, I.R.; Tambourgi, D.V.; Ramos, O.H.; Perales, J. & Chudzinski-Tavassi, A.M. (2008). Immunochemical and proteomic technologies as tools for unravelling toxins involved in envenoming by accidental contact with *Lonomia obliqua* caterpillars. *Toxicon*. Vol. 51, No. 6, pp. 1017-28.

Rodrigues-Sgrignolli, L.; Florido-Mendes, G.E.; Carlos, C.P.; Burdmann, E.A. (2011). Acute kidney injury caused by *Bothrops* snake venom. *Nephron Clinical Practice*. Vol. 119, No. 2 pp. c131-7.

Rucavado, A.; Soto, M.; Escalante, T.; Loría, G.D.; Arni, R. & Gutiérrez, J.M. (2005). Thrombocytopenia and platelet hypoaggregation induced by *Bothrops asper* snake venom. Toxins involved and their contribution to metalloproteinase-induced pulmonary hemorrhage. *Thrombosis and Haemostasis*. Vol. 94, No. 1, pp. 123-31.

Sampaio, S.C.; Hyslop, S.; Fontes, M.R.; Prado-Franceschi, J.; Zambelli, V.O.; Magro, A.J.; Brigatte, P.; Gutiérrez, V.P. & Cury, Y. (2010). Crotoxin: novel activities for a classic beta-neurotoxin. *Toxicon*. Vol. 55, No. 6, pp. 1045-60.

Santoro, ML. & Sano-Martins, I.S. (2004). Platelet dysfunction during *Bothrops jararaca* snake envenomation in rabbits. *Thrombosis and Haemostasis*. Vol. 92, No. 2, pp.369-83.

Seibert, C.S.; Oliveira, M.R.; Gonçalves, L.R.; Santoro, M.L. & Sano-Martins, I.S. (2004). Intravascular hemolysis induced by *Lonomia obliqua* caterpillar bristle extract: an experimental model of envenomation in rats. *Toxicon*. Vol. 44, No. 7, pp. 793-9.

Seibert, C.S.; Tanaka-Azevedo, A.M.; Santoro, M.L.; Mackessy, S.P.; Soares-Torquato, R.J.; Lebrun, I.; Tanaka, A.S. & Sano-Martins, I.S. (2006). Purification of a phospholipase A2 from *Lonomia obliqua* caterpillar bristle extract. *Biochemical and Biophysical Research Communications*. Vol. 342, No. 4, pp. 1027-33.

Sezerino, U.M.; Zannin, M.; Coelho, L.K.; Gonçalves-Júnior, J.; Grando, M.; Mattosinho, S.G.; Cardoso, J.L.; von Eickstedt, V.R.; França, F.O.; Barbaro, K.C. & Fan, H.W. (1998). A clinical and epidemiological study of *Loxosceles* spider envenoming in Santa Catarina, Brazil. *Transactions of the Royal Society of Tropical Medicine and Hygiene*. Vol. 92, No. 5, pp. 546-8.

Silveira, P.V. & Nishioka, A. (1992). South American rattlesnake bite in a Brazilian teaching hospital. Clinical and epidemiological study of 87 cases, with analysis of factors predictive of renal failure. *Transactions of the Royal Society of Tropical Medicine and Hygiene*. Vol. 86, No. 5, pp. 562-4.

Sitprija, V. (2006). Snakebite nephropathy. *Nephrology (Carlton)*. Vol. 11, No. 5, pp. 442-8.

Soares, A.M.; Mancin, A.C.; Cecchini, A.L.; Arantes, E.C.; França, S.C.; Gutiérrez, J.M. & Giglio, J.R. (2001). Effects of chemical modifications of crotoxin B, the phospholipase A(2) subunit of crotoxin from *Crotalus durissus terrificus* snake venom, on its enzymatic and pharmacological activities. *International Journal of Biochemistry and Cell Biology*. Vol. 33, No. 9, pp. 877-88.

Swanson, D.L.; Vetter, R.S. (2006). Loxoscelism. *Clinics in Dermatology*. Vol. 24, pp. 213-221.

Terra, R.M.; Guimarães, J.A. & Verli, H. (2007). Structural and functional behavior of biologically active monomeric melittin. *Journal of Molecular Graphics and Modelling*. Vol. 25, No. 6, pp. 767-72.

Trevisan-Silva, D.; Gremski, L.H.; Chaim, O.M.; da Silveira, R.B.; Meissner, G.O.; Mangili, O.C.; Barbaro, K.C.; Gremski, W.; Veiga, S.S. & Senff-Ribeiro, A. (2010). Astacin-like metalloproteases are a gene family of toxins present in the venom of different species of the brown spider (genus *Loxosceles*). *Biochimie*. Vol. 92, No. 1, pp. 21-32.

Veiga, A.B.; Blochtein, B. & Guimarães, J.A. (2001a). Structures involved in production, secretion and injection of the venom produced by the caterpillar *Lonomia obliqua* (Lepidoptera, Saturniidae). *Toxicon*. Vol. 39, No., 9, pp. 1343-51.

Veiga, A.B.; Pinto, A.F. & Guimarães, J.A. (2003). Fibrinogenolytic and procoagulant activities in the hemorrhagic syndrome caused by *Lonomia obliqua* caterpillars. *Thrombosis Research*. Vol. 111, No. 1-2, pp. 95-101.

Veiga, A.B.; Ribeiro, J.M.; Guimarães, J.A. & Francischetti, I.M. (2005). A catalog for the transcripts from the venomous structures of the caterpillar *Lonomia obliqua*: identification of the proteins potentially involved in the coagulation disorder and hemorrhagic syndrome. *Gene*. Vol. 355, pp. 11-27.

Veiga, A.B.; Berger, M. & Guimarães, J.A. (2009). *Lonomia obliqua* venom: pharmaco-toxicological effects and biotechnological perspectives. In: *Animal toxins: the state of the art. Perspectives on health and biotechnology*. De Lima, M.E.; Pimenta, A.M; Martin-Eauclaire, M.F.; Zingali, R.B. & Rochat, H. (editors), pp. 371-390, UFMG, ISBN 978-85-7041-735-0, Belo Horizonte, Brazil.

Veiga, S.S.; Feitosa, L.; dos Santos, V.L.; de Souza, G.A.; Ribeiro, A.S.; Mangili, O.C.; Porcionatto, M.A.; Nader, H.B.; Dietrich, C.P.; Brentani, R.R. & Gremski, W. (2000). Effect of brown spider venom on basement membrane structures. *Histochemical Journal*. Vol. 32, No. 7, pp. 397-408.

Veiga, S.S.; Zanetti, V.C.; Franco, C.R.; Trindade, E.S.; Porcionatto, M.A.; Mangili, O.C.; Gremski, W.; Dietrich, C.P. & Nader, H.B. (2001b). *In vivo* and *in vitro* cytotoxicity of brown spider venom for blood vessel endothelial cells. *Thrombosis Research*. Vol. 102, No. 3, pp. 229-37.

Vetter, R.S.; Visscher, P.K. & Camazine, S. (1999). Mass envenomations by honey bees and wasps. *Western Journal of Medicine*. Vol. 170, No. 4, pp. 223-7.

Warrell, D.A. (2010). Snake bite. *Lancet*. Vol. 375, No. 9708, pp. 77-88.

White, J. (2005). Snake venoms and coagulopathy. *Toxicon*. Vol. 45, No. 8, pp. 951-67.

Williams, D.; Gutiérrez, J.M.; Harrison, R.; Warrell, D.A.; White, J.; Winkel, K.D. & Gopalakrishnakone, P. (2010). Global Snake Bite Initiative Working Group; International Society on Toxinology. The Global Snake Bite Initiative: an antidote for snake bite. *Lancet*. Vol. 375, No. 9708, pp. 89-91.

WHO, 2007. Rabies and Envenomings. A Neglected Public Health Issue. World Health Organization, Geneva. Available from: www.who.int/rabies/relevant_documents/en/index.html

WHO, 2010a. Guidelines for the management of snake-bites. World Health Organization, Geneva. Available from: apps.who.int/medicinedocs/en/m/abstract/Js17111e/

WHO, 2010b. Guidelines for the Production, Control and Regulation of Snake Antivenom Immunoglobulins. World Health Organization, Geneva. Available from: www.who.int/bloodproducts/snake_antivenoms/snakeantivenomguide/en/index.html

Xuan, B.H.; Mai, H.L.; Thi, T.X.; Thi, M.T.; Nguyen, H.N. & Rabenou, R.A. (2010). Swarming hornet attacks: shock and acute kidney injury - a large case series from Vietnam. *Nephrology, Dialysis, Transplantation*. Vol. 25, No. 4, pp. 1146-50.

Yamasaki, S.C.; Villarroel, J.S.; Barone, J.M.; Zambotti-Villela, L. & Silveira, P.F. (2008). Aminopeptidase activities, oxidative stress and renal function in *Crotalus durissus terrificus* envenomation in mice. *Toxicon*. Vol. 52, No. 3, pp. 345-54.

Zager, R.A. (1996). Rhabdomyolysis and myohemoglobinuric acute renal failure. *Kidney International*. Vol. 49, No. 2, pp. 314-26.

Zambrano, A.; González, J. & Callejas, G. (2005). Severe loxoscelism with lethal outcome. Report of one case. *Revista Médica de Chile*. Vol. 133, No. 2, pp. 219-23.

Zannin, M.; Lourenço, D.M.; Motta, G.; Dalla Costa, L.R.; Grando, M.; Gamborgi, G.P.; Noguti, M.A. & Chudzinski-Tavassi, A.M. (2003). Blood coagulation and fibrinolytic factors in 105 patients with hemorrhagic syndrome caused by accidental contact with *Lonomia obliqua* caterpillar in Santa Catarina, southern Brazil. *Thrombosis and Haemostasis*. Vol. 89, No. 2, pp. 355-64.

Zelanis, A.; Tashima, A.K.; Rocha, M.M.; Furtado, M.F.; Camargo, A.C.; Ho, P.L. & Serrano, S.M. (2010). Analysis of the ontogenetic variation in the venom proteome/peptidome of *Bothrops jararaca* reveals different strategies to deal with prey. *Journal of Proteome Research*. Vol. 9, No. 5, pp. 2278-91.

Zingali, R.B.; Ferreira, M.S.; Assafim, M.; Frattani, F.S. & Monteiro RQ. (2005). Bothrojaracin, a *Bothrops jararaca* snake venom-derived (pro)thrombin inhibitor, as an anti-thrombotic molecule. *Pathophysiology of Haemostasis and Thrombosis*. Vol. 34, No. 4-5, pp. 160-3.

Zhang, R.; Meleg-Smith, S. & Batuman, V. (2001). Acute tubulointerstitial nephritis after wasp stings. *American Journal of Kidney Diseases*. Vol. 38, No. 6, pp. E33.

10

Contrast Nephropathy: A Paradigm for Cardiorenal Interactions in Clinical Practice

Michele Meschi[1], Simona Detrenis[1], Laura Bianchi[2] and Alberto Caiazza[1]
[1]*Department of Medicine and Diagnostics, Borgo Val di Taro Hospital, Azienda USL Parma,*
[2]*Postgraduate School of Paediatrics, University of Parma*
Italy

1. Introduction

Contrast-induced nephropathy (CIN) is defined as acute deterioration of renal function after intravascular administration of iodinated contrast agents, in the absence of other causes. Laboratory diagnosis is expressed as an increase in serum creatinine levels of 0.5 mg/dL (or 44 µmol/L) or a 25% or greater relative increase from baseline 48-72 hours after a diagnostic or interventional procedure, even if the clinical significance of this definition in the absence of pre-existing renal failure is questionable (Thomsen & Morcos, 2006).

The Acute Kidney Injury (AKI) Network was estabilished in 2007 to study the improvement of outcomes associated with various forms of acute renal failure; recently, it has expressed the hope that the diagnostic criteria for all cases of acute kidney injury are standardized in sudden reduction (within 48 hours) of renal function with a serum creatinine increase ≥ 0.3 mg/dL or a 50% or greater increase from baseline, or after onset of oligoanuria (urinary output < 0.5 mL/kg/hour for 6 hours) (Mehta et al., 2007).

However, there is no consensus in bringing CIN parameters in AKI criteria, because contrast medium damage usually causes a serum creatinine peak on the third-fifth day after contrast medium exposure, and rarely occurs with oligoanuria, except in patients with advanced impairment of renal function (Detrenis et al., 2007a). Nevertheless, recent literature uses the term "radiocontrast-induced acute kidney injury" (RCI-AKI) rather than CIN, although the clinical implications of different definitions have never been tested on a large scale (Goldfarb et al., 2009).

2. Epidemiology

RCI-AKI is today the third nosographic entity related to hospital-acquired acute renal failure, after organ hypoperfusion and nephrotoxic drugs (eg, nonsteroidal anti-inflammatory drugs) (Nash et al, 2002). RCI-AKI incidence is significantly greater in the case of intra-arterial (from 10-20% for moderate to 25-70% for high-risk patients; 0.15-2.30% in general population) compared to intravenous administration (~5%) (Detrenis et al., 2007a).

The probability of renal replacement therapy is closely related to individual patient comorbidities, but it is reasonable to assume that it varies from less than 1% of all patients undergoing percutaneous coronary intervention to 10%of those with pre-existing alteration in renal function parameters who have RCI-AKI after coronary angiography (Meschi et al., 2006). In other words, the probability of RCI-AKI requiring dialysis increases from 0.04 to 48% if measured glomerular filtration rate is reduced from 50 to 10 mL/min; on the other hand, 13-50% of subjects undergoing dialysis after RCI-AKI tends to prolong renal replacement therapy definitively (Toprak, 2007).

As in general for nephropatic patients, even for those affected by RCI-AKI the incidence of associated cardiovascular events or major adverse cardiac effects was assessed: a study on 16.000 hospitalized subjects who underwent coronary angiography (Levy et al., 1996) shows that those with RCI-AKI develop a risk for complications and death 5-fold higher than in controls, even after data correction for any existing comorbidities. Even for the majority of cases, with benign clinical course (pre-existing serum creatinine values restoration in 1-3 weeks, no symptoms or dialysis), there was a significant increase in 1- and 5-years mortality (Rihal et al., 2002). This evidence is greater for cases with unfavourable renal prognosis requiring temporary renal replacement therapy (McCullough et al., 1997).

Consequently, even if the pathophysiological relationship between contrast nephropathy, morbidity and mortality it is not clear, RCI-AKI is today definitely considered an independent predictor for long term mortality. It is possible to hypothesize that the pathogenic process underlying RCI-AKI may interfere with pro-atherogenic mechanisms of cardiovascular disease, although there are no definitive studies on this issue (Detrenis et al., 2005).

3. Risk markers for contrast nephropathy

The pathogenetic events underlying RCI-AKI are still not completely understood and the identification of "risk factors" for disease is difficult, because the term usually refers to a medical condition or nosographic entity associated with a therapeutic intervention or preventive approach. It is therefore considered that the term "marker" is more useful to identify patients predisposed to acute deterioration of renal function in this context, due to specific pathophysiological features (Toprak, 2007).

In one third of cases, these markers do not correspond to changeable conditions. Instead, the early recognition of remaining situations becomes a prerequisite to the use of prophylactic protocols. Even in the absence of incontrovertible evidence, these protocols have shown a variable reduction in the incidence of RCI-AKI during prospective or retrospective studies (Toprak, 2007) **(Fig. 1)**.

3.1 Advancing age, chronic nephropathy and accurate assessment of renal function

Between markers of risk, the reduction in renal function before the administration of iodinated contrast medium plays a predominant significance, particularly if baseline glomerular filtration rate values are < 60 mL/min/1.73 m^2, that is in the course of chronic kidney disease at stage 3, 4, 5 for the National Kidney Foundation (Nelson & Tuttle, 2007).

The decrease of renal function can not be revealed by routine measurement of serum creatinine, because there is an inverse, non-linear relationship between serum creatinine (varying with the muscle mass, age and sex of the patient) and corresponding glomerular filtration rate. In any case, glomerular filtration rate tends to decrease progressively with increasing age and can be measured indirectly by creatinine clearance (Detrenis et al., 2007b). A recent analysis of more than 20000 patients undergoing coronary angiography showed that there is a significantly higher incidence of RCI-AKI in the elderly, especially women, who usually have a net reduction of glomerular filtration rate even when there is an apparently normal serum creatinine. Indeed, a relative reduction in muscle mass is frequently observed in these subjects (Sidhu et al., 2008) **(Fig. 2)**.

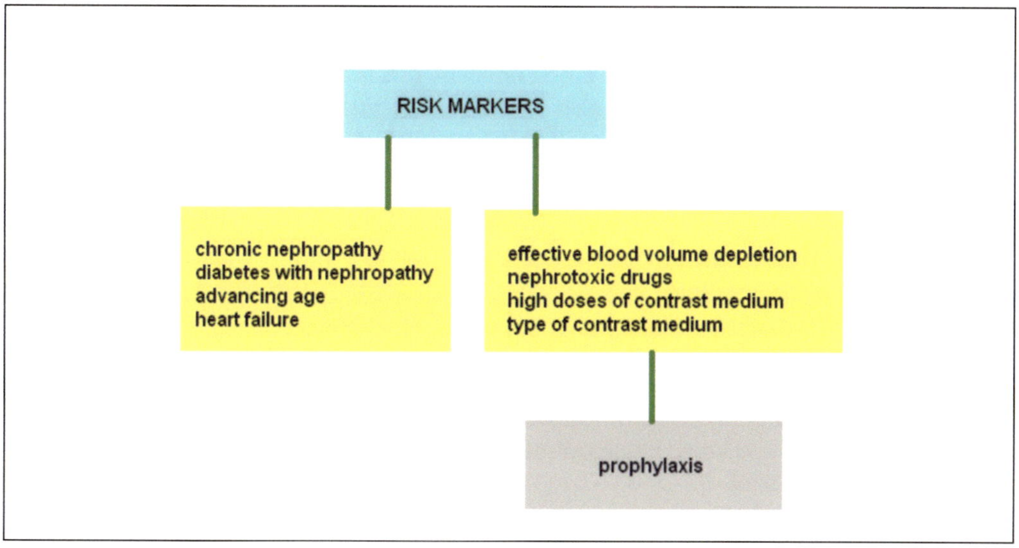

Fig. 1. Risk markers for contrast nephropathy

When the creatinine clearance **(1)** is not easily achieved trough the urinary output collection, so-called MDRD or Levey equation (from the Modification of Diet in Renal Disease Study) **(2)** can be used to estimate glomerular filtration rate (Levey et al., 1999). However, the simple evaluation of creatinine clearance by classical Cockcroft and Gault formula **(3)**, which consider daily urinary creatinine and only requires knowledge of body weight, age and sex of the patient, it is appropriate to clinical practice (Cockcroft & Gault, 1976).

$$\text{creatinine clearance} = \frac{\text{urine creatinine} \times \text{daily urinary output}}{\text{serum creatinine} \times 1440} \quad (1)$$

$$\text{creatinine clearance} = \frac{(140 - \text{age}) \times \text{body weight}}{\text{serum creatinine} \times 72} \times 0.85 \text{ (if female)} \quad (2)$$

$$\begin{aligned} \text{estimated GFR} &= 186 \times (\text{serum creatinine})^{-1.154} \times (\text{age})^{-0.203} \times 0.742 \text{ (if female)} \\ &= 186 \times (\text{serum creatinine})^{-1.154} \times (\text{age})^{-0.203} \times 1.210 \text{ (if afro-american)} \quad (3) \\ &\text{(for } 1.76 \text{ m}^2 \text{ body surface area)} \end{aligned}$$

Cystatin C, produced at a constant rate by nucleated cells and released into circulation (normal values <0.95 mg/L in subjects aged < 45 years, up to 1.2 mg/L in older), was recently identified as a marker of renal injury early and easily measurable. It is freely filtered by the glomerulus and completely reabsorbed and metabolized, but not secreted by cells of the proximal tubule. Furthermore, it is not subject to significant urinary excretion, and is not affected by gender or muscle mass of the patient (Perkins et al., 2005).

Some studies have used direct measurements of glomerular filtration rate as a gold standard to compare the use of cystatin C with serum creatinine and serum creatinine-based assessments, demostrating the superiority of the former especially in diabetic patients (Perkins et al., 2005).

The data on clinical use of this method, however, are controversial. The serum concentrations of cystatin C identify a condition of preclinical renal damage earlier than other laboratory parameters, and are also a possible risk marker for heart failure and other cardiovascular events in elderly patients. On the contrary, is not yet clear the real influence of other factors (cigarette smoking, thyroid disease, high levels of C-reactive protein, corticosteroid therapy) on these measurements (Burkhardt et al., 2002).

In other words, the accuracy of this diagnostic test has been documented when the sensitivity of serum creatinine measurement is reduced. However, cystatin C can be interpreted not only as a marker of renal function, but also as generic indicator of inflammatory processes (Burkhardt et al., 2002). In addition, quantitative data on extrarenal clearance of the molecule are not available. Therefore, because its early serum increase (within 24 hours after contrast administration) it could be a useful parameter for RCI-AKI after angiographic procedures, but requires further prospective evaluation for large-scale use (Detrenis et al., 2007b).

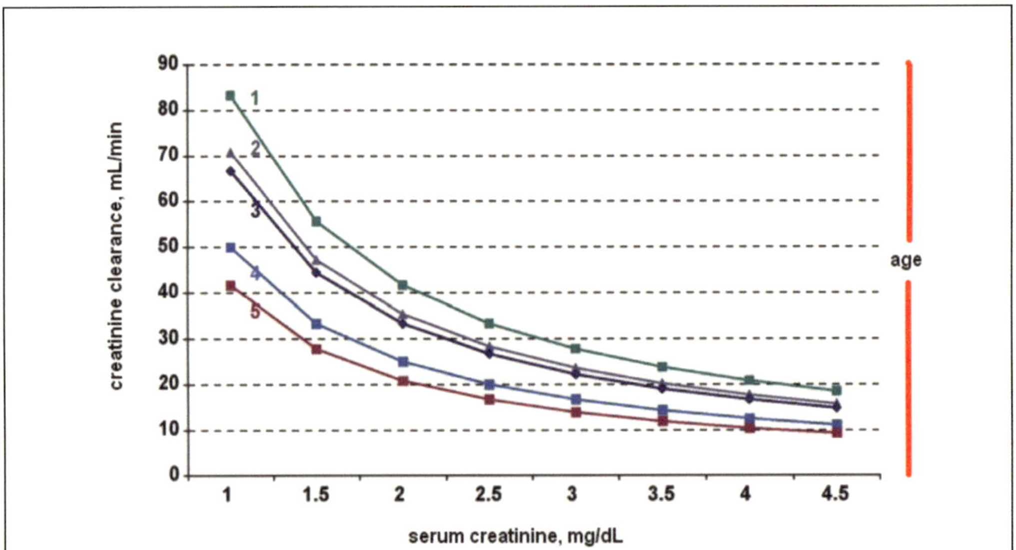

Fig. 2. Serum creatinine, creatinine clearance and age. 1: male, 60 kg, 40 years. 2: female, 60 kg, 40 years. 3: male, 60 kg, 60 years. 4: male, 60 kg, 80 years. 5: male, 60 kg, 90 years

3.2 Impaired fasting glucose, diabetes mellitus and its complications

Between changes in carbohydrate, lipid and protein profile (dyslipidemia, hyperuricemia, metabolic syndrome), diabetes mellitus - according to definition in use, two measurements of fasting plasma glucose > 126 mg/dL - does not seem constitute an additional risk for RCI-AKI in itself, but only if there is consequent impairment of renal function (Parfrey PS et al., 1989).

Conversely, a prospective evaluation suggests a slight, but significant increase in the incidence of RCI-AKI in diabetic, non-nephropatic subjects, and even for those with impaired fasting glucose, compared to the general population (Toprak et al., 2007).

This is consistent with the hypothesis that the so-called endothelial dysfunction contributes to development of disease. In fact, it is present in all the above conditions of dysglycemia. At the level of the renal glomerulus, it leads to reduced availability of vasodilatory substances, such as nitric oxide and prostaglandins, which are synthesized in the endothelium. In this way, the renal ischemia associated with administration of iodinated contrast is encouraged, through the role of oxygen free radicals, which are able to induce the formation of reactive species in enzymes and membrane protein structures, using mechanisms of nitrosylation and oxidation (Detrenis et al., 2005).

3.3 Dehydration and relative hypovolemia

Even patients with heart failure and low cardiac output leading to reduced renal perfusion should be considered at increased risk for RCI-AKI (Thomsen & Morcos, 2003). This condition may worsen hypoxia and ischemia of the kidney caused by iodinated contrast agents. After an initial vasodilation, contrast media lead to a prolonged vasoconstriction in the medulla of the nephron, which already is less perfused than the cortex (Detrenis et al., 2005).

Subjects with the effective blood volume depletion, peripheral hypoperfusion, hypotension can be found under the same conditions. A similar trend is observed during sepsis, liver disease with severe hypoalbuminemia and dysproteinaemia, or in severe protein loss from any cause (Savazzi et al., 1997).

Periprocedural hydration and consequent volume expansion of the patient appear as the only safe options for RCI-AKI prophylaxis. They stimulate physiological diuresis and dilute concentrations of contrast medium and circulating mediators of vasoconstriction (adenosine, endothelin, angiotensin II). Therefore, true effectiveness of parenteral infusion protocols does not depend on the characteristics of the fluids used, or peculiar infusion rate. The use of solutions of sodium bicarbonate (154 mEq/L, 3 mL/kg/hour to 1 hour before the procedure, 1 mL/kg/ hour in the next 6 hours) (Merten et al., 2004) or isotonic saline (1 mL/kg/hour, 12 hours before and 12 hours after the procedure) (Mueller et al., 2002) is designed to correct the evident or latent depletion of the extra- and intracellular body compartments (Meschi et al., 2006).

4. Iodinated contrast media and other drugs

High-osmolal appear to be more nephrotoxic than current low-osmolal contrast media and recent iso-osmolal dimers, which did not demonstrate a favorable cost-effectiveness ratio (Savazzi et al., 2005; Detrenis et al., 2007c).

Although the CM-induced renal damage is dose-dependent, the volume below which the risk is reduced has not been identified, particularly when there is a preexisting decrease in renal function associated with diabetes (Meschi et al., 2006).

The intra-arterial route of administration (eg, interventional cardiology) is associated with an increased risk of RCI-AKI that the intravenous (eg, computed tomography), especially when examinations are repeated in succession at an interval of time less than 72 hours (Detrenis et al., 2007a).

In the case of concomitant use of contrast media, it is mandatory to avoid traditional nephrotoxic drugs (eg aminoglycosides), as well as nonsteroidal anti-inflammatory drugs, which can reduce the filtrate due to inhibition of intrarenal vasodilatation (Meschi et al., 2006).

The continuous treatment with agents that interfere with the renin-angiotensin system (angiotensin converting enzyme inhibitors, angiotensin receptor antagonists) contribute to the increase in the incidence of RCI-AKI in patients with chronic kidney disease. In fact, they cause efferent arteriolar vasodilation and thus the relative reduction of pressure within the glomerulus. According to some evidence, angiotensin converting enzyme inhibitors, angiotensin receptor blockers and diuretics should be discontinued the day before and day of the procedure with contrast, and should be taken after 2 days, unless contraindicated (Komenda et al., 2007; Cirit et al., 2006). However, more recent studies refute the efficacy of withdrawal (Rosenstock et al., 2008); on the contrary, telmisartan may play a protective role, at least in animals (Duan et al., 2009).

Extreme caution must be observed in the administration of contrast media in patients with diabetes treated with metformin. In fact, renal failure caused or worsened by concomitant AKI-RCI tends to result in a significant accumulation of biguanide, with possible development of lactic acidosis (Thomsen & Morcos, 1999).

5. The myth of monoclonal gammopathies

Until a few years ago, many clinicians prescribing the so called "screening for Bence Jones proteinuria" before performing an examination with contrast medium (Strada et al., 2008). Many laboratories provided (and still provide) a report in mg/dL, compared with a normal range (0 – 0.8 mg/dL). With this system, "Bence Jones proteinuria" greater than 0.8 mg/dL was defined as positive.

Many criticisms can be conducted in this model. Under normal conditions, immunoglobulin light chains (kappa, lambda) are freely filtered by the glomerulus and subsequently reabsorbed from the tubule to 99%. A normal urinary excretion of light chains is estimated at 20-40 mg per day (Strada et al., 2008). This amount increases significantly in case of impaired tubular reabsorption, for example during tubule-interstitial nephropathy, but concerns polyclonal light chains that are not of neoplastic origin.

On the contrary, the real Bence Jones protein was first described in 1962 as "consisting of monoclonal light chains" and produced by a single clone of B lymphocytes. It appears in the urine when the efficiency of tubular reabsorption is saturated, as in the course of diseases such as multiple myeloma, Waldenstrom's macroglobulinemia and lymphoproliferative disorders (Strada et al., 2008). For this reason, a pathological parameter (M monoclonal component), which under normal conditions should not be detected, can not be expressed in a range defined as physiological (0 - 0.8 mg/dL).

Moreover, despite the monoclonal gammopathies have been reported as risk markers for RCI-AKI for a long time, all the reviews of the scientific literature indicate that the association between the two comorbidities occurs only if a severe depletion of water and blood volume of the patient is demonstrated, or when the hematological malignancy has led to renal failure or hypercalcemic syndrome.

Thus, the monoclonal gammopathies should not be considered as primary contributing factors of the RCI-AKI, and screening of the so-called Bence Jones proteinuria has no clinical significance in patients undergoing contrast media (Meschi et al., 2006; Toprak, 2007). The presence of monoclonal gammopathy should be considered critically and the procedure with contrast medium, when necessary, can be implemented after evaluating volume, fluid and electrolyte status and renal function of the patient **(Fig. 3)**.

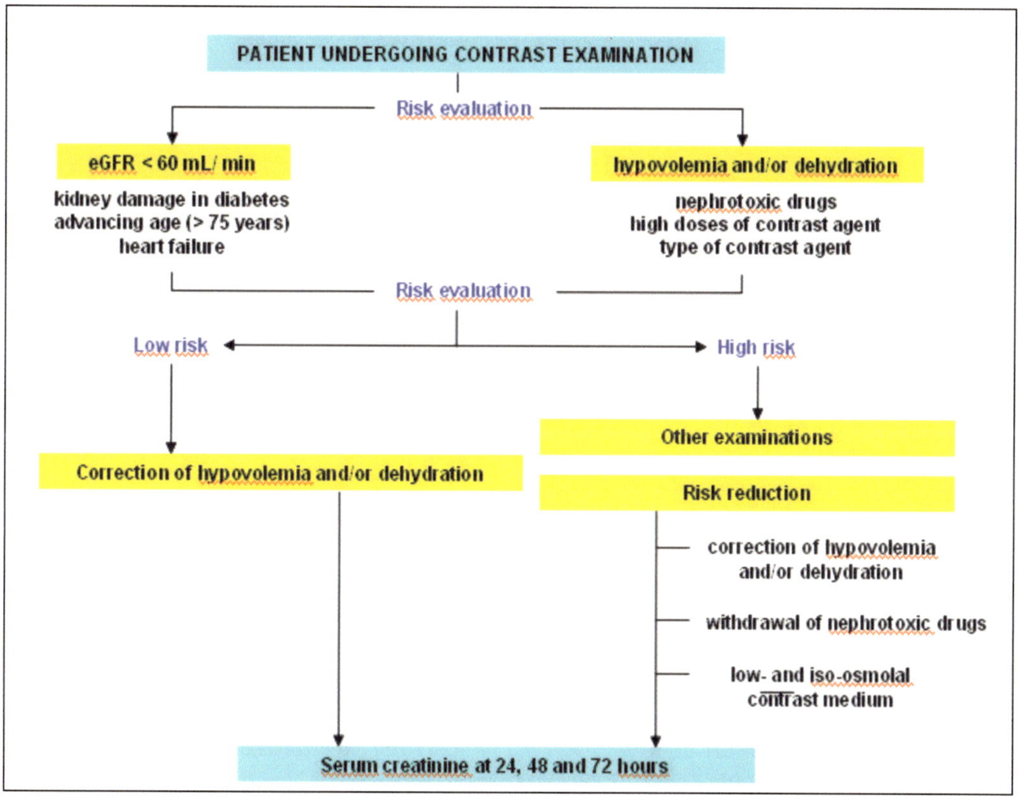

Fig. 3. Management of the patient undergoing contrast medium examination.

6. Acknowledgment

Our sincere thanks to Giorgio Savazzi, MD, associate professor of Internal Medicine and Nephrology, for his teachings and inspiration of this work.

7. References

Burkhardt, H., Bojarsky, G., & Gladisch, R. (2002). Diagnostic efficiency of cystatin C and serum creatinine as markers of reduced glomerular filtration rate in the elderly. *Clinical Chemistry and Laboratory Medicine*, Vol. 40, N. 11, pp. 1135-1138

Cirit, M.; Toprak, O.; Yesil, M.; Bayata, S.; Postaci, N.; Pupim, L., & Esi E. (2006). Angiotensin-converting enzyme inhibitors as a risk factor for contrast-induced nephropathy. *Nephron Clinical Practice*, Vol. 104, N. 1, pp. c20-c27

Cockcroft, D.W, & Gault, M.H. (1976). Prediction of creatinine clearance from serum creatinine. *Nephron*, Vol. 16, N. 1, pp. 31-41

Detrenis, S.; Meschi, M., & Savazzi, G. (2007). Contrast nephropathy: isosmolar and low-osmolar contrast media. *Journal of the American College of Cardiology*, Vol. 49, N. 8, pp. 922-923 (c)

Detrenis, S.; Meschi, M.; Bertolini, L., & Savazzi, G. (2007). Contrast medium administration in the elderly patient: is advancing age an independent risk factor for contrast nephropathy after angiographic procedures? *Journal of Vascular and Interventional Radiology*, Vol. 18, N. 2, pp. 177-185 (b)

Detrenis, S.; Meschi, M.; Jordana-Sanchez, M., & Savazzi, G. (2007). Contrast medium induced nephropathy in urological practice. *The Journal of Urology*, Vol. 178, N. 4, pp. 1164-1170 (a)

Detrenis, S.; Meschi, M.; Musini, S., & Savazzi, G. (2005). Lights and shadows on the pathogenesis of contrast-induced nephropathy: state of the art. *Nephrology, Dialysis, Transplantation*, Vol. 20, N. 8, pp. 1542-1550

Duan, S.B.; Wang, Y.H.; Liu, F.Y.; Xu, X.Q.; Wang, P.; Zou, Q., & Peng, Y.M. (2009). The protective role of telmisartan against nephrotoxicity induced by X-ray contrast media in rat model. *Acta Radiologica*, Vol. 50, N. 7, pp. 754-759

Goldfarb, S.; McCullough, P.A.; McDermott, J., & Gay, S.B. (2009). Contrast-induced acute kidney injury: speciality-specific protocols for interventional radiology, diagnostic computed tomography radiology, and interventional cardiology. *Mayo Clinic Proceedings*, Vol. 84, N. 2, pp. 170-179

Komenda., P; Zalunardo, N.; Burnett, S.; Love, J.; Buller, C.; Taylor, P.; Duncan, J.; Djurdjev, O., & Levin, A. (2007). Conservative outpatient renoprotective protocol in patients with low GFR undergoing contrast angiography: a case series. *Clinical and Experimental Nephrology*, Vol. 11, N. 3, pp. 209-213

Levey, A.S.; Stevens, L.A.; Schmid, C.H.; Zhang, Y.L.; Castro, A.F. 3rd; Feldman, H.I. ; Kusek, J.W. ; Eggers, P. ; Van Lente, F. ; Greene, T., & Coresh, J. (2009). A new equation to estimate glomerular filtration rate. *Annals of Internal Medicine*, Vol. 150, N. 9, pp. 604-612

Levy, E.M.; Viscoli, C.M., & Horwitz, R.I. (1996). The effect of acute renal failure on mortality. A cohort analysis. *Journal of American Medical Association (JAMA)*, Vol. 275, N. 19, pp. 1489-1494

Marenzi, G.; Lauri, G.; Assanelli, E.; Campodonico, J.; De Metrio, M.; Marana, I.; Grazi, M.; Veglia, F., & Bartorelli, A.L. (2004). Contrast-induced nephropathy in patients undergoing primary angioplasty for acute myocardial infarction. *Journal of the American College of Cardiology*, Vol. 44, N. 9, pp. 1780-1785

McCullough, P.A.; Wolyn, R.; Rocher, L.L.; Levin, R.N., & O'Neill, W.W. (1997). Acute renal failure after coronary intervention: incidence, risk factors, and relationship to mortality. *American Journal of Medicine*, Vol. 103, N. 5, pp. 368-375

Mehta, R.L.; Kellum, J.A.; Shah, S.V.; Molitoris, B.A.; Ronco, C.; Warnock, D.G., & Levin, A. (2007). Acute Kidney Injury Network: report of an initiative to improve outcomes in acute kidney injury. *Critical Care*, Vol. 11, N. 2, pp. R 31

Merten, G.J.; Burgess, W.P.; Gray, L.V.; Holleman, J.H.; Roush, T.S.; Kowalchuk, G.J.; Bersin, R.M.; Van Moore, A.; Simonton, C.A. 3rd; Rittase, R.A.; Norton, H.J., & Kennedy, T.P. (2004). Prevention of contrast-induced nephropathy with sodium bicarbonate: a randomized controlled trial. *Journal of the American Medical Association (JAMA)*, Vol. 291, N. 19, pp. 2328-2334

Meschi, M.; Detrenis, S.; & Savazzi, G. (2008). Contrast-induced nephropathy. Current concepts and propositions for Italian guidelines. *Recenti Progressi in Medicina*, Vol. 99, N. 3, pp. 155-162

Meschi, M.; Detrenis, S.; Musini, S; Strada, E., & Savazzi, G. (2006). Facts and fallacies concerning the prevention of contrast medium-induced nephropathy. *Critical Care Medicine*, Vol. 34, N. 8, pp. 2060-2068

Mueller, C.; Buerkle, G.; Buettner, H.J.; Petersen, J.; Perruchoud, A.P.; Eriksson, U.; Marsch, S., & Roskamm, H. (2002). Prevention of contrast media-associated nephropathy: randomized comparison of 2 hydration regimens in 1620 patients undergoing coronary angioplasty. *Archives of Internal Medicine*, Vol. 162, N. 3, pp. 329-336

Nash, K.; Hafeez, A., & Hou, S. (2002). Hospital-acquired renal insufficiency. *American Journal of Kidney Diseases*, Vol. 39, N. 5, pp. 930-936

Nelson, R.G., & Tuttle, K.R. (2007). The new KDOQI clinical practice guidelines and clinical practice recommendations for diabetes and CKD. *Blood Purification*, Vol. 25, N. 1, pp. 112-114

Parfrey, P.S.; Griffiths, S.M.; Barrett, B.J.; Paul, M.D.; Genge, M.; Withers, J.; Farid, N., & McManamon, P.J. (1989). Contrast material-induced renal failure in patients with diabetes mellitus, renal insufficiency, or both. A prospective controlled study. *New England Journal of Medicine*, Vol. 320, N. 3, pp. 143-149

Perkins, B.A.; Nelson, R.G.; Ostrander, B.E.; Blouch, K.L.; Krolewski, A.S.; Myers, B.D., & Warram, J.H. (2005). Detection of renal function decline in patients with diabetes and normal or elevated GFR by serial measurements of serum cystatin C concentration: results of a 4-year follow-up study. *Journal of the American Society of Nephrology*, Vol. 16, N. 5, pp. 1404-1412

Rihal, C.S.; Textor, S.C.; Grill, D.E.; Berger, P.B.; Ting, H.H.; Best, P.J.; Singh, M.; Bell, M.R.; Barsness, G.W.; Mathew, V.; Garratt, K.N., & Holmes, D.R. Jr. (2002). Incidence and prognostic importance of acute renal failure after percutaneous coronary intervention. *Circulation*, Vol. 105, N. 19, pp. 2259-226

Rosenstock, J.L.; Bruno, R.; Kim, J.K.; Lubarsky, L.; Schaller, R.; Panagopoulos, G.; DeVita, M.V., & Michelis, M.F. (2008) The effect of withdrawal of ACE inhibitors or angiotensin receptor blockers prior to coronary angiography on the incidence of contrast-induced nephropathy. *International Urology and Nephrology*, Vol. 40, N. 3, pp. 749-755

Savazzi, G.; Detrenis, S.; Meschi, M., & Musini S. (2005). Low-osmolar and iso-osmolar contrast media in contrast-induced nephropathy. *American Journal of Kidney Diseases*, Vol. 45, N. 2, pp. 435-436

Savazzi, G.; Cusmano, F.; Allegri, L., & Garini, G. (1997). Physiopathology, clinical aspects and prevention of renal insufficiency caused by contrast media. *Recenti Progressi in Medicina*, Vol. 88, N. 3, pp. 109-114

Sidhu, R.B.; Brown, J.R.; Robb, J.F.; Jayne J.E.; Friedman, B.J.; Hettleman, B.D.; Kaplan, A.V.; Niles, N.W., & Thompson, C.A. (2008). Interaction of gender and age on post cardiac catheterization contrast-induced acute kidney injury. *American Journal of Cardiology*, Vol. 102, N. 11, pp. 1482-1486

Strada, E.; Battistelli, L., & Savazzi, G. (2008). Bence-Jones proteinuria and kidney's damages. *Recenti Progressi in Medicina*, Vol. 99, N. 7, pp. 389-394

Thomsen, H.S. & Morcos, SK. (2003). Contrast media and the kidney: European Society of Urogenital Radiology (ESUR) guidelines. *British Journal of Radiology*, Vol. 76, N. 908, pp. 513-518

Thomsen, H.S. & Morcos, SK. (2006). Contrast medium induced nephropathy: is there a new consensus? A review of published guidelines. *European Radiology*, Vol. 16, N. 8, pp. 1835-1840

Thomsen, H.S., & Morcos, S.K. (1999). Contrast media and metformin: guidelines to diminish the risk of lactic acidosis in non-insulin-dependent diabetics after administration of contrast media. ESUR Contrast Media Safety Committee. *European Radiology*, Vol. 9, N. 4, pp. 738-740

Toprak, O. (2007). Conflicting and new risk factors for contrast induced nephropathy. *The Journal of Urology*, Vol. 178, N. 6, pp. 2277-2283

Toprak, O. (2007). Risk markers for contrast-induced nephropathy. *American Journal of Medical Sciences*, Vol. 334, N. 4, pp. 283-290

Toprak, O.; Cirit, M.; Yesil, M.; Bayata, S.; Tanrisev, M.; Varol, U.; Ersoy, R.; Esi, & E. (2007). Impact of diabetic and pre-diabetic state on development of contrast-induced nephropathy in patients with chronic kidney disease. *Nephrology, Dialysis, Transplantation*, Vol. 22, N. 3, pp. 819-826

11

The Outcome of HIV-Positive Patients Admitted to Intensive Care Units with Acute Kidney Injury

J. D. Nel and M. R. Moosa
Division of Nephrology, Department of Medicine, University of Stellenbosch and Renal Unit, Tygerberg Hospital, Cape Town South Africa

1. Introduction

Acute kidney injury is a serious clinical problem with significant morbidity and mortality. Several factors are recognized to aggravate the outcome including advanced age, gender, oliguria and the serum creatinine level. What is currently unknown is whether the presence of the human immunodeficiency virus (HIV) aggravates the outcome of patients who develop acute kidney injury (AKI). Sub-Saharan Africa currently bears the brunt of the global HIV pandemic. In South Africa alone more than 5.7 million people are infected ((UNAIDS 2008 report on the global AIDS epidemic, 2009), creating substantial additional pressure on already inadequate social and healthcare infrastructures. Acute kidney injury occurs commonly in HIV-infected patients admitted to hospital and carries with it substantial mortality. In a resource-poor environment clinicians are often forced to select patients with a better chance of survival for admission to the intensive care unit (ICU). A rigorous evaluation of the outcomes of HIV-positive patients admitted to ICU with AKI may assist in identifying factors associated with better survival, and thus aid in the cost-effective management of these patients.

2. Description of the conditions involved

2.1 Acute kidney injury

Acute kidney injury is characterized by a sudden reduction in glomerular filtration rate and is expressed clinically as azotemia with or without accompanying oliguria. Research on the outcomes of patients with AKI has been hampered by the absence of uniformity in the definition of the condition. With more than 35 different definitions being used before 2002, clinicians battled a bewildering array of reports varying in severity and mortality rates for patients (Ronco et al, 2010). In order to create some uniformity, the Acute Dialysis Quality Initiative formulated a consensus definition, the RIFLE criteria which were published in 2004. In a subsequent review, The Acute Kidney Injury network (AKIN) proposed minor modifications to the RIFLE system. This included the use of the term *acute kidney injury* instead of *acute renal failure,* recognizing that kidney injure does not always result in failure or the need for renal replacement therapy, but that even minor injury can have severe consequences, especially in severely ill patients, including HIV-infected patients.

The mortality of AKI remains high and is of the order of 50% in hospitalized patients who require dialysis (Metcalfe et al, 2002). ICU patients with multi-organ failure have mortality rates approaching 90%, despite improvements in the management of these patients (Uchino et al, 2005).

AKI is common in HIV-infected patients admitted to hospital, with a published occurrence rate of 5.9 per 100 person years in developed countries (Franceschini et al, 2005). More than 50% of episodes are attributed to infection. Most patients have pre-renal failure, often resulting in acute tubular necrosis from sepsis and fluid depletion because of vomiting, diarrhea and poor intake (Williams et al, 1998). There are little reliable data available on the causes and incidence of acute HIV-related kidney injury in Africa, but it is clear that a different pattern of presentation from the developed world is observed. Patients are frequently previously well young black adults who present with overwhelming opportunistic infections. In a Cape Town-based study this has lead to a 500% escalation in the provision of acute dialysis to HIV-infected patients over a 6 year period (Arendse et al, 2011). This study found acute tubular necrosis as the clinical and biopsy-determined cause for AKI requiring urgent dialysis in 58% of the HIV-infected patients between 2002 and 2007. These findings are almost identical to a study by Williams reported in 1998. In contrast, the main causes of AKI in HIV patients in developed countries are predominantly nephrotoxicity, rhabdomyolysis, ischemia and dehydration (Izzedine et al, 2007). Other common causes include interstitial nephritis due to infections and drugs commonly used to treat or prevent opportunistic infections, as well as obstructive uropathy, crystalluria and other insults from the antiretroviral drugs.

2.2 Human Immunodeficiency virus (HIV) infection and the kidney

The profound immunodeficiency from HIV infection is well described, and results primarily from the progressive deficiency of the subset of CD4-helper T cells. The CD4 receptor is vital for HIV entry, and the subsequent immune dysfunction, results in a high risk of developing opportunistic infections and neoplasms. The progression from infection to seroconversion, latent disease, early symptomatic infection and eventually advanced AIDS disease is well documented. Human Immunodeficiency Virus-associated nephropathy (HIVAN) is a common cause of end-stage renal failure, predominantly in black patients. Though timely interventions with antiretroviral (ARV) therapy and angiotensin converting enzyme inhibitors (ACEI) can reduce the progression of the disease, this aggressive glomerulopathy can advance to endstage kidney disease (ESKD) within weeks to months. It may be difficult to distinguish the effects of an acute insult to the kidneys from underlying HIVAN. The kidneys are typically normal or even increased in size even in advanced HIVAN, in contrast to the small kidneys found sonographically in most other forms of ESKD. To compound the issue, conditions frequently co-exist: in biopsies performed in a study on HIV-positive patients with presumed acute renal failure, 20% of the patients had HIVAN as the predominant underlying pathology (Arendse et al, 2011).

Given the complexity of HIV-associated renal failure and the impact of this increasing burden of disease on countries in sub-Saharan Africa, it would be important to be able to identify patients with potentially better outcomes from the severe case-load of critically ill HIV-positive patients, and apply limited resources in such a way that would offer the most benefit.

3. Objectives

With this literature review we planned to assess the survival of HIV-positive patients with AKI admitted to ICU, compared to the survival of those who were HIV-negative. If possible, we also wanted to identify factors which may predict poorer outcomes. The primary outcome to be assessed was survival in ICU, with our secondary outcomes being 30-day and 90-day post ICU survival, provided that sufficient data were available.

4. Methods

We searched the following databases: Pubmed (incorporating Medline), Web of Science (including Science Citation Index), Academic Search Premier, the Cochrane Library and Scopus (incorporating Embase) for all relevant literature up to June 2011. We used a controlled vocabulary of Medical Subject Headings terms, and free text, appropriately modified for the different databases. Included in the string sentence were the terms "acute renal failure" OR "ARF" AND "human immunodeficiency virus" OR "HIV" AND "Intensive Care Unit" OR "ICU". The electronic search results yielded a total of 84 articles which were screened liberally from titles and abstracts and followed by the selection of full papers for inclusion in the review. Particular attention was paid to the possible inclusion of duplicate publications or overlap of databases in order to avoid the multiple inclusions of the same study.

All randomised control trials, case-control, and cohort studies investigating the survival of HIV-positive patients with acute renal failure compared to the survival of the general population with acute renal failure in ICU were to be included. Only studies published in the English language were included. In order to include the largest number of published articles, the definition of acute renal failure/acute injury was not limited to the RIFLE/AKIN criteria. We decided to distinguish clearly on mortality in ARV-naïve patients as compared to patients on ARV therapy if possible. Studies correcting for confounding factors were to be given preference.

5. Results

Our search yielded articles from 1988 to 2010. Of the 84 articles identified by our databases, 5 were identified by more than one database. One article was written in German and thus excluded, 5 were identified as posters, abstracts at congresses or personal correspondence and thus not available for scrutiny, and one article could not be accessed by the electronic resources from our library.

Seventy-two articles remained and were scrutinised carefully. Of these, 22 were dismissed as not being relevant to our review. Individual case studies numbered 8, all of which were discarded reducing the total of relevant articles to 42. Of these 3 dealt with HIV infection and respiratory illness; 1 reviewed the survival of HIV-positive paediatric patients in ICU without mentioning acute renal failure; 8 addressed HIV-positive patients in ICU due to respiratory failure or *Pneumocystis jiroveci* infection; 2 focused solely on acute respiratory failure without addressing HIV infection; 8 articles covered other systemic infections in patients with HIV without addressing ICU outcomes or AKI; 6 articles covered aspects of HIV infection with AKI but without assessing any Intensive Care aspect; 3 articles dealt with

AKI in the ICU but did not address any aspect of HIV infection, and 5 of the identified articles dealt with aspects of AKI only without addressing ICU or HIV infection.

Only 5 articles addressed all three of our key search items: HIV infection, intensive care and ARF/AKI. Of these, one listed the number of HIV-positive patients as 1% of their total study population without discussing outcome or comparison to the HIV-negative ICU patients with renal failure, and was thus discarded (Mehta et al, 2004). Another assessed the application of the RIFLE criteria for acute renal failure in critically ill HIV-infected patients, as well as their survival, but failed to compare it to the uninfected patients in their ICU, and was discarded as well (Lopes et al, 2007a). An article evaluating long-term risk of mortality after AKI in patients with sepsis was discarded because it only assessed the mortality of the group surviving ICU admission two years after their discharge (Lopes et al, 2010). The remaining two articles assessed the impact of acute renal failure on the HIV population in ICU retrospectively as single unit studies and identified it as a cause for increased mortality, but failed again to compare their outcomes with outcomes of patients from the general population with acute renal failure in ICU (Coquet et al, 2010; Lopes et al, 2007b).

6. Conclusion

There are insufficient publications available comparing the outcomes of HIV-positive patients with AKI admitted to ICU directly with that of the general population in ICU with acute renal failure in randomised control trials, cohort studies or retrospective studies to provide clear answers.

7. Discussion

Significant progress has been made in the treatment of HIV-disease since the early days of the pandemic, when the issues regarding acquired immunodeficiency syndrome patients and dialysis were still being debated (Pennel & Bourgoignie, 1988). It is commonly accepted that the outcome of patients with HIV is no different to other patients admitted to ICU (Rosen et al, 2006). Several publications have reported that critically ill patients with HIV infection have similar outcomes to other patients with a comparable severity of illness (Casalino et al, 1988; Forrest et al, 1988). Although outcome studies in patients with HIV infection are limited by retrospective analyses and subsequent selection bias a South African study (albeit with significant methodological limitations) confirmed this (Bhagwanjee et al, 1997).

In the ARV era, ICU survival of critically ill HIV-patients has increased significantly, despite unchanged disease severity (Coquet et al, 2010). Whereas ICU management of these patients was widely perceived as futile in the 1980s, mortality rates steadily declined as shown by a single-centre study, where co-morbidities and organ dysfunctions - but not HIV-variables were associated with mortality (Coquet et al, 2010). In this study, AKI was still independently associated with death, as it is in non HIV-infected ICU patients (Odds ratio 4.21; 95% Confidence interval). In a study on the long-term risk of mortality after AKI in patients with sepsis, HIV infection was not associated with increased 2-year mortality after discharge from the ICU (Lopes et al, 2010). This study, however, made no comparison between the in-ICU survival of HIV-infected patients who developed AKI associated with sepsis, and HIV non-infected patients.

Little prospective data are available on the survival of the subgroup of HIV-infected patients in ICU who develop AKI. A small single-centre study demonstrated a significantly higher mortality rate in ICU in HIV-infected patients who develop AKI compared to HIV-infected patients who do not. Sepsis was the most common associated aetiology (Lopes et al, 2007b). In a publication examining the same data, the authors assessed the RIFLE criteria for acute renal failure in these patients, and found that mortality increased significantly from normal to RIFLE class F (normal, 23.5%; class R, 50%; class I, 66.6% and class F, 72%; $P<0.0001$). The majority of their patients died within one month of ICU admission, but all survivors had complete recovery of renal function (Lopes et al, 2007a). When compared to a retrospective cohort study in seven intensive care units where the mortality rates for RIFLE class R was 8.8%, class I, 11.4% and class F 26% (Hoste et al, 2006), it would seem that HIV-infected patients have significantly worse outcomes. This comparison is however problematic, since neither differences in the severity of illness of the patients nor their subsequent renal management was corrected for.

In conclusion, there are no prospective studies available comparing the outcomes of HIV-positive patients with AKI admitted to ICU directly with that of HIV uninfected ICU patients with comparable severities of illness. The available literature on patients with HIV infection in the ICU is most often confounded by single centre experience, reflecting local ICU admission criteria, and management, practice patterns and especially management of renal failure. Prospective studies are needed to provide further answers.

8. References

Arendse, CG. Okpechi, I. Swanepoel, CR. (2011). Acute dialysis in HIV-positive patients in Cape Town, South Africa. *Nephrology* 16:39-44

Bhagwanjee, S. Muckart, DJJ. Jeena, PM.; et al. (1997). Does HIV status influence the outcome of patients admitted to a surgical intensive care unit? A prospective double blind study. *BMJ* 314:1077–1084.

Casalino, E. Mendoza-Sassi, G. Wolff, M. et al. (1998). Predictors of short-and long-term survival in HIV-infected patients admitted to the ICU. *Chest* 113:421–429

Coquet, I. Pavie, J. Palmer, P. Barbier, F. Legriel, S. Mayaux, J. et al. (2010). Survival trends in critically ill HIV-infected patients in the highly active antiretroviral therapy era. *Crit Care* 14(3):R107

Forrest, DM. Djurdjev, O. Zala, C. et al. (1998). Validation of the multisystem organ failure score as a predictor of mortality in patients with AIDS-related *Pneumocystis carinii* pneumonia and respiratory failure. *Chest* 114:199–206

Franceschini, N. Napravnik, S. Eron, JJ. Szcezech, LA. Finn, WF. (2005). Incidence and aetiology of acute renal failure among ambulatory HIV-infected patients. *Kidney Int.* 2005; 67: 1526–31.

Hoste, EAJ. Clermont, G. Kersten, A. et al. (2006). RIFLE criteria for acute kidney injury are associated with hospital mortality in critically ill patients: a cohort analysis. *Crit Care* 10(3) R73

Izzedine, H. Baumelou, A. Deray, G. Acute renal failure in HIV patients. (2007). *Nephrol Dial Transpl.* 22: 2757-62

Lopes, JA. Fernandes, J. Jorge, S. Neves, J. Antunes, F. Prata, MM. (2007a). An assessment of the RIFLE criteria for acute renal failure in critically ill HIV-infected patients. *Crit Care* 11(1):401

Lopes, JA. Fernandes, J. Jorge, S. Neves, J. Antunes, F. Prata, MM. (2007b). Acute renal failure in critically ill HIV-infected patients. *Crit Care* 11(1)404

Lopes, JA. Fernandes, J. Jorge, S. Resina, C. Santos, C. Pereira, A. et al. (2010). Long-term risk of mortality after acute kidney injury in patients with sepsis: a contemporary analysis. *BMC Nephrol* June 2, 2011; 11:9.

Mehta, RL. Ipascual, MT. Soroko, S. Savage, BR. Himmelfarb, J. Alp Ikizler, T. et al. (2004) Spectrum of acute renal failure in the intensive care unit: The PICARD experience. *Kidney Int.* 10; 66(4): 1613-1621

Metcalfe, W. Simpson, M. Khan, IH. et al. (2002) Acute renal failure requiring renal replacement therapy: Incidence and outcome. *Q. J. Med.* 95: 579–83.

Pennel, JP. Bourgoignie, JJ. (1988) Should AIDS patients be dialyzed? ASAIO Transactions 34 (4):907-911

Ronco, C. Bellomo, R. Kellum, JA. (Editors) (2010). *Critical Care Nephrology*, 2nd edition, Saunders Elsevier, p840-844

Rosen, MJ. Narasimhan, M. (2006). Critical care of immunocompromised patients: Human immunodeficeincy virus. *Crit Care Med.* 34:9 S425-429

The Joint United Nations Programme on HIV/AIDS (UNAIDS) 2008 report on the global AIDS epidemic. 2008 (12 July 2009). Available at: http://data.unaids.org/pub/GlobalReport/2008/JC1510_2008GlobalReport_en.zip.

Uchino, S. Kellum, JA. Bellomo, R. et al . (2005). Acute renal failure in critically ill patients: A multinational, multicentre study. *JAMA* 294: 813–18.

Williams, DI. Williams, DJ. Williams, IG. Unwin, RJ. Griffiths, MH. Miller, RF. (1998). Presentation, pathology, and outcome of HIV associated renal disease in a specialist centre for HIV/AIDS. *Sex Transm. Inf.* 74: 179–84.

12

Management of Heparin-Induced Thrombocytopenia in Uremic Patients with Hemodialysis

Takefumi Matsuo
Hyogo Prefectural Awaji Hospital, Sumoto
Japan

1. Introduction

Unfractionated heparin is the most commonly used anticoagulant for hemodialysis (HD) (Sonawane et al., 2006). It is well-known that heparin can cause immune-mediated thrombocytopenia due to immunoglobulin antibody formation against the complex of platelet factor 4 (PF4) and heparin. Heparin may also contribute to HD-associated platelet activation, thrombocytopenia, and increased PF4 release from platelets during a heparin dialytic session (Matsuo et al., 1986). Typically, IgG isotype HIT antibodies develop after 5-14 days of heparin exposure. The incidence of heparin-induced thrombocytopenia (HIT) was estimated at 3.9% in newly treated hemodialysis patients (Yamamoto et al., 1996). Also, dialysis is often complicated by clotting of the dialysis lines and/or dialyzer due to hypercoagulation regardless of the etiology. When a diagnosis of HIT based on clinical symptoms of thrombocytopenia and immunoassay for PF4/heparin complex antibodies is employed, it remains unclear whether a few patients have HIT. An antigen-based immunoassay to detect the presence of antibodies in a patient's circulation that binds to the PF4/heparin complex is highly sensitive but less specific. Thus, the serological diagnosis of HIT needs to be confirmed by employing a functional assay such as ^{14}C-serotonin release assay and heparin-induced platelet aggregation test. The enzyme-linked immunosorbent assay (ELISA) usually detects antibodies of three classes of isotype (IgG, IgA, and IgM) regardless of the capability of these antibodies to activate platelets. There is a way to improve the specificity based on only IgG class antibodies having the capability of inducing platelet activation by heparin (Chang et al., 2006; Syed & Reilly, 2009).

There are two kinds of dialysis-related complication: unexpected clotting in the circuit and abrupt fistula thrombosis. The former seems to be more frequent in HIT patients than that in non-HIT patients. Visible clotting in the extracorporeal circulation can provide a clue to suspect HIT. AVF thrombosis is also observed in both HIT and non-HIT patients. After starting heparin, the sudden onset of fistula closure is rare as HIT-complicated thrombosis (O'Shea et al., 2002; Nakamoto et al., 2005).

HD patients who develop HIT require not only the discontinuation of heparin, but essentially also the introduction of alternative anticoagulant therapy. An alternative anticoagulant, such as citric acid, and some therapeutic methods, such as heparin-free dialysis and peritoneal dialysis, have been employed for patients who require dialysis. However, these therapeutic modalities are unlikely to be beneficial because of the absence of evidence for long-term management.

Regarding clinical evidence to support HIT, a non-heparin anticoagulant should be started with an alternative to heparin. Argatroban rather than lepirudin is recommended as elimination is not via the kidneys, but mainly via the billiary system. As the elimination of lepirudin mainly depends on the renal function, it is not easy to monitor the optimal dose of lepirudin in each session. However, the dose of argatroban in hepato-renal failure is recognized variably to reduce while avoiding major bleeding in a critical setting (Hurting & Murray et al., 2007). Nafamostat mesilate, a polyvalent protease inhibitor, is sometimes used as an alternative to heparin in Japan. Although a few patients showed the effective resolution of clotting and a gradual increase of the platelet count to the baseline level in a subsequent session receiving nafamostat mesilate, no clinical trial has ever been carried out to evaluate the efficacy in the management of HIT (Matsuo & Wanaka, 2008b). Although hemodialysis-related HIT appears in an early session after starting HD with heparin, some patients with the anti-PF4/heparin complex antibodies have a risk of delayed-onset HIT, and they may suffer from HIT after cardiovascular intervention.

2. Frequency of HIT in dialysis patients

The frequency of HIT is suggested to be from 1 to 5% of patients exposed to unfractionated heparin, and significantly lower in patients exposed to low-molecular-weight heparin. As one of the reasons for the various frequencies of HIT, assays used to detect HIT antibodies vary in their specificity and sensitivity. An assay for HIT antibody usually detects both non-pathogenic and pathogenic antibodies irrespective of the presence of thrombocytopenia. The clinical significance without thrombocytopenia in which a patient exhibits a stable titer of long-term HIT antibodies remains unclear, but there is an ongoing survey on whether or not subjects have a risk of thrombosis (Asmis et al., 2008).

Few reports on the frequency of HIT in dialysis patients are known, although heparin is employed as the most useful anticoagulant during dialysis. It was believed that the frequency of HIT would be low in a survey targeting to all dialytic patients including both acute and chronic stages (Hutchison et al., 2005). Two surveys involving different subjects show quite different figures on the frequency of HIT. A relatively high frequency of 3.2% was reported for newly treated subjects receiving dialysis in three months (Yamamoto et al., 1996), and a low rate frequency of 0.6% is described in chronic dialysis patients treated for over 3 months (Matsuo et al., 2006). Thus, the frequency of HIT in a dialysis population is different between newly treated and chronic maintained dialytic groups. HIT in the former shows a similar incidence to the heparin-sensitive group, and HIT in the later group is rarely identified as HIT or recurrence of HIT when a patient experiences changes in the immunological tolerance brought about by cardiovascular surgery, orthopedic surgery, and high-dose administration of erythropoietin with an adverse platelet-stimulating reaction.

3. Clinical manifestations and laboratory testing in HD-HIT patients

Major clinical manifestations are primary thrombocytopenia and new thrombosis. The onset of thrombocytopenia and/or thrombosis which sometimes complicates before thrombocytopenia usually occurs 5-10 days after starting heparin anticoagulation. Although thrombocytopenia is ordinarily defined as a >50% fall in the platelet count and below 100×10^9 /L, the definition of HD-HIT is less strict, in the range of a >30% fall in the platelet count and below 150×10^9 /L due to the intermittent use of heparin. Timing of the fall of platelet counts also is likely to delay due to the intermittent heparin use. Thus, no dialytic session day may give a chance of recovering the platelet count, and the timing is usually delayed over 10 days. However, heparin flushing to maintain the patency of the inserted catheter in non-session days sometimes leads to the conventional formation of HIT antibodies (Table 1).

Step	Clinical and Lab. assessment	Action plan
1	suspicion of HIT	thrombocytopenia (<150×10^9 /L, unexplained decrease of > 30%), timing of over 5 days, no other cause of thrombocytopenia or thrombosis
2	ELISA (IgG, A, M)	no likelihood of HIT due to a negative qualitative assay
3	specific IgG-ELISA	high specificity for platelet-activating antibodies
4	^{14}C serotonin release assay (platelet aggregation test)	confirmation of HIT as a gold standard test (not preferable due to being less sensitive)
5	reassessment of HIT if necessary	recheck other causes of thrombocytopenia and thrombosis, assess with alternative therapy

Table 1. Diagnostic approach to HIT

HIT symptoms may occur more rapidly within 24 hr or less in patients who have had a previous exposure to heparin within the prior 3 months. However, a dialytic patient can experience the onset of acute systemic reaction associated with circuit clotting and a marked drop in the platelet count immediately after a bolus heparin injection at start of the session. In chronic intermittent dialysis, HIT is unlikely to occur after several weeks of heparin exposure.

HIT testing is grouped into two types: 1) detection of immunoglobulin antibody against heparin/PF4 complexes by ELISA as a standard technique, and ELISA is simple to perform, can be done in a few hours, is highly sensitive and less specific for antibody detection. Owing in part to its high sensitivity, ELISA often detects antibodies that would not be positive in ^{14}C serotonin release and may be clinically insignificant. ELISA provides much information about the likelihood that a patient has HIT (Shaheed et al., 2007; Aster RH. 2010), and 2) functional assays for the detection of platelet-activating immunoglobulin G by ^{14}C serotonin release. ELISA permits the identification of three subclasses of immunoglobulin: IgG, IgA, and IgM, reacting with PF4/heparin complexes in a solid-phase plate. To avoid the overdiagnosis of HIT, the pathogenic impact of HIT antibodies should be considered if the optical density is ≥ 0.4 (Warkentin et al., 2008). Therefore, a negative result excludes the diagnosis of HIT. ELISA detects together with IgA and IgM antibodies that do not react on FcγIIA-mediated platelet activation. Specific IgG-HIT antibodies can contribute to the interaction of the HIT antibody/PF4/heparin complexes with the FcγIIA receptor, and subsequently induce platelet activation and the release of microparticles. A high-titer of IgG antibodies is accountable for HIT as well (EI-Shahawy et al., 2007; Carrier et al., 2008).

The ^{14}C serotonin release assay is the gold standard because of its high sensitivity and specificity. Thus, the ^{14}C serotonin release assay should be performed to confirm the diagnosis if a weak positive result is obtained using ELISA (Sheriden et al., 1986; Pouplard et al., 1999). For the assessment of HD-HIT, the pretest probability of the diagnosis of HIT (4T's test) has not been elucidated whether clot formation in the extracorporeal circulation is the first sign of HIT (Weiss et al., 2007). Sudden unexpected clotting in the circuit often provides an important clue for HIT diagnosis despite of there being many causes of clotting during dialysis. After changing the clotted dialyzer and circuit to new ones, dialysis must be restarted with an alternative to heparin, and the planned treatment modality can be uneventfully completed. Subsequent sessions will never affect re-clotting and the recurrence of thrombocytopenia under adequate switching to non-heparin anticoagulation. Furthermore, the patient is more likely to have HIT in the presence of a comparable HIT-antibody seroconversion. Clotting of the extracorporeal circuit seems to be a manifestation of HIT in the context of primary thrombocytopenia, the visible resolution of clotting with an alternative anticoagulant, HIT antibody formation, and timing within 3 months of starting HD.

Step 1. Recognition of HIT is most important: 1. Unexpected clotting of dialyzer/circuit, and thrombotic occlusion of arteriovenous fistula/grafting despite optimal dose of heparin infusion 2. Absence of other cause of clotting: slow blood flows, high hematocrit, high ultrafiltration rate, intradialytic blood and blood product transfusion, intradialytic lipid transfusion 3. Check thrombocytopenia
Step 2. Emergent protocol for suspected HIT patient: 1. Stop dialysis immediately, and replace whole extracorporeal circuit with a new one 2. Restart dialysis with argatroban (lepirudin) 3. Confirm by visible inspection that there is no clot in the circuit once starting an alternative to heparin 4. Avoid heparin flush on non-session days

Table 2. Management strategy for HIT in dialytic patients

The clinical features of HIT in dialysis patients includes acute thrombocytopenia that is associated with renal insufficiency except HIT (Oliveria et al., 2008), and repeated clotting of extracorporeal circulation undergoing heparin administration (Lasocki et al., 2008), and the clear disappearance of clots on using an alternative anticoagulant to heparin, and/or, rarely, thrombotic occlusion in AV fistula/grafting (O'Shea et al., 2002, Nakamoto et al., 2005). Circuit clotting occasionally occurs in a routine dialysis procedure, caused by non-HIT factors. The causes of clotting are slow blood flow, high hematocrit, high ultrafiltration rate, intradialytic blood and blood product transfusion, intradialytic lipid transfusion. In clinical settings, it is difficult to decide whether the clotted circuit is derived from HIT or not. No differences in the platelet count's fall and timing between clotting-circuit and non-clotting circuit groups have been found in clinical settings. However, a higher level of optical density in ELISA is noted in the clotting patient group. This suggests that HIT antibody formation may be active in the clotting rather than non-clotting patent group (Table 2).

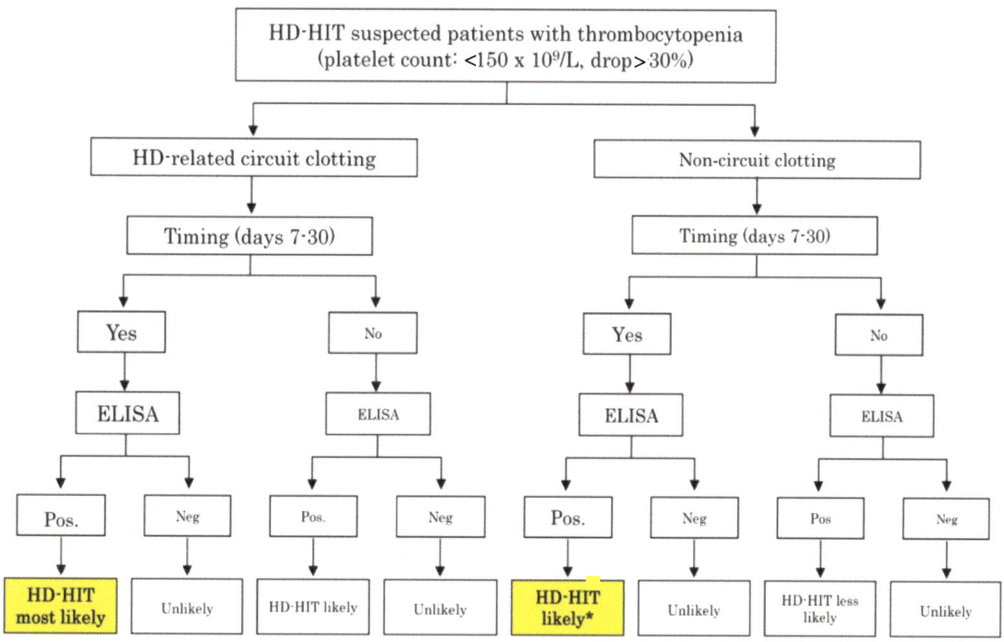

Fig. 1. Algorithm for the diagnosis of HIT in hemodialysis by adding the results of ELISA

4. Diagnostic approach to HD-HIT patients

An HD patient associated with HIT is recognized by stepwise assessment. The first step is the evaluation of the platelet count with the definition ($<150\times10^9$ /L and > 30%). If the patient shows circuit clotting with no other causes, the next step would be to evaluate the timing of thrombocytopenia over days 7-30. The timing of HD-HIT is generally applied over a wider range than usual due to the duration of heparin use always being limited in dialysis of 4-6 hours per day. Positive ELISA added to platelet reduction, the presence of a clotting circuit, and reasonable timing, should be considered as revealing HIT. Thirty six (92.3%) of 39 patients with four-factor combinations of thrombocytopenia, clotted circuit, optimal timing of platelet count fall, and positive ELISA had a positive ^{14}C serotonin release assay (Matsuo et al., accepted in Clin Appl Throm/Hemost). According to the algorithm under the condition of no circuit clotting, five (71.4%) of 7 patients with thrombocytopenia, reasonable timing, and positive ELISA also had a positive ^{14}C serotonin release assay. In the algorithm (Fig. 1), four groups can be identified: HD-HIT is most likely due to a highest positive rate of ^{14}C serotonin release among the four groups, 'HD-HIT most likely'; secondly, HD-HIT is likely to show a relatively high rate on a functional assay, 'HD-HIT likely'. Timing outside the range and a negative ELISA despite the presence of a clotting circuit should be identified as 'unlikely'. 'HD-HIT less likely' without any clotting is rare even though ELISA is positive.

The sudden occurrence of clots in the dialyzer and/or circuit with an unexpected fall in the platelet count between 7 and 30 days are dramatic symptoms of HIT in HD patients undergoing appropriate anticoagulation with heparin. In an HD patient with suspected HIT, the clinical implication of clotting in the circuit as HIT can easily be supported in combination with thrombocytopenia, timing of the platelet fall, and result of ELISA.

5. Management of HD-HIT patients

Visible clotting in the circuit, including blood chambers, tubes, and dialyzer, are easily recognized by medical staff in the session, so HIT management can be initiated immediately when the clotting is likely to arise from HD-HIT. Once the HIT diagnosis has been established from high clinical suspicion alone before laboratory confirmation, it is essential that all sources of heparin, including low-molecular-weight-heparin, heparin flushing, and heparin-coated catheters or devices, must be discontinued. The early recognition of HIT in the presence of clot formation in the extracorporeal circuit is critical, and any additional infusion of heparin on the misunderstanding of heparin shortage must be contraindicated to resolve the clot. When the dialytic procedure cannot be continued with circuit clotting, a new dialyzer and devices of the extracorporeal circuit must be set up, and the session must be immediately restarted with an alternative anticoagulant. Then, the diagnosis of HIT can be verified using the algorithmic assessment in Fig. 1 and Table 2.

Established alternative anticoagulation in HD patients with HIT is conducted with danaparoid, lepirudin, and argatroban. Danaparoid is a low- molecular-weight heparinoid. Although danaparoid is the most widely used for HD-HIT patients, it does not exhibit proper anticoagulation for HD-HIT due to clinically relevant cross-reactivity. Lepirudin is a recombinant hirudin preparation. Adequate dose adjustment is very difficult in for HD-HIT patients, in which it is cleared mainly by the kidneys and its half-life is markedly long in uremic patients.

Argatroban (formerly called MD805), a synthetic direct thrombin inhibitor, is non-immunogenic and does not show cross-reactivity with HIT antibodies. In contrast to lepirudin, argatroban is primarily hepatically metabolized, and its half-life is moderately extended in HD patients (Matsuo et al., 1988; Matsuo et al., 1990). Argatroban as an alternative anticoagulant is predominantly used for the prevention of extracorporeal circuit clotting in HD-HIT patients at the initial dose of 250μg/kg at the start of dialysis, and followed by a continuous infusion of at 2μg/kg/min while the hepatic function is normal. Dose adjustment is conducted for an empirical target of a 1.5-3.0-fold prolongation of the activated partial thromboplastin time (APTT) test, as an equivalent to the prolongation of heparin therapy. This dose can be reduced to <2μg/kg/min with a 1.5-2.5-fold prolongation of the APTT after the acute phase of HIT has subsided. The dose should also be reduced to

<2μg/kg/min depending on the severity hepatic dysfunction to avoid unexpected hemorrhagic complications. Only the replacement of heparin with argatroban in dialysis can lead to recovery from symptoms of HIT (Gozdzikiewicz et al., 2007; Roncon-Albuquerque et al., 2010; Matsuo & Wanaka, 2008a). Despite there being no apparent evidence for the systemic administration of argatroban on non-session days, argatroban anticoagulation may be useful to prevent the risk of new and worsening thrombotic events. When an HD-HIT patient is in a hypercoagulable state, such as with an elevated level of plasma D-dimer, argatroban therapy seems to be essential. The empirical dose of the drug is estimated to 0.7μg/kg/min in patients with a normal liver function and 0.2μg/kg/min in those with hepatic dysfunction or a risk of bleeding. Future studies should be done on how to apply the drug on non-session days (Hursting & Murray et al., 2008).

Nafamostat mesilate, a polyvalent synthetic protease inhibitor, is employed as a regional anticoagulant in dialysis patients with bleeding risks as an alternative to heparin in Japan. The drug has no influence on the systemic blood coagulation cascade due to its very short half-life, within 10 min, about 40% of the drug is removed from the dialyzer, and there is no cross-reactivity with HIT antibodies. Despite the fact that the HD-HIT session is uneventfully completed using nafamostat mesilate, it remains why the drug has a therapeutic benefit on the resolution of HIT over the effect of heparin cessation (Matsuo et al., 2001; Matsuo & Wanaka, 2008b)

	Age/sex	Type of surgery	Thrombocytopenia (50%fall, 5-10 days from pre-op. level)	Immunoassay (pos >0.4 OD)			Functional assay (pos >20%)		
				Pre	7days	14days	Pre	7days	14days
1	58/M	aortic aneurysm grafting	–*	–**	1.82	2.39	–***	–	96
2	67/M	aortic aneurysm grafting	+ (56.6%)	–	–	–	–	–	–
3	63/M	CABG	–	–	–	–	–	–	–
4	69/M	CABG	+ (69.6%)	–	–	–	–	–	–
5	55/M	CABG	–	–	–	–	–	–	–
6	60/F	CABG	+ (73.5%)	–	–	–	–	–	–
7	63/M	valve op.	–	–	–	–	–	–	–
8	70/M	CABG	–	1.28	1.87	2.01	-	65	68

* not consistent with platelet criteria
**optical density < 0.4 by ELISA
***radioactive serotonin release under 20%

Table 3. Seroconversion in cardiac surgery patients with chronic hemodialysis

6. Cardiovascular surgery with chronic hemodialysis

Chronic dialysis patients who repeatedly exposed to heparin rarely are at risk of developing HIT, show high-level mortality due to atherosclerotic cardiovascular events (Mureebe et al., 2004). Sometimes they have indications for cardiovascular surgery on non-dialysis sessions. There are few data available on whether long-term heparin usage affects post-operative seroconversion, and the development of HIT. Surgical procedures usually stimulate the release of PF4 from platelets and the endothelium. PF4 does certainly facilitate complex formation in the presence of a dynamic equilibrium with external heparin. Macromolecular PF4/heparin complexes stimulate the immunomediated production of anti-PF4/heparin complex antibodies. Increased levels of immunomediated HIT-antibody production are occasionally recognized in the post-operative period. Although a high rate of seroconversion appears to be involved in the development of HIT, most seroconversion shows a lack of thrombocytopenia, and very few patients with seroconversion develop HIT.

In cardiovascular patients receiving regular dialysis, the risk of HIT is presumed to increase in certain situations, such as cardiac interventions, by the modification of immunological tolerance to PF4/heparin complexes. Eight of 79 patients with cardiovascular surgery were treated with dialysis (Table 2). Two patients with neither thrombocytopenia nor thrombosis experienced seroconversion with the development of positive ELISA and SRA. One patient was negative in the pre-operative state despite heparin dialysis for 3.5 years. He may have undergone a resetting of the immunologic response to PF4/heparin complexes due to the influence of perioperative surgical procedures (case #1 in Table 3). The other patient had pre-existing HIT antibodies on ELISA, and the positive SRA would be induced by accelerating the production of HIT antibodies due to cardiac intervention (case #8 in Table 3). Although no 'true HIT' patient could be found in the series, this suggests that reactivation of the immune system could be functioning in the perioperative period, and the risk of developing HIT may be continuing until subsidence of HIT antibody production. Any thrombocytopenia corresponding to HIT criteria could not be detected with the monitoring of platelet counts in post-operation, despite a marked fall within 4 postoperative days, and steeply increasing platelet counts in the following days were observed regardless of whether or not the patients experienced seroconversion.

Post-operative thrombocytosis, in contrast to HIT-related thrombocytopenia, can influence the results of platelet counts, because marked thrombocytosis must compensate for thrombocytopenia derived from immune-mediate platelet consumption. When the recovery of platelet counts remains low over the 5th post-operative day and an abrupt platelet fall is induced by the reuse of heparin, HIT should be considered in patients with no other cause of thrombocytopenia.

HD patients with both positive ELISA and serotonin release assay and without defined thrombocytopenia may have a risk of developing HIT through re-exposure to heparin in a restarted dialysis session. A clotting circuit recognized as atypical HIT-related thrombosis is causally linked to the onset of thrombocytopenia, and the event will be certainly resolved by employing an alternative to heparin. HIT may occur even after years of uneventful chronic intermittent hemodialysis due to resetting of the immune mechanism triggered in cardiac surgery, catheter intervention, and, rarely, a platelet-activating procedures and agents.

	Symptoms of acute systemic reaction	Circuit clotting	AVF thrombus	Platelet count ($\times10^9$/L) at ASR	Maximum fall (%) in platelet count	Timing of platelet fall (days)
1	Dyspnea, chills, fever	+**	-	53	85	14
2	Nausea, vomiting	-	+	25	88	12
3*	Dyspnea, flushing, chills, fever,	-	-	16	90	13
4	Dyspnea, chest pain	+	-	28	94	7
5	Dyspnea, chest pain, hypotension, nausea, vomiting	-	+	84	72	13
6*	Dyspnea, fever	+	-	57	67	8
7***	Dyspnea, chills, nausea	+	-	92	80	11
8	Dyspnea, chills, fever, chest pain, nausea	+	-	74	73	11

*diagnosed with pseudo-pulmonary embolism, ** unexpected closure of hollow fibers of dialyzer with fibrin-platelet aggregates in two consecutive sessions, ***heparin flushing on non-session day.

Table 4. Eight patients with HIT-induced acute systemic reaction from twenty-seven dialytic patients who experienced some acute systemic reactions

7. Characteristics of acute systemic reaction in dialytic patients

Infrequently, an acute systemic reaction (ASR) as a manifestation of HIT occurs 5-30 min after heparin bolus administration at the start of dialysis. The symptoms are fever, chills, and flushing as acute inflammatory reactions, and hypertension, tachycardia, dyspnea, chest pain, and cardiopulmonary arrest. Although hypertension is usually associated with ASR (Warkentin et al., 2009), in contrast, acute hypotension often occurs as a sign of cardiovascular collapse during dialysis. When dyspnea as the cardiorespiratory reaction in ASR is prominent, it is considered to be a pseudo-pulmonary embolism (Tejedor Alonso et al., 2005; Hartman et al., 2006; Matsuo et al., 2007). However, the signs and symptoms are very similar to those in dialyzer reactions, dialytic complications as disequilibrium syndrome, and circuit clotting during the HD procedure. Except for platelet reduction by heparin, it is difficult to determine whether symptoms of ASR are most likely to be due to HIT in clinical settings. There are two causes of hypotension: HIT-induced hypotension may associate with cardiorespiratory collapse due to pseudo-pulmonary embolism, and HD-induced hypotension often with nausea and vomiting, and occasionally with back pain and syncope.

As the clinical features of eight patients defined with HIT-induced ASR from twenty-seven patients who experienced some ASR, seven of the eight patients suffered from dyspnea, and two ASR patients (case #3, #6 in Table 4) showing hypoxia, no radiological evidence, and the quick recovery of symptoms after the cessation of heparin were defined as pseudo-pulmonary embolism. Hypotension was implicated when pulmonary collapse was noted in a patient (case #5 in Table 4). Thus, hypotension was not a primary feature of the HIT-induced acute systemic reaction. However, no hypertension appeared in eight HIT-induced ASR patients. Either complications of circuit clotting or AVF thrombus formation appeared in seven patients excluding a case (case #3 in Table 4) of pseudo-pulmonary embolism. The platelet fall rate and timing in HIT-induced ASR cannot be differentiated from those of HD-induced ASR (Table 4). Complications during dialysis including dialyzer reactions, clotting circuit, anticoagulation failure, and hypotension may mimic the signs and symptoms of HIT-induced ASR except hypotension. Thus, a platelet count and assays for HIT antibodies should be considered for diagnosing acute HIT when HD patients show an abrupt fall in platelet counts and clinical symptoms of ASR with an unknown cause during dialysis. The results of the HIT-antibody assay showed that the differential diagnosis would be straightforward regarding whether HD patients with thrombocytopenia suffered from HIT-induced or HD-complicated ASR.

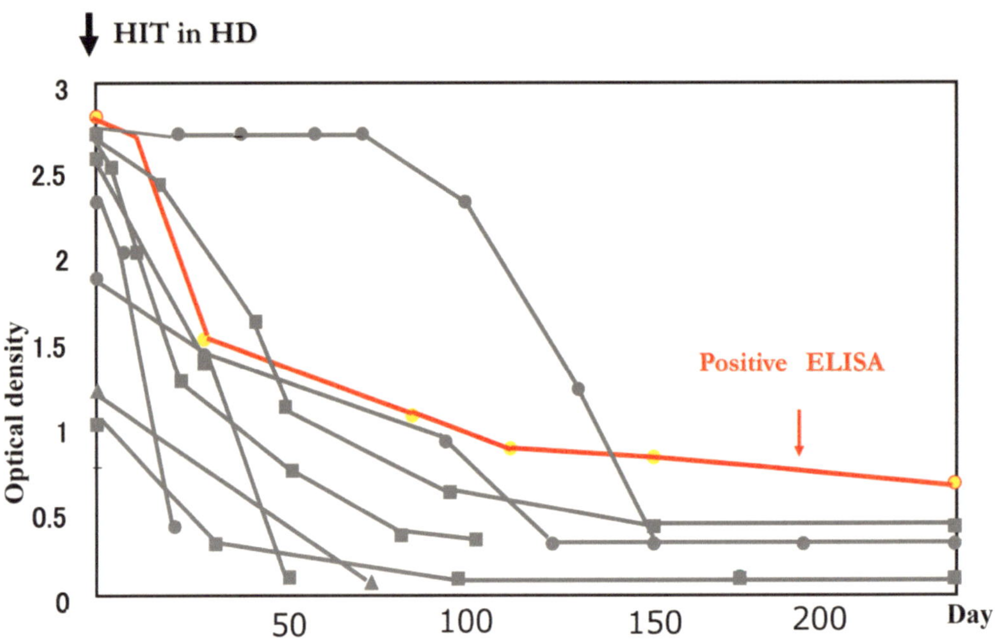

Fig. 2. Reduction in optical density of ELISA after heparin cessation in HD-HIT

8. Reexposure to heparin

The principal of heparin reexposure is based on a characteristic immune response in T-cell independent B-cell activation because of lack of a strong memory response, perhaps explaining transience and lack of anamnesis of the anti PF4/heparin immune response (Selleng et al., 2010). The reexposure can be carried out with lack of immune memory for the PF4/heparin complex antigen in patients with previous episodes of HIT when their HIT antibodies become negative. Currently, there is no clinical consensus regarding reexposure to heparin for HIT. However, it reexposure is needed at least 100 days after no detection of

HIT antibodies by ELISA. Reductions in the optical density of ELISA are quite variable after the cessation of heparin (Fig. 2). While a positive ELISA continues long-term over years marked as positive ELISA is also recognizable in Fig.2, a short span type is also contained. Since the various half-life of HIT antibodies may reflect the existence of different properties of HIT antibodies, each patient should be followed by ELISA until there is no longer a detection of HIT antibodies. Reexposure to heparin should be introduced under negative ELISA where adequate emergent measures are adopted including platelet counting tests (Matsuo et al., 2003; Davenport et al., 2009; Wanaka et al., 2010). A majority of heparin-reexposure patients show no recurrence of HIT unless they undergo cardiovascular surgery, catheter intervention, and, rarely, receive platelet-stimulating drugs. Reexposure to heparin in HD patients carrying a stable titer with an optical density over 0.4 may not be allowed because the risk of recurrence of HIT is likely to increase on heparin reuse.

9. Conclusion

HD-HIT is a drug-induced, immunoglobulin-mediated disorder that it is suspected in dialytic patients with an unexpected fall in the platelet count, and/or unexplained thrombotic events, particularly visible clotting in the circuit under an adequate heparin dose, and that begins between 5 and 10 days (nadir between 7 and 30 days, mostly by the third to fifth session) after heparin initiation. Although a positive result of HIT antibodies is presumably detected by sensitive ELISA, the diagnosis should be confirmed, whenever possible, using a functional assay. Immediately after the clinical suspicion of HIT, all sources of heparin should be discontinued including heparin used to flush or lock catheters. Alternative non-heparin anticoagulants, preferentially in a direct thrombin inhibitor, should be restarted for dialysis. Early treatment is important as thrombus formation including a clotting circuit may complicate at a high rate in 30 days after the cessation of heparin. Argatroban as an alternative to heparin must contribute to the quick recovery of the platelet count and immediate disappearance of circuit clotting. A steady decrease of the ELISA titers can be expected after heparin discontinuation. A negative seroconversion of HIT antibodies is usually observed by ~30 to more than 100 days after the discontinuation. Reexposure to heparin can be selected at the same dose of heparin as used before the onset of HIT. Small peak of HIT antibodies may often appear after exposure, but a follow-up of the antibody titers does not reach a threshold to induce the recurrence of HIT. When HD-HIT patients exhibit a high risk of thrombotic formation or worsening thrombosis, the same alternative anticoagulant therapy may be needed in non-session days.

10. References

Asmis LM, Segal JB, Plantnga LC, Fink NE, Kerman JS, Kickler TS, Coresh J, Gardner LB. (2008) Heparin-induced antibodies and cardiovascular risk in patients on dialysis. Thromb Haemost 100: 498-504.

Aster RH. Improving specificity in HIT testing. Blood 2010; 116: 1632-1633.

Chang JJ, Parikh CR. (2006) When heparin causes thrombosis: significance, recognition, and management of heparin-induced thrombocytopenia in dialysis patients. Semin Dial 19: 297-304.

Carrier M, Rodger MA, Fergusson D, Doucette S, Kovacs MJ, Moore J, Kelton JG, Knoll GA. (2008) Increased mortality in hemodialysis patients having specific antibodies to the platelet factor 4-heparin complex. Kidney Int 73: 213-219.

Davenport A. Sudden collapse during haemodialysis due to immune-mediated heparin-induced thrombocytopenia. (2006) Nephrol Dial Transplant 21: 1721-1724.

Davenport A. (2009) Antibodies to heparin–platelet factor 4 complex: pathogenesis, epidemiology, and management of heparin-induced thrombocytopenia in hemodialysis. Am J Kidney Dis, 54; 361-374

El-Shahawy, M, Noureddin M, Abdullah H, Mack WJ, Calverley DC. (2007) Platelet FcgammaRIIA receptor surface expression is increased in patients with ESRD and is associated with atherosclerotic cardiovascular events. Am J Kidney Dis 49: 127-134.

Gozdzikiewicz J, Borawski J, Mysliwiec M. (2007) Treatment of heparin-induced thrombocytopenia type II in hemodialysis patients: the search for a holy grail continues. Clin Appl Thromb/Hemost 13:110-111.

Holmes CE, Huang JC, Cartelli C, Howard A, Rimmer J, Cushman M. (2009) The clinical diagnosis of heparin-induced thrombocytopenia in patients receving continuous renal replacement therapy. J Thromb Thromboly 27:406-412.

Hartman V, Malbrain M, Daelemans R, Meersman P, Zachee P. (2006) Psudo-pulmonary embolism as a sign of acute heparin-induced thrombocytopenia in hemodialysis patients: safety of resuming heparin after disappearnance of HIT antibodies. Nephron Clin Pract 104:c143-148.

Hursting M, Murray P. (2008) Argatroban anticoagulation in renal dysfunction: a literature analysis. Nephron Clin Pract 109:c80-c94.

Hutchison CA, Dasgupta I. (2005) National survey of heparin-induced thrombocytopenia in the haemodialysis population of the UK population. Nephrol Dial Transplant 20: 444-446.

Lasocki S, Piednoir P, Ajzenberg N, Geffroy A, Benbara A, Montravers P. (2008) Anti-PF4/heparin antibodies associated with repeated hemofiltration-filter clotting: a retrospective study. Crit Care 12(3) R84 Epub.

Matsuo T, Chikahira Y, Yamada Y, Nakao K, Uesima S, Matsuo O. (1988) Effect of synthetic thrombin inhibitor (MD805) as an alternative drug on heparin induced thrombocytopenia during hemodialysis. Thromb Res 52; 165-171.

Matsuo T, Yamada T, Yamanashi T, Ryo R. (1990) Anticoagulant therapy with MD805 of a hemodialysis patient with heparin-induced thrombocytopenia. Thromb Res 58; 663-666.

Matsuo T, Matsuo M, Ouga-Maruyama S. Can nafamostat mesilate be used for temporary management of hemodialysis in a patient with heparin-induced thrombocytopenia (HIT)? (2001) Thromb Haemost 86; 1115-1116.

Matsuo T, Matsuo M, Wanaka, K, Sakai R. (2003) Heparin re-exposure after heparin-induced thrombocytopenia in a chronic hemodialysis patient. Clin Lab Haematol 25: 333-334.

Matsuo T, Kobayashi H, Matsuo M, Wanaka K, Nakamoto H, Matsusima H, Sakai R. (2006) Frequency of anti-heparin-PF4 complex antibodies (HIT antibodies) in uremic patients on chronic intermittent hemodialysis. Pathphysiol Haemost Thromb; 35:445-450.

Matsuo T, Kusano H, Wanaka K, Ishihara M, Oyama A. (2007) Heparin-induced thrombocytopenia in a uremic patient requiring hemodialysis: an alternative treatment and reexposure to heparin. Clin Appl Thromb Hemost. 13:182-7

Matsuo T, Wanaka K. Hemodialysis and argatroban. (2008a) Semin Thromb Hemost 34 (Suppl 1); 56-61.

Matsuo T, Wanaka K. Management of uremic patients with heparin-induced thrombocytopenia requiring hemodialysis. (2008b) Clin Appl Thromb Hemost 14; 459-464.

Mureebe L, Coats RD, Silliman WR, Shouster TA, Nichols WK, Silver D. (2004) Heparin-associated antiplatelet antibodies increase morbidity and mortality in hemodialysis patients. Surgery 136:848-853.

Nakamoto H, Shimada Y, Kanno T, Wanaka K, Matsuo T, Suzuki H.(2005) Role of platelet factor 4-heparin complex antibody (HIT antibody) in the pathogenesis of thrombotic episodes in patients on hemodialysis. Hemodial Int 9(suppl 1):s2-5.

O'Shea SI, Sands JJ, Nudo SA, Ortel TL. (2002) Frequency of anti-heparin-platelet factor 4 antibodies in hemodialysis patients and correlation with recurrent vascular thrombosis. Am J Hematol 69:72-73.

Oliveria GBF, Crespo EM, Becker RC, Honeycutt EF, Abrams CS, Anstrom KJ, Berger PB, Davidson-Ray LD, Eisenstein EL, Kleiman NS, Moliterno DJ, Moll S, Rice L, Rodgers JO, Steinhubl SR, Tapson VF, Ohman EM, Granger CB. (2008) Incidence and prognostic significance of thrombocytopenia in patients treated with prolonged heparin therapy. Arch Intern Med 168:94-102.

Pouplard C, Amiral J, Borg JY, Laporte-Simitsidis S, Delahousse B, Gruel Y. (1999) Decision analysis for use of platelet aggregation test, carbon 14-serotonin release assay, and heparin-platelet factor 4 enzyme-linked immunosorbent assay for diagnosis of heparin-induced thrombocytopenia. Am J Clin Pathol 111:700-706.

Roncon-Albuquerque R, Beco A, Ferreira AL, Gomes-Carvalho C, Costa A, Frazao J, Pestana M, von Hafe P. (2010) Therapeutic implications of heparin-induced thrombocytopenia complicating acute hemodialysis. Clin Nephrol 73: 326-330.

Selleng K, Schutt A, Selleng S, Warkentin TE, Greinacher A. Studies of the anti-PF4/heparin immune response: adapting the enzyme-linked immunosorbent spot assay for detection of memory B cells antigens. (2010) Transfusion 50; 32-39.

Shaheed G, Malkovska V, Mendoza J, Patel M, Rees J, Wesley R, Merryman P, Horne M. (2007) PF4 ENHANCD assay for the diagnosis of heparin-induced thrombocytopenia in complex medical and surgical patients. Crit Care Med 35:1784-1785.

Sheriden D, Carter C, Kelton JG. (1986) A diagnostic test for heparin-induced thrombocytopenia. Blood 67: 27-30.

Sonawane S, Kasbekar N, Berns JS. (2006) The safety of heparins in end-stage renal disease. Semin Dial 19:305-310.

Syed S, Reilly RF. (2009) Heparin-induced thrombocytopenia: a renal perspective. Nat Rev Nephrol 5: 501-511.

Tejedor Alonso, MA, Revuelta Lopez K, Garcia Bueno MJ, Casas L,Osada ML, Ingelmo Rosado A, Gruss Vergara E, Vila Albelda C, Moro Moro M. (2005) Thrombocytopenia and anaphylaxis secondary to heparin in a hemodialysis patient. Clin Nepherol 63: 236-240

Warkentin TE, Sheppaed JI, Moore JC, Sigouin CS, Kelton JG. (2008) Quantitative interpretation of optical density measurements using PF4-dependent enzyme-immunoassays. J Throm Haemost 6: 1304-1312.

Warkentin TE, Greinacher A. (2009) Heparin-induced anaphylactic and anaphylactoid reactions: two distinct but overlapping syndromes. Expert Opin Drug Saf 8; 129-144.

Wanaka K, Matsuo T, Matsuo M, Kaneko C, Miyasita K, Asada R, Matsusima H, Nakajima Y. (2010) Re-exposure to heparin in uremic patients requiring hemodialysis with heparin-induced thrombocytopenia. J Thromb Haemost 8; 616-618.

Weiss BM, Shumway NM, Howard RS, Ketchum LK, Reid TJ. (2008) Optical density values correlate with the clinical probability of heparin-induced thrombocytopenia. J Thromb Thrombolysis 26; 26: 243-247.

Yamamoto S, Koide M, Matsuo M, Suzuki S, Ohtaka M, Saika S, Matsuo T. (1996) Heparin-induced thrombocytopenia in hemodialysis patients. Am J Kidney Dis 28:82-85.

13

The Psychological Impact of Hemodialysis on Patients with Chronic Renal Failure

Liang-Jen Wang[1,2] and Chih-Ken Chen[1,2]
[1]Department of Psychiatry, Chang Gung Memorial Hospital, Keelung,
[2]Chang Gung University School of Medicine, Taoyuan
Taiwan

1. Introduction

Renal disease is common throughout the world. In the United States alone, almost 100,000 people began renal replacement therapy (RRT) for end-stage renal disease (ESRD) in 2001(Kimmel & Peterson, 2005); by 2008, this number had increased to 485,000 patients (Collins et al., 2009). More than 90% of these patients were started on hemodialysis (HD), while only 8.5% began RRT with peritoneal dialysis (PD)(Kimmel & Peterson, 2005). In Korea, the number of dialysis centers and machines has continuously increased, and 62.1% of patients receiving RRT were being treated with HD (Son et al., 2009). An international comparison showed that Taiwan has the greatest incidence and second-greatest prevalence of ESRD (Kuo et al., 2007). Furthermore, renal disease is one of the top 10 causes of death in Taiwan, and roughly 95% of ESRD patients are on HD (Hsieh et al., 2007).

While HD does not cure renal disease, its use does allow patients with ESRD to survive (Weisbord et al., 2007a). Nevertheless, HD is a lifelong treatment that significantly and sometimes adversely affects patients both physically and mentally (Kimmel, 2001). Common psychological effects include depression, anxiety, fatigue, decreased quality of life (QoL) and increased suicide risk (Chen et al., 2010). The global effects of continual treatment lead to changes in patients' family roles and ability to work, with feelings of loss of control and fear of death. These very real psychological consequences of treatment may affect survival in HD patients (Chilcot et al., 2011; Kimmel & Peterson, 2005). Therefore, it is imperative to identify and treat these psychological symptoms among HD patients.

2. Depression

2.1 Prevalence and influence of depression

Depression is one of the most common psychological problems among HD patients. We still lack reliable data that can be used to directly compare the prevalence of depression between HD patients and the general population. However, extant investigations generally agree that the rate of depression is high among HD patients.

In the general population, the lifetime prevalence of major depressive disorder is about 16.2% (Kessler et al., 2003). However, the rates vary widely across countries, ranging from

1.5% in Taiwan to 19% in Beirut, Lebanon (Weissman et al., 1996). Chilcot et al. (2008) reported that the prevalence of major depression among ESRD patients is approximately 20% to 30%. When we reviewed the recent literature, depression rates among HD patients ranged from 19.3% (Araujo et al., 2011) to 60.5% (Kao et al., 2009). These studies are summarized in **Table 1**.

Study	Number of patients	Assessment tools	Prevalence	Additional outcomes
Kurella et al. (2005)	465,563	Medical evidence form in Medicare and Medicaid Services	Withdrew from dialysis: 9.6% Died from suicide: 0.005%	Persons with ESRD had significantly higher suicide rates than in the general population. Independent predictors of suicide: age >75 yr, male gender, geographic region, alcohol or drug dependence, and recent hospitalization with mental illness.
Taskapan et al. (2005)	40	HDRS, HARS, PRIME-MD, MMSE, SF-36	Depression: 30% Anxiety: 35% Somatoform disorder: 32.5%	All patients' MMSE were normal. No relationship between any psychiatric disorder and demographic characteristics. Negative correlation between weight gain and QoL during dialysis.
Drayer et al. (2006)	62	PRIME-MD, KDQOL-SF	Depression: 28%	Depressed patients were younger and had lower health-related QoL. Depression predicted mortality in a mean duration of 29 months.
Kalender et al. (2007a)	HD: 68 PD: 47	BDI, SF-36	Depression in HD: 33.8% Depression in PD: 12.8%	Significant negative correlation between QoL and depression. Significant positive correlation between the QoL and the Hct value and serum albumin levels. Inverse correlation between the QoL and the serum CRP level in the HD patients.

Study	Number of patients	Assessment tools	Prevalence	Additional outcomes
Cukor et al. (2008)	70	SCID, HADS, KDQOL-SF	Depression: 29% Anxiety: 45.7%	Patients with persistent depression showed marked decreases in QoL and self-reported health status, compared with the nondepressed and intermittently depressed patients.
Hedayati et al. (2008)	98	SCID, BDI, CDI, CESD	Depression: 26.7% Major depression: 17.3%	There were no differences between reasons for hospitalization for the depressed vs. non-depressed. Patients with depression had increased risk of death or hospitalization in one year.
Ibrahim & Salamony (2008)	60	BDI, SF-36, DSI, MIS	Depression: 33.3%	Depression was affected by employment and marital status. DSI and MIS showed positive correlations with BDI scores and negative correlations with SF-36 scores
Hsu et al. (2009)	51	HADS	Depression: 35%	Depression was less common in patients who used polysulfone dialyzers than among those who used cellulose derivative dialyzers. Depression was also associated with, gender, albumin, and number of comorbidities.
Kao et al. (2009)	861	SF-36, BDI	Depression: 60.5% Insomnia: 31.0% Fatigue: 30.6%	Depression scores were negatively correlated with QoL. Higher monthly income and increased social activities were associated with better health-related QoL.
Son et al. (2009)	146	BDI, PHQ-9, KDQOL	Depression: 25.3%	There were more symptoms and poorer QoL reported in depressed patients than in non-depressed ones.
Bossola et al. (2010)	80	BDI, HARS, SF-36, SCL-90-R ,CCI; MMSE	Depression: 52.5% Mild anxiety: 47.5% Moderate to severe anxiety: 48.7%	BDI score correlated significantly with age, the CCI, SF-36 Vitality Subscale, MMSE, creatinine, albumin, plasma 25-hydroxy vitamin D, and IL-6 levels.

Study	Number of patients	Assessment tools	Prevalence	Additional outcomes
Chen et al. (2010)	200	MINI, HADS, CFS, SF-36	Depression: 35% Anxiety: 21%	In the previous month, 21.5% patients had suicidal ideation. Depressed patients had higher rates of fatigue, and lower QoL. Suicide risk was strongly related to depression and anxiety.
Montinaro et al. (2010)	HD: 30 Control (patients with CKD stage 1-2): 20	HADS, KDQOL	Depression: HD = 50%, controls = 20% Anxiety: HD = 43%, controls =45%.	Cytokine production (IL-1, IL-6 and TNF-α) was significantly higher in HD patients than controls. KDQOL correlated inversely with levels of IL-6, TNF-α and IL-10. IL-6 was associated with anxiety.
Keskin & Engin (2011)	92	BDI, SBQ, COPE	Depression: 40.2%	Suicidal ideation increased as the severity of depression increased. Depression and suicidal ideation were increasing with age and lower education status.
Araujo et al. (2011)	400	BDI	Depression: 19.3%	Depression was associated with female gender, poor sleep quality, unemployment, diabetes, hypoalbuminemia, low education, and pruritus.

KEY: BDI: Beck Depression Inventory; CCI: Charlson Comorbidity Index; CESD: Center of Epidemiological Studies Depression Scale; CFS: Chalder Fatigue Scale; CKD: chronic kidney disease; COPE: Coping Orientation to Problems Experienced Inventory; CRP: C-reactive protein; DSI: Dialysis Symptom Index; HADS: Hospital Anxiety and Depression Rating Scale; ESRD: end-stage renal disease; HARS: Hamilton Anxiety Rating Scale; HD: hemodialysis; HDRS: Hamilton Depression Rating Scale; IL: interleukin; KDQoL: Kidney Disease Quality of Life; KDQoL-SF: Kidney Disease and Quality of Life Short Form; MINI: Mini International Neuropsychiatric Interview; MIS: Malnutrition-Inflammation Score; MMSE: Mini Mental State Examination; PD: peritoneal dialysis; PHQ-9: Patient Health Questionnaire; PRIME-MD: Primary Care Evaluation of Mental Disorders; SBQ: Suicide Behaviours Questionnaire; SCID: Structured Clinical Interview for DSM; SCL-90-R: Hopkins Symptom Checklist 90 Revised; SF-36: The Short-form Health-related Quality of Life; TNF: tumor necrosis factor

Table 1. Psychological impacts in hemodialysis patients demonstrated in recent studies

The variation in prevalence rates of depression might be accounted for by differences in sample sizes and assessment tools (Watnick et al., 2005). Despite such discrepancies, depression is unquestionably one of the most important mental illnesses among HD patients. Strong correlations have been noted between depression and longitudinal outcome among HD patients, including poor treatment adherence and higher mortality rates (Drayer et al., 2006; Kimmel et al., 1993). In addition, depression in HD patients is associated with higher rates of hospital admission, and a greater likelihood of emergency department visits (Abbas Tavallaii et al., 2009; Hedayati et al., 2008).

2.2 Biological factors underlying depression

The etiology of dialysis-related depression is multifactorial, and is related to biological, psychological, and social mechanisms (Chilcot et al., 2008). Some of the biological mechanisms include increased cytokine levels, possible genetic predisposition, and neurotransmitters affected by uremia (Kimmel, 2001; Smogorzewski et al., 1995).

For decades it's been known that immunologic factors have potent influences on neurotransmitter metabolism and neuroendocrine function (Irwin & Miller, 2007; Wichers & Maes, 2002). A growing number of studies have investigated the relationships between cytokines and depression (Howren et al., 2009; Loftis et al., 2010; Sonikian et al., 2010). During hemodialysis, the blood-dialyzer interaction has the potential to activate mononuclear and dendritic cells, leading to production of inflammatory cytokines (Agrawal et al., 2010; Pertosa et al., 2000). Several researchers support the supposition that pro-inflammatory cytokines are involved with depression in renal patients. In particular, there is evidence that depression is associated with interleukin (IL)-1, IL-6, tumor necrosis factor-alpha (TNF-α), and C-reactive protein (CRP) in both the general and ESRD populations (Gill et al., 2010; Simic Ogrizovic et al., 2009; Sonikian et al., 2010). These pro-inflammatory cytokines also appear to be associated with survival rate in HD patients (Kimmel et al., 1998). The underlying biological mechanisms have been proposed as a defect in serotonergic function and hypercortisolemia associated with stimulation of the hypothalamic-pituitary-adrenal (HPA) axis (Capuron & Miller, 2011; Leonard, 2010), thus leading to depression and affecting mortality.

Malnutrition, which is commonly observed in dialysis patients, is related to chronic inflammation (Pertosa et al., 2000). It has also been reported that malnutrition is associated with emotional symptoms among HD patients (Bossola et al., 2009; Czira et al., 2011; Huang & Lee, 2007; Ibrahim & El Salamony, 2008; Koo et al., 2003). These authors also determined that patients with depression had lower-than-normal body mass indices (BMI) (Chen et al., 2010).

There is evidence of an association between malnutrition, inflammation, and atherosclerosis (MIA) in ESRD patients, and some researchers have suggested that depression might be involved in the MIA syndrome (Simic Ogrizovic et al., 2009). Others have demonstrated frequent and close relationships between serum albumin levels and depression (Huang & Lee, 2007; Hung et al., 2011; Koo et al., 2003). However, a correlation between hemoglobin, ferritin, and emotional symptoms is less clear-cut (Bossola et al., 2009; Czira et al., 2011; Huang & Lee, 2007). Hopefully the causal relationships in the complexity of psychoneuroimmune mechanisms will be further elucidated in future studies.

Racial effects on depression and anxiety have been studied in HD patients, once again with conflicting results (Feroze et al., 2010). Higher prevalence rates of major depressive disorders have been noted among Caucasians than among African-Americans or Mexican-Americans (Riolo et al., 2005). In contrast, the results of some studies revealed no differences in the prevalence of depression among races (Chen et al., 2011; Weisbord et al., 2007b). Balakrishnan et al. (2004) demonstrated that single nucleotide polymorphisms in the promoter region of the proinflammatory cytokines appear to have a strong association with indices of comorbidity, biological and nutritional markers. Whether depression is associated with a genetic predisposition for racial differences or cytokine gene polymorphisms warrants further investigation.

Other studies have evaluated the possible effects of dialysis materials on depression. Peritoneal dialysis (PD) patients have been noted to have less severe anxiety, insomnia, and depression than do HD patients (Ginieri-Coccossis et al., 2008; Noshad et al., 2009). It has been suggested that the rate of depression is greater among patients using cellulose-derivative dialyzers than among those using polysulfone dialyzers (Hsu et al., 2009). Using PD or more biocompatible dialyzers thus might be associated with better mental health in HD patients.

2.3 Psychological and social factors for depression

A number of studies have focused upon the effects of HD patients, including feelings of hopelessness, perceptions of loss and lack of control, job loss, and altered family and social relationships (Kimmel, 2001). Because ESRD is a lifelong disease, feelings of lack of control and perceptions of overwhelming illness might be inevitable. The intrusiveness of these thoughts is related to depression (Christensen & Ehlers, 2002; Devins et al., 1997).

More recent work has focused upon the possible effects of underlying illness upon depressive symptoms among ESRD patients (Guzman & Nicassio, 2003). Perception of loss has been regarded as a strong predictor of depression (Chan et al., 2009), which in turn predicts mortality (Chilcot et al., 2011). In terms of the risk by demographic characteristics, results have been inconsistent (Taskapan et al., 2005). It was reported that depression among dialysis patients increased with increasing age and lower educational levels (Keskin & Engin, 2011). In some studies, depressive symptoms were more common among women, and increased with unemployment and also rose among patients with higher comorbidity of physical diseases (Araujo et al., 2011; Chen et al., 2010; Ibrahim & El Salamony, 2008). Thus, negative cognition and lack of social support might exacerbate patients' negative feelings, and thus further contribute to depression.

3. Anxiety

Anxiety is also commonly seen in HD patients (Kring & Crane, 2009). Cukor et al. demonstrated a 27% incidence of anxiety among 70 urban HD patients, which was somewhat higher than the 18% incidence reported in a national survey (Kessler et al., 2005). During a 16-month follow-up study, 9% of patients had both anxiety and depression at baseline; the incidence of both conditions rose to 13% by the end of the study. At the end of the study, two-thirds of individuals with comorbid depression and anxiety at baseline had both diagnoses (Cukor et al., 2008b). Furthermore, Cukor et al. (2008a) reported that 45.7%

of a group of dialysis patients recruited from a single center met criteria for an anxiety disorder. The most prevalent disorders were specific phobias (26.6%) and panic disorder (21.0%). Bossola et al. (2010) indicated that 47.5% of 80 HD patients had mild symptoms of anxiety, while 48.7% had moderate or severe symptoms of anxiety. In addition, the anxiety scores correlated significantly with age and comorbidities, and anxiety were commonly noted in patients with poor appetite (Bossola et al., 2011). A review of 55 studies that investigated symptoms of anxiety in ESRD patients found that 12% to 52% of patients with ESRD had substantial anxiety (Murtagh et al., 2007).

In one of our previous studies, 21% of dialysis patients had symptoms of anxiety. In addition, 15.5% of these subjects had comorbid depression and anxiety, and 44.3% of depressed patients had comorbid anxiety (Chen et al., 2010). Furthermore, suicide risk was not only attributed to depression, but also to anxiety.

The call for depression screening in HD patients is growing, but screening for anxiety in patients with ESRD population is relatively disregarded. This is an indication that many clinicians underestimate the importance of anxiety among HD patients. O'Donovan et al. (2010) reported that clinically anxious participants exhibited significantly lower levels of morning cortisol and significantly higher levels of IL-6, compared with non-anxious participants. Uncertainty about the future and fear of losing control of one's life are important factors associated with anxiety that adversely impact emotional stability (Haenel et al., 1980). Notably, anxiety is a common psychological problem that may emerge during the initial course of dialysis (Cukor et al., 2008b), and is a reminder to clinicians to pay close attention to this issue.

4. Fatigue

Fatigue is a subjective symptom characterized by tiredness, weakness, and lack of energy.(Lee et al., 1991) Fatigue is also one of the most debilitating symptoms reported by HD patients, and roughly 60% to 97% of patients on HD experience some degree of it (Jhamb et al., 2008). People with chronic renal disease, regardless of whether they are pre-dialysis or receiving either HD or PD, are reported having high levels of fatigue and are often unable to engage in normal daily activities (Bonner et al., 2010). In addition, fatigue is positively correlated with depression (Chen et al., 2010; Sklar et al., 1996), and negatively correlated with QoL (Lee et al., 2007). In one study, researchers noted a significant relationship between the duration of treatment and the level of fatigue. The experience of fatigue was more commonly reported in respondents who had been receiving treatment for more than 2 years, compared to those treated for less than 2 years (Letchmi et al., 2011). In a longitudinal analysis of 917 incident HD and PD patients, those with lower levels of fatigue at baseline survived longer (Jhamb et al., 2009).

Factors that may contribute to fatigue in dialysis patients include anemia, malnutrition, inflammation, depression and/or sleep disorders (Jhamb et al., 2008). Anemia resulting from reduced erythropoietin production has been cited as an important cause of fatigue in this population (Singh et al., 2006). Additionally, patients undergoing chronic HD show evidence of accelerated protein catabolism, which might be due to the significant loss of amino acids induced by dialysis (Pertosa et al., 2000). Thus, it is reasonable to presume that lower levels of albumin can be significantly correlated with greater levels of fatigue (Bonner et al., 2010). Malnutrition in dialysis patients might also be related to poor intake, or the result of chronic inflammation (Stenvinkel et al., 1999). Cytokines productions, particularly IL-6, might induce protein catabolism and lipolysis (Memoli et al., 2002), and cytokines have a strong negative correlation with serum albumin levels in HD patients (Montinaro et al., 2010). Thus, chronic inflammation and malnutrition might result in fatigue by either directly activating the central nervous system through adrenal axis or by indirectly triggering multisystem deregulation (Jhamb et al., 2008).

5. Decreased Quality of Life (QoL)

Health-related QoL is an important measure of how a disease affects the lives of patients. The QoL domains include physical, psychological, and social functioning and general satisfaction with life (Tsay & Healstead, 2002). Once patients with ESRD start to receive HD, they must face the chronic stress related to restrictions on their time, the economical and vocational costs related to treatment, functional limitations, dietary constraints, and possible adverse effects of medications (Son et al., 2009). Numerous studies have demonstrated that these patients have a lower QoL than that of healthy populations (Kao et al., 2009; Perlman et al., 2005; Wolcott et al., 1988). Depression is strongly correlated with decreased health-related QoL, especially in mental dimensions (Chen et al., 2010; Kao et al., 2009). Furthermore, several studies have shown that patients with poorer QoL had a higher incidence of anxiety and fatigue (Kring & Crane, 2009), and longitudinal follow-up showed increased mortality (Drayer et al., 2006; Wolcott et al., 1988).

Biological function, mental illnesses, general health perception, and characteristics of the individual and environment may contribute to the variability in patients' QoL (Kring & Crane, 2009). Biological factors that have been associated with QoL include altered hemoglobin, albumin, ferritin, CRP, IL-6, IL-8, and TNF-α levels (Farag et al., 2011; Kalender et al., 2007a; Montinaro et al., 2010; Perlman et al., 2005). Poor exercise tolerance and muscle weakness may limit daily activity, again causing poor QoL (Hsieh et al., 2007; Sakkas et al., 2003). However, Barros et al. (2011) suggested there was no association of nutritional status with malnutrition-inflammation, QoL, or depressive symptoms. There is still debate about whether patients' QoL can be directly correlated to malnutrition-inflammation markers.

Among psychological issues, uncertainty about the future and lack of energy emerged as the major contributors to poor QoL (Tsay & Healstead, 2002). A patient's dependency on treatment may negatively impact his or her QoL and exacerbate feelings of a loss of control (Chilcot et al., 2008). Improved QoL is correlated with higher self-esteem and lower levels of mood disturbances (Wolcott et al., 1988). Furthermore, time of diagnosis of chronic renal failure may be an important factor related to the QoL of patients receiving dialysis. Late diagnosis of renal failure and the consequent lack of predialysis care adversely affect QoL among these patients (Sesso & Yoshihiro, 1997). Therefore, early detection of renal failure and identification of underlying mental illnesses might be important issues for establishing better QoL in HD patients.

6. Suicide

Suicide may be the most serious result of mental illness among HD patients. Kurella et al. (2005) reported the death rate from suicide was 0.24% per 1000 dialysis patients-years at risk. Patients with ESRD had a significantly higher rate of suicide compared with the general population in the United States. Chen et al. (2010) demonstrated that among 200 patients with HD, 21.5% had suicidal ideation; 3.5% had planned a suicide attempt in prior months; and 3.5% had attempted suicide during their lifetime. It is noteworthy that an increased number of patients with ESRD had withdrawn from dialysis before their death. Nevertheless, only a small proportion (12%) of the respondents were unsure or believed that discontinuing dialysis was the equivalent of suicide (Cohen et al., 2002). If the data on withdrawal from dialysis were factored into current epidemiologic investigations, the suicide rate among HD patients might be much greater.

Suicide was associated with several demographic characteristics among HD patients. Independent predictors of suicide included old age, male gender, lower educational status, alcohol or drug dependence, and recent hospitalization for mental illness (Keskin & Engin, 2011; Kurella et al., 2005). Having strong religious beliefs has been suggested as one protective factor of suicide risk among HD patients (Martiny et al., 2011). Preexisting depression and anxiety disorders have been identified as independent risk factors for subsequent onset of suicidal ideation and attempts in the general population (Martiny et al., 2011; Sareen et al., 2005). Specific for HD patients, suicide risk was also significantly predicted by anxiety and depression. On the other hand, fatigue and QoL may not directly affect suicide risk (Chen et al., 2010). Because suicide might be preventable via early detection of warning signs, it is crucial to identify the psychological impact and possible risk of suicide among dialysis patients.

7. Managing the psychological impact on dialysis patients

Numerous studies investigated the managements for mental illness in HD patients, including pharmacological and non-pharmacological interventions (Table 2).

7.1 Pharmacological interventions

Today, selective serotonin reuptake inhibitors (SSRIs) are the treatment of choice for HD patients with depression or anxiety (Raymond et al., 2008). Fluoxetine has been effective and safe in HD patients, although trials have thus far involved only small numbers of patients (Blumenfield et al., 1997). Citalpram, which is similar to fluoxetine in treatment effects, is thought to be safe (Cohen et al., 2004), and it has been beneficial for improving QoL in HD patients (Kalender et al., 2007b). Paroxetine, combined with supportive psychotherapy, has been shown to be not only successful for treating depression, but also for improving nutritional status in chronic HD patients with depression (Koo et al., 2005). Sertraline has safe pharmacokinetics in patients with ESRD, and treatment with sertraline in PD patients is associated with improved of QoL and fewer symptoms of depression (Atalay et al., 2010). Duloxetine and venlafaxine, which are categorized as serotonin-norepinephrine reuptake inhibitors, are beneficial for patients with major depressive disorder (Ye et al., 2011). However, these agents' safety and efficacy have not been specifically established for HD patients. Bupropion, a dopamine-norepinephrine reuptake inhibitor, and mirtazapine, a noradrenergic and specific serotonergic, have also been widely used for patients with depression. However, once again, it is not clear whether the beneficial effects of these agents can be generalized to dialysis patients. Generally, older tricyclic medications have an adverse cardiac profile and anticholinergic effects, which limits their use for HD patients

(Cohen et al., 2004). In the case of trazodone and nefazodone, treatment effects have only been demonstrated in case reports (Doweiko et al., 1984; Seabolt & De Leon, 2001).

Treatment	Target Symptoms	Side Effects	Clinical Considerations
Pharmacological interventions			
Selective serotonin reuptake inhibitors (fluoxetine, citalopram, paroxetine, sertraline)	Depression Anxiety	Gastrointestinal symptoms, sexual dysfunction, risk of bleeding, suicidal ideation	Fluoxetine: long half-life Citalopram: use cautiously in severe renal impairment patients. Paroxetine: use lower dose.
Serotonin-norepinephrine reuptake inhibitors (venlafaxine, duloxetine)	Depression	Accumulation of toxic metabolites, sexual dysfunction, hypertension	Decrease total daily dose by 50% in mild-to-moderate renal impairment.
Dopamine-norepinephrine reuptake inhibitors (bupropion)	Depression Fatigue	Insomnia, agitation, seizure, accumulation of toxic metabolites	Use with caution and consider a reduction for dose in renal impairment.
Noradrenergic and specific serotonergics (mirtazapine)	Depression	Sedation, somnolence, weight gain	Reduce dose, give before sleep.
Tricyclics and tetracyclics (amitriptyline, desipramine,doxepin, nortriptyline)	Depression	Anticholinergic effects, sedation, QTc prolongation, cardiac arrhythmias, orthostatic hypotension	Avoid if possible given cardiac side effects.
Serotonin modulators (netazodone, trazodone)	Depression	Accumulation of toxic metabolites, liver failure (for nefazodone), sedation, hypotension, cardiac arrhythmias	Avoid use in patients with cardiac disease or hypotension.
Erythropoietin	Fatigue Quality of life	Seizures, increased clotting, and influenza-like syndromes	No significant difference between once-weekly versus thrice-weekly subcutaneous administration.

Treatment	Target Symptoms	Side Effects	Clinical Considerations
Pharmacological interventions			
Partial Serotonin 5HT(1A) receptor agonists (buspirone)	Anxiety	Dizziness, nausea, headache, insomnia, tremor	Usually 25% to 50% dose reduction
Benzodiazepines (alprazolam, lorazepam, diazepam, midazolam, chlordiazepoxide)	Anxiety Insomnia	Prolong sedation, physical and psychological dependence, cognition impairment, withdrawal symptoms	High rate of side effects Alprazolam and diazepam: increased free fraction of plasma protein bound drug in ESRD.
Non-pharmacological interventions			
Cognitive behavior therapy (CBT)	Depression Quality of life	Takes longer time to reach effects than pharmacological treatment	Group therapy, weekly sessions, need well-trained therapists
Exercise training	Depression Quality of life	No serious adverse effects were reported	10-month to 1-year exercise training program. Also improves the heart rate variability (HRV) indices
Acupuncture	Quality of life	No serious adverse effects were reported	Individualized acupuncture treatments provided twice a week for 6 consecutive weeks
Social support, marital, family counseling	Depression Spousal depression	No serious adverse effects were reported.	Treatment programs need to be comprehensive.

5HT: 5-hydroxytryptamine; QTc: corrected QT interval

Table 2. Treatment options for psychological impact on hemodialysis patients

In summary, with the exception of the SSRIs, the efficacy and safety of antidepressant drug therapy in dialysis patients have not been clearly established, although these medications are believed to improve depression empirically. Notably, the relative activity and mode of excretion of metabolites of antidepressants in dialysis patients are as yet unknown and may complicate the use of these drugs if adverse events occur. It also remains unclear whether there are potential drug-drug interactions between antidepressants and other drugs commonly used in HD patients. Therefore, the general rule for prescribing antidepressants among HD patients is to start at a lower dose and increase the dosage gradually (Cohen et al., 2004).

There is evidence that the use of erythropoietin-stimulating agents might reduce fatigue and improve QoL among ESRD patients (Jones et al., 2004). Benzodiazepines (BZD), such as diazepam, alprazolam, and lorazepam, have been successfully used to relieve acute episodes of panic and anxiety. In addition, BZD are also widely prescribed for HD patients with insomnia (Wyne et al., 2011). In recent years, the use of non-BZD drugs such as zolpidem, zopiclone, and zaleplon for insomnia patients has rapidly increased. However, it is noteworthy that the liability for abuse and dependence exist in both BZD and non-BZD drugs, especially with long-term use (Victorri-Vigneau et al., 2007). Buspirone, a partial serotonin agonist that acts on the 5HT(1A) receptor, is often recommended for patients with anxiety, and it is generally is considered to have fewer unfavorable side effects than does BZD. Generally, it is not necessary to adjust the dosage of most of the erythropoietin-stimulating agents we have mentioned for the level of the glomerular filtation rate, for these agents are metabolized in the liver (Hedayati & Finkelstein, 2009). However, buspirone and lorazepam may take longer to be eliminated in ESRD patients, and thus the dosage of these two drugs should be carefully titrated. Notably, Winkelmayer et al. (2007) reported that BZD or zolpidem are commonly used for incident dialysis patients and may be associated with greater mortality in this group. Although the causal reference to this effect warrants further investigation, it is also a warning that clinicians need to consider the necessity of long-term use of BZD in dialysis patients.

7.2 Non-pharmacological interventions

Psychotherapy has been used for a wide range of chronic illnesses, including patients with HD (Hedayati & Finkelstein, 2009). Of these approaches, cognitive behavioral therapy (CBT), a well-documented evidence-based therapy for depression, has been shown to be effective (Chen et al., 2011; Duarte et al., 2009). CBT is based on the assumption that one's dysfunctional "automatic thoughts" in response to a situation can result in strong negative feelings/emotions, and thus lead to depression. Correction of those faulty dysfunctional constructs can lead to clinical improvement. Duarte et al. (2009) demonstrated that CBT performed during 3-month-long group therapy is effective for improving depression and many dimensions of QoL in chronic HD patients. Chen et al. (2011) conducted a randomized controlled interventional study of 72 sleep-disturbed HD patients. Compared with the control group (who received sleep health education), patients who received CBT had significant improvements in sleep quality, fatigue, depression, and anxiety. Interestingly, CRP, IL-18, and oxidized low-density lipoprotein levels also significantly declined among those receiving CBT in comparison to those in the control group (Chen et al., 2011). Thus, these studies suggest that CBT might be effective for improving mental health, and for reducing inflammation and oxidative stress in HD patients.

Exercise programs may have a beneficial effect on depressive symptoms in patients with ESRD. Ouzouni et al. (2009) reported that 10-month intradialytic exercise training improved QoL in both physical functioning and psychological status in HD patients, and decreased in self-reported depression. In another study, a 1-year exercise training program reduced emotional distress and concomitantly improved cardiac autonomic modulation measured by heart rate variability (HRV) indices (Kouidi et al., 2010). For alternative therapy, Kim et al. (2011) reported that 24 HD patients who received individualized acupuncture treatments over 6 consecutive weeks showed significant improvements in some QoL subscales.

Social support has been shown to help improve emotional disturbances in a variety of chronic illnesses. Support and education, either individually to patients or including their caregivers and family members, may be helpful (Symister & Friend, 2003). A patient's depression could be influenced by the psychosocial status of his or her spouse, and the spouse might be amenable to interventions that could improve patient outcome (Daneker et al., 2001). Social support has been shown to decrease depression by improving the self-esteem of patients with ESRD, which led to increased optimism (Symister & Friend, 2003). Treatment programs that address problems with social interactions of patients need to be comprehensive, and should explore use of family and marital counseling, and involvement of the community, along with consideration of the patient's social life (Cohen et al., 2007).

8. Conclusion

HD is a life-sustaining treatment for patients with ESRD; however, it adversely affects patients' mental status. Increasingly, depression is being recognized as a substantial comorbid illness in these patients. Anxiety, feelings of fatigue, and decreasing QoL are also significant psychological symptoms, and they may be interrelated. Depression and anxiety particularly increase patients' suicide risk. Mental illnesses may have underlying biological and psychological causes. There is considerable evidence that these psychological effects are associated with adverse outcomes in HD patients with ESRD. It is important, therefore, to develop systematic approaches to screening patients for mental illness, and then planning treatment strategies. To improve treatment outcome and patient Qol, a comprehensive management plan that includes pharmacological and psychosocial interventions, is essential.

9. References

Abbas Tavallaii, S., Ebrahimnia, M., Shamspour, N. & Assari, S. (2009). Effect of depression on health care utilization in patients with end-stage renal disease treated with hemodialysis. *Eur J Intern Med*, 20, 411-414

Agrawal, S., Gollapudi, P., Elahimehr, R., Pahl, M.V. & Vaziri, N.D. (2010). Effects of end-stage renal disease and haemodialysis on dendritic cell subsets and basal and LPS-stimulated cytokine production. *Nephrol Dial Transplant*, 25, 737-746

Araujo, S.M., De Bruin, V.M., Daher, E.D., Almeida, G.H., Medeiros, C.A. & De Bruin, P.F. (2011). Risk factors for depressive symptoms in a large population on chronic hemodialysis. *Int Urol Nephrol* (In press)

Atalay, H., Solak, Y., Biyik, M., Biyik, Z., Yeksan, M., Uguz, F., et al. (2010). Sertraline treatment is associated with an improvement in depression and health-related quality of life in chronic peritoneal dialysis patients. *Int Urol Nephrol*, 42, 527-536

Balakrishnan, V.S., Guo, D., Rao, M., Jaber, B.L., Tighiouart, H., Freeman, R.L., et al. (2004). Cytokine gene polymorphisms in hemodialysis patients: association with comorbidity, functionality, and serum albumin. *Kidney Int*, 65, 1449-1460

Barros, A., Da Costa, B.E., Poli-De-Figueiredo, C.E., Antonello, I.C. & D'avila, D.O. (2011). Nutritional status evaluated by multi-frequency bioimpedance is not associated with quality of life or depressive symptoms in hemodialysis patients. *Ther Apher Dial*, 15, 58-65

Blumenfield, M., Levy, N.B., Spinowitz, B., Charytan, C., Beasley, C.M., Jr., Dubey, A.K., et al. (1997). Fluoxetine in depressed patients on dialysis. *Int J Psychiatry Med*, 27, 71-80

Bonner, A., Wellard, S. & Caltabiano, M. (2010). The impact of fatigue on daily activity in people with chronic kidney disease. *J Clin Nurs*, 19, 3006-3015

Bossola, M., Ciciarelli, C., Di Stasio, E., Conte, G.L., Vulpio, C., Luciani, G., et al. (2010). Correlates of symptoms of depression and anxiety in chronic hemodialysis patients. *Gen Hosp Psychiatry*, 32, 125-131

Bossola, M., Ciciarelli, C., Di Stasio, E., Panocchia, N., Conte, G.L., Rosa, F., et al. (2011). Relationship between Appetite and Symptoms of Depression and Anxiety in Patients on Chronic Hemodialysis. *J Ren Nutr* (In press)

Bossola, M., Luciani, G. & Tazza, L. (2009). Fatigue and its correlates in chronic hemodialysis patients. *Blood Purif*, 28, 245-252

Capuron, L. & Miller, A.H. (2011). Immune system to brain signaling: neuropsychopharmacological implications. *Pharmacol Ther*, 130, 226-238

Chan, R., Brooks, R., Erlich, J., Chow, J. & Suranyi, M. (2009). The effects of kidney-disease-related loss on long-term dialysis patients' depression and quality of life: positive affect as a mediator. *Clin J Am Soc Nephrol*, 4, 160-167

Chen, C.K., Tsai, Y.C., Hsu, H.J., Wu, I.W., Sun, C.Y., Chou, C.C., et al. (2010). Depression and suicide risk in hemodialysis patients with chronic renal failure. *Psychosomatics*, 51, 528-528 e526

Chen, H.Y., Cheng, I.C., Pan, Y.J., Chiu, Y.L., Hsu, S.P., Pai, M.F., et al. (2011). Cognitive-behavioral therapy for sleep disturbance decreases inflammatory cytokines and oxidative stress in hemodialysis patients. *Kidney Int*, 80, 415-422

Chilcot, J., Wellsted, D., Da Silva-Gane, M. & Farrington, K. (2008). Depression on dialysis. *Nephron Clin Pract*, 108, c256-264

Chilcot, J., Wellsted, D. & Farrington, K. (2011). Illness perceptions predict survival in haemodialysis patients. *Am J Nephrol*, 33, 358-363

Christensen, A.J. & Ehlers, S.L. (2002). Psychological factors in end-stage renal disease: an emerging context for behavioral medicine research. *J Consult Clin Psychol*, 70, 712-724

Cohen, L.M., Dobscha, S.K., Hails, K.C., Pekow, P.S. & Chochinov, H.M. (2002). Depression and suicidal ideation in patients who discontinue the life-support treatment of dialysis. *Psychosom Med*, 64, 889-896

Cohen, L.M., Tessier, E.G., Germain, M.J. & Levy, N.B. (2004). Update on psychotropic medication use in renal disease. *Psychosomatics*, 45, 34-48

Cohen, S.D., Sharma, T., Acquaviva, K., Peterson, R.A., Patel, S.S. & Kimmel, P.L. (2007). Social support and chronic kidney disease: an update. *Adv Chronic Kidney Dis*, 14, 335-344

Collins, A.J., Foley, R.N., Herzog, C., Chavers, B., Gilbertson, D., Ishani, A., et al. (2009). United States Renal Data System 2008 Annual Data Report. *Am J Kidney Dis*, 53, S1-374

Cukor, D., Coplan, J., Brown, C., Friedman, S., Cromwell-Smith, A., Peterson, R.A., et al. (2007). Depression and anxiety in urban hemodialysis patients. *Clin J Am Soc Nephrol*, 2, 484-490

Cukor, D., Coplan, J., Brown, C., Friedman, S., Newville, H., Safier, M., et al. (2008a). Anxiety disorders in adults treated by hemodialysis: a single-center study. *Am J Kidney Dis*, 52, 128-136

Cukor, D., Coplan, J., Brown, C., Peterson, R.A. & Kimmel, P.L. (2008b). Course of depression and anxiety diagnosis in patients treated with hemodialysis: a 16-month follow-up. *Clin J Am Soc Nephrol*, 3, 1752-1758

Czira, M.E., Lindner, A.V., Szeifert, L., Molnar, M.Z., Fornadi, K., Kelemen, A., et al. (2011). Association between the Malnutrition-Inflammation Score and depressive symptoms in kidney transplanted patients. *Gen Hosp Psychiatry*, 33, 157-165

Daneker, B., Kimmel, P.L., Ranich, T. & Peterson, R.A. (2001). Depression and marital dissatisfaction in patients with end-stage renal disease and in their spouses. *Am J Kidney Dis*, 38, 839-846

Devins, G.M., Beiser, M., Dion, R., Pelletier, L.G. & Edwards, R.G. (1997). Cross-cultural measurements of psychological well-being: the psychometric equivalence of Cantonese, Vietnamese, and Laotian translations of the Affect Balance Scale. *Am J Public Health*, 87, 794-799

Doweiko, J., Fogel, B.S. & Goldberg, R.J. (1984). Trazodone and hemodialysis. *J Clin Psychiatry*, 45, 361

Drayer, R.A., Piraino, B., Reynolds, C.F., 3rd, Houck, P.R., Mazumdar, S., Bernardini, J., et al. (2006). Characteristics of depression in hemodialysis patients: symptoms, quality of life and mortality risk. *Gen Hosp Psychiatry*, 28, 306-312

Duarte, P.S., Miyazaki, M.C., Blay, S.L. & Sesso, R. (2009). Cognitive-behavioral group therapy is an effective treatment for major depression in hemodialysis patients. *Kidney Int*, 76, 414-421

Farag, Y.M., Keithi-Reddy, S.R., Mittal, B.V., Surana, S.P., Addabbo, F., Goligorsky, M.S., et al. (2011). Anemia, inflammation and health-related quality of life in chronic kidney disease patients. *Clin Nephrol*, 75, 524-533

Feroze, U., Martin, D., Reina-Patton, A., Kalantar-Zadeh, K. & Kopple, J.D. (2010). Mental health, depression, and anxiety in patients on maintenance dialysis. *Iran J Kidney Dis*, 4, 173-180

Gill, J., Luckenbaugh, D., Charney, D. & Vythilingam, M. (2010). Sustained elevation of serum interleukin-6 and relative insensitivity to hydrocortisone differentiates posttraumatic stress disorder with and without depression. *Biol Psychiatry*, 68, 999-1006

Ginieri-Coccossis, M., Theofilou, P., Synodinou, C., Tomaras, V. & Soldatos, C. (2008). Quality of life, mental health and health beliefs in haemodialysis and peritoneal dialysis patients: investigating differences in early and later years of current treatment. *BMC Nephrol*, 9, 14

Group, T.W. (1998). Development of the World Health Organization WHOQOL-BREF quality of life assessment. The WHOQOL Group. *Psychol Med*, 28, 551-558

Guzman, S.J. & Nicassio, P.M. (2003). The contribution of negative and positive illness schemas to depression in patients with end-stage renal disease. *J Behav Med*, 26, 517-534

Haenel, T., Brunner, F. & Battegay, R. (1980). Renal dialysis and suicide: occurrence in Switzerland and in Europe. *Compr Psychiatry*, 21, 140-145

Hedayati, S.S., Bosworth, H.B., Briley, L.P., Sloane, R.J., Pieper, C.F., Kimmel, P.L., et al. (2008). Death or hospitalization of patients on chronic hemodialysis is associated with a physician-based diagnosis of depression. *Kidney Int*, 74, 930-936

Hedayati, S.S. & Finkelstein, F.O. (2009). Epidemiology, diagnosis, and management of depression in patients with CKD. *Am J Kidney Dis*, 54, 741-752

Howren, M.B., Lamkin, D.M. & Suls, J. (2009). Associations of depression with C-reactive protein, IL-1, and IL-6: a meta-analysis. *Psychosom Med*, 71, 171-186

Hsieh, R.L., Lee, W.C., Huang, H.Y. & Chang, C.H. (2007). Quality of life and its correlates in ambulatory hemodialysis patients. *J Nephrol*, 20, 731-738

Hsu, H.J., Chen, C.K. & Wu, M.S. (2009). Lower prevalence of depression in hemodialysis patients who use polysulfone dialyzers. *Am J Nephrol*, 29, 592-597

Huang, T.L. & Lee, C.T. (2007). Low serum albumin and high ferritin levels in chronic hemodialysis patients with major depression. *Psychiatry Res*, 152, 277-280

Hung, K.C., Wu, C.C., Chen, H.S., Ma, W.Y., Tseng, C.F., Yang, L.K., et al. (2011). Serum IL-6, albumin and co-morbidities are closely correlated with symptoms of depression in patients on maintenance haemodialysis. *Nephrol Dial Transplant*, 26, 658-664

Ibrahim, S. & El Salamony, O. (2008). Depression, quality of life and malnutrition-inflammation scores in hemodialysis patients. *Am J Nephrol*, 28, 784-791

Irwin, M.R. & Miller, A.H. (2007). Depressive disorders and immunity: 20 years of progress and discovery. *Brain Behav Immun*, 21, 374-383

Jhamb, M., Argyropoulos, C., Steel, J.L., Plantinga, L., Wu, A.W., Fink, N.E., et al. (2009). Correlates and outcomes of fatigue among incident dialysis patients. *Clin J Am Soc Nephrol*, 4, 1779-1786

Jhamb, M., Weisbord, S.D., Steel, J.L. & Unruh, M. (2008). Fatigue in patients receiving maintenance dialysis: a review of definitions, measures, and contributing factors. *Am J Kidney Dis*, 52, 353-365

Jones, M., Ibels, L., Schenkel, B. & Zagari, M. (2004). Impact of epoetin alfa on clinical end points in patients with chronic renal failure: a meta-analysis. *Kidney Int*, 65, 757-767

Kalender, B., Ozdemir, A.C., Dervisoglu, E. & Ozdemir, O. (2007a). Quality of life in chronic kidney disease: effects of treatment modality, depression, malnutrition and inflammation. *Int J Clin Pract*, 61, 569-576

Kalender, B., Ozdemir, A.C., Yalug, I. & Dervisoglu, E. (2007b). Antidepressant treatment increases quality of life in patients with chronic renal failure. *Ren Fail*, 29, 817-822

Kao, T.W., Lai, M.S., Tsai, T.J., Jan, C.F., Chie, W.C. & Chen, W.Y. (2009). Economic, social, and psychological factors associated with health-related quality of life of chronic hemodialysis patients in northern Taiwan: a multicenter study. *Artif Organs*, 33, 61-68

Keskin, G. & Engin, E. (2011). The evaluation of depression, suicidal ideation and coping strategies in haemodialysis patients with renal failure. *J Clin Nurs* (In press)

Kessler, R.C., Berglund, P., Demler, O., Jin, R., Koretz, D., Merikangas, K.R., et al. (2003). The epidemiology of major depressive disorder: results from the National Comorbidity Survey Replication (NCS-R). *JAMA*, 289, 3095-3105

Kessler, R.C., Chiu, W.T., Demler, O., Merikangas, K.R. & Walters, E.E. (2005). Prevalence, severity, and comorbidity of 12-month DSM-IV disorders in the National Comorbidity Survey Replication. *Arch Gen Psychiatry*, 62, 617-627

Kim, K.H., Kim, T.H., Kang, J.W., Sul, J.U., Lee, M.S., Kim, J.I., et al. (2011). Acupuncture for symptom management in hemodialysis patients: a prospective, observational pilot study. *J Altern Complement Med*, 17, 741-748

Kimmel, P.L. (2001). Psychosocial factors in dialysis patients. *Kidney Int*, 59, 1599-1613

Kimmel, P.L. & Peterson, R.A. (2005). Depression in end-stage renal disease patients treated with hemodialysis: tools, correlates, outcomes, and needs. *Semin Dial*, 18, 91-97

Kimmel, P.L., Phillips, T.M., Simmens, S.J., Peterson, R.A., Weihs, K.L., Alleyne, S., et al. (1998). Immunologic function and survival in hemodialysis patients. *Kidney Int*, 54, 236-244

Kimmel, P.L., Weihs, K. & Peterson, R.A. (1993). Survival in hemodialysis patients: the role of depression. *J Am Soc Nephrol*, 4, 12-27

Koo, J.R., Yoon, J.W., Kim, S.G., Lee, Y.K., Oh, K.H., Kim, G.H., et al. (2003). Association of depression with malnutrition in chronic hemodialysis patients. *Am J Kidney Dis*, 41, 1037-1042

Koo, J.R., Yoon, J.Y., Joo, M.H., Lee, H.S., Oh, J.E., Kim, S.G., et al. (2005). Treatment of depression and effect of antidepression treatment on nutritional status in chronic hemodialysis patients. *Am J Med Sci*, 329, 1-5

Kouidi, E., Karagiannis, V., Grekas, D., Iakovides, A., Kaprinis, G., Tourkantonis, A., et al. (2010). Depression, heart rate variability, and exercise training in dialysis patients. *Eur J Cardiovasc Prev Rehabil*, 17, 160-167

Kring, D.L. & Crane, P.B. (2009). Factors affecting quality of life in persons on hemodialysis. *Nephrol Nurs J*, 36, 15-24, 55

Kuo, H.W., Tsai, S.S., Tiao, M.M. & Yang, C.Y. (2007). Epidemiological features of CKD in Taiwan. *Am J Kidney Dis*, 49, 46-55

Kurella, M., Kimmel, P.L., Young, B.S. & Chertow, G.M. (2005). Suicide in the United States end-stage renal disease program. *J Am Soc Nephrol*, 16, 774-781

Lee, B.O., Lin, C.C., Chaboyer, W., Chiang, C.L. & Hung, C.C. (2007). The fatigue experience of haemodialysis patients in Taiwan. *J Clin Nurs*, 16, 407-413

Lee, K.A., Hicks, G. & Nino-Murcia, G. (1991). Validity and reliability of a scale to assess fatigue. *Psychiatry Res*, 36, 291-298

Leonard, B.E. (2010). The concept of depression as a dysfunction of the immune system. *Curr Immunol Rev*, 6, 205-212

Letchmi, S., Das, S., Halim, H., Zakariah, F.A., Hassan, H., Mat, S., et al. (2011). Fatigue experienced by patients receiving maintenance dialysis in hemodialysis units. *Nurs Health Sci*, 13, 60-64

Loftis, J.M., Huckans, M. & Morasco, B.J. (2010). Neuroimmune mechanisms of cytokine-induced depression: current theories and novel treatment strategies. *Neurobiol Dis*, 37, 519-533

Martiny, C., De Oliveira, E.S.A.C., Neto, J.P. & Nardi, A.E. (2011). Factors associated with risk of suicide in patients with hemodialysis. *Compr Psychiatry*, 52, 465-468

Memoli, B., Minutolo, R., Bisesti, V., Postiglione, L., Conti, A., Marzano, L., et al. (2002). Changes of serum albumin and C-reactive protein are related to changes of interleukin-6 release by peripheral blood mononuclear cells in hemodialysis patients treated with different membranes. *Am J Kidney Dis*, 39, 266-273

Montinaro, V., Iaffaldano, G.P., Granata, S., Porcelli, P., Todarello, O., Schena, F.P., et al. (2010). Emotional symptoms, quality of life and cytokine profile in hemodialysis patients. *Clin Nephrol*, 73, 36-43

Murtagh, F.E., Addington-Hall, J. & Higginson, I.J. (2007). The prevalence of symptoms in end-stage renal disease: a systematic review. *Adv Chronic Kidney Dis*, 14, 82-99

Noshad, H., Sadreddini, S., Nezami, N., Salekzamani, Y. & Ardalan, M.R. (2009). Comparison of outcome and quality of life: haemodialysis versus peritoneal dialysis patients. *Singapore Med J*, 50, 185-192

O'donovan, A., Hughes, B.M., Slavich, G.M., Lynch, L., Cronin, M.T., O'farrelly, C., et al. (2010). Clinical anxiety, cortisol and interleukin-6: evidence for specificity in emotion-biology relationships. *Brain Behav Immun*, 24, 1074-1077

Ouzouni, S., Kouidi, E., Sioulis, A., Grekas, D. & Deligiannis, A. (2009). Effects of intradialytic exercise training on health-related quality of life indices in haemodialysis patients. *Clin Rehabil*, 23, 53-63

Perlman, R.L., Finkelstein, F.O., Liu, L., Roys, E., Kiser, M., Eisele, G., et al. (2005). Quality of life in chronic kidney disease (CKD): a cross-sectional analysis in the Renal Research Institute-CKD study. *Am J Kidney Dis*, 45, 658-666

Pertosa, G., Grandaliano, G., Gesualdo, L. & Schena, F.P. (2000). Clinical relevance of cytokine production in hemodialysis. *Kidney Int Suppl*, 76, S104-111

Raymond, C.B., Wazny, L.D. & Honcharik, P.L. (2008). Pharmacotherapeutic options for the treatment of depression in patients with chronic kidney disease. *Nephrol Nurs J*, 35, 257-263; quiz 264

Riolo, S.A., Nguyen, T.A., Greden, J.F. & King, C.A. (2005). Prevalence of depression by race/ethnicity: findings from the National Health and Nutrition Examination Survey III. *Am J Public Health*, 95, 998-1000

Sakkas, G.K., Sargeant, A.J., Mercer, T.H., Ball, D., Koufaki, P., Karatzaferi, C., et al. (2003). Changes in muscle morphology in dialysis patients after 6 months of aerobic exercise training. *Nephrol Dial Transplant*, 18, 1854-1861

Sareen, J., Cox, B.J., Afifi, T.O., De Graaf, R., Asmundson, G.J., Ten Have, M., et al. (2005). Anxiety disorders and risk for suicidal ideation and suicide attempts: a population-based longitudinal study of adults. *Arch Gen Psychiatry*, 62, 1249-1257

Seabolt, J.L. & De Leon, O.A. (2001). Response to nefazodone in a depressed patient with end-stage renal disease. *Gen Hosp Psychiatry*, 23, 45-46

Sesso, R. & Yoshihiro, M.M. (1997). Time of diagnosis of chronic renal failure and assessment of quality of life in haemodialysis patients. *Nephrol Dial Transplant*, 12, 2111-2116

Simic Ogrizovic, S., Jovanovic, D., Dopsaj, V., Radovic, M., Sumarac, Z., Bogavac, S.N., et al. (2009). Could depression be a new branch of MIA syndrome? *Clin Nephrol*, 71, 164-172

Singh, A.K., Szczech, L., Tang, K.L., Barnhart, H., Sapp, S., Wolfson, M., et al. (2006). Correction of anemia with epoetin alfa in chronic kidney disease. *N Engl J Med*, 355, 2085-2098

Sklar, A.H., Riesenberg, L.A., Silber, A.K., Ahmed, W. & Ali, A. (1996). Postdialysis fatigue. *Am J Kidney Dis*, 28, 732-736

Smogorzewski, M., Ni, Z. & Massry, S.G. (1995). Function and metabolism of brain synaptosomes in chronic renal failure. *Artif Organs*, 19, 795-800

Son, Y.J., Choi, K.S., Park, Y.R., Bae, J.S. & Lee, J.B. (2009). Depression, symptoms and the quality of life in patients on hemodialysis for end-stage renal disease. *Am J Nephrol*, 29, 36-42

Sonikian, M., Metaxaki, P., Papavasileiou, D., Boufidou, F., Nikolaou, C., Vlassopoulos, D., et al. (2010). Effects of interleukin-6 on depression risk in dialysis patients. *Am J Nephrol*, 31, 303-308

Stenvinkel, P., Heimburger, O., Paultre, F., Diczfalusy, U., Wang, T., Berglund, L., et al. (1999). Strong association between malnutrition, inflammation, and atherosclerosis in chronic renal failure. *Kidney Int*, 55, 1899-1911

Symister, P. & Friend, R. (2003). The influence of social support and problematic support on optimism and depression in chronic illness: a prospective study evaluating self-esteem as a mediator. *Health Psychol*, 22, 123-129

Taskapan, H., Ates, F., Kaya, B., Emul, M., Kaya, M., Taskapan, C., et al. (2005). Psychiatric disorders and large interdialytic weight gain in patients on chronic haemodialysis. *Nephrology (Carlton)*, 10, 15-20

Tsay, S.L. & Healstead, M. (2002). Self-care self-efficacy, depression, and quality of life among patients receiving hemodialysis in Taiwan. *Int J Nurs Stud*, 39, 245-251

Victorri-Vigneau, C., Dailly, E., Veyrac, G. & Jolliet, P. (2007). Evidence of zolpidem abuse and dependence: results of the French Centre for Evaluation and Information on Pharmacodependence (CEIP) network survey. *Br J Clin Pharmacol*, 64, 198-209

Watnick, S., Wang, P.L., Demadura, T. & Ganzini, L. (2005). Validation of 2 depression screening tools in dialysis patients. *Am J Kidney Dis*, 46, 919-924

Weisbord, S.D., Fried, L.F., Mor, M.K., Resnick, A.L., Kimmel, P.L., Palevsky, P.M., et al. (2007a). Associations of race and ethnicity with anemia management among patients initiating renal replacement therapy. *J Natl Med Assoc*, 99, 1218-1226

Weisbord, S.D., Fried, L.F., Unruh, M.L., Kimmel, P.L., Switzer, G.E., Fine, M.J., et al. (2007b). Associations of race with depression and symptoms in patients on maintenance haemodialysis. *Nephrol Dial Transplant*, 22, 203-208

Weissman, M.M., Bland, R.C., Canino, G.J., Faravelli, C., Greenwald, S., Hwu, H.G., et al. (1996). Cross-national epidemiology of major depression and bipolar disorder. *JAMA*, 276, 293-299

Wichers, M. & Maes, M. (2002). The psychoneuroimmuno-pathophysiology of cytokine-induced depression in humans. *Int J Neuropsychopharmacol*, 5, 375-388

Winkelmayer, W.C., Mehta, J. & Wang, P.S. (2007). Benzodiazepine use and mortality of incident dialysis patients in the United States. *Kidney Int*, 72, 1388-1393

Wolcott, D.L., Nissenson, A.R. & Landsverk, J. (1988). Quality of life in chronic dialysis patients. Factors unrelated to dialysis modality. *Gen Hosp Psychiatry*, 10, 267-277

Wyne, A., Rai, R., Cuerden, M., Clark, W.F. & Suri, R.S. (2011). Opioid and benzodiazepine use in end-stage renal disease: a systematic review. *Clin J Am Soc Nephrol*, 6, 326-333

Ye, W., Zhao, Y., Robinson, R.L. & Swindle, R.W. (2011). Treatment patterns associated with Duloxetine and Venlafaxine use for Major Depressive Disorder. *BMC Psychiatry*, 11, 19

14

Renal Replacement Therapy in Uremic Diabetic Patients – Experience from The Republic of Macedonia

Momir H. Polenakovic
Macedonian Academy of Sciences and Arts, Skopje,
Department of Nephrology, Medical Faculty, Ss. Cyril and Methodius University, Skopje
Republic of Macedonia

1. Introduction

In many countries, diabetic renal disease has become, or will soon become, the single most common cause of end-stage renal disease (ESRD). End stage renal failure (ESRF) in type 2 diabetic patients is increasing worldwide (1).

Diabetic nephropathy (DN) is the most prevalent cause of ESRD in the USA. The proportion of ESRD patients who are diabetic is increasing by more than 1% each year in the USA. The rate of admission of uraemic patients with diabetes as a co-morbid condition in the USA was 107 per million population (p.m.p.) per year in 1994 (2) and is currently approximately 120 p.m.p. The corresponding figures in other countries are lower: 66 p.m.p. in Japan and 52 p.m.p. in southwestern Germany (1). The incidence of ESRD in Europe due to diabetes, hypertension and renal vascular disease has nearly doubled over 10 years; in 1998-99, it varied between countries from 10.2 to 39.3 p.m.p. for diabetes, from 5.8 to 21.0 for hypertension, and from 1.0 to 15.5 for renal vascular disease (3). The figures are lower in the Mediterranean countries, as well as in Macedonia (4), although an increase has recently been reported from Spain (5) and Italy (6). ESRD and ESRF caused by DN was 10%, 5-15% in different haemodialysis

Centres for adults in 2000 in the Republic of Macedonia (4), as well as 22% in 2006 (4a).

The great majority of diabetic patients admitted suffer from type 2 diabetes.

The increasing trend may be explained by a number of factors:

1. the increasing prevalence of type II diabetes in the general population;
2. improved survival of diabetic patients, particularly diabetic patients with nephropathy, because of better treatment of hypertension and coronary heart disease, so that they live long enough to experience renal failure;
3. less restriction of admission to renal replacement therapy.

One major problem continues to be late referral.

The poor prognosis of patients with diabetic nephropathy is well known in both in type 1 and type 2 diabetes. The high mortality and morbidity, especially in type 2 diabetic patients with nephropathy, are mainly caused by coronary artery, cerebrovascular and peripheral vascular disease (7).

The survival of type 1 diabetic patients requiring renal replacement therapy has been dramatically improved during the last decade; however, prognosis for type 2 diabetic patients with ESRD continues to be extremely poor (1).

2. Evaluation of the diabetic patient with preterminal renal failure

Evaluation of the diabetic patients with preterminal renal failure has the following aims:

1. to assess the course of renal failure (progression);
2. to recognize the presence of acute renal failure, or acute or chronic renal failure;
3. to recognize renal problems other than diabetic nephropathy, for example ischaemic nephropathy, diabetic cystopathy, urinary tract infection;
4. to monitor the patient for clinical evidence of extrarenal microvascular and macrovascular complications, for example retinopathy or polyneuropathy and coronary heart disease or arterioocclusive disease.

Some of these coincident kidney diseases are listed below.

2.1 Ischaemic renal disease

Renal ischaemia or atherosclerotic renal artery stenosis is much more common in diabetics than previously assumed (8). In this case one should be cautious regarding ACE-inhibitors or angiotensin receptor blocking antihypertensives. Frequent control of s-creatinin, s-potassium and bodyweight are mandatory. A two-fold increase in s-creatinine should prompt the physician to stop this type of medication.

2.2 Urinary tract infection

Urinary tract infection (UTI) has frequently led to renal parenchymatous infection with purulent papillary necrosis and intrarenal abscess formation. UTI may be frequent in diabetics, especially when residual urine is present.

2.3 Glomerulonephritis

Glomerulonephritis (GN), particularly membranous GN, is thought to be more frequent in diabetics, but this has not been supported by other studies.

2.4 Acute renal failure

Diabetic patients with nephropathy are exceptionally susceptible to acute renal failure (ARF) after the administration of radiocontrast media, the risk being similar with ionic and non-ionic materials. The risk may be reduced by fluid administration and a temporary withdrawal of diuretics. In patients with severely elevated serum-creatinine a dialysis procedure immediately after the radiographic procedure is warranted, without any delay in time.

Hydroxyethyl starch and ACE inhibitors also cause deterioration of renal function in diabetic patients, especially in those with congestive heart failure.

The points relating to treatment strategies and decision-making in diabetic patients with renal failure present are: evaluation (and treatment) of risk factors for progression, monitoring of progression, evaluation of patient for renal replacement therapy (dialysis, transplantation), informing patient both and care about renal replacement therapy, preparing patients for renal replacement therapy (vascular access, check-up for transplantation) and adjustment of diet and insulin or oral hypoglycaemic agents.

In the table 1 is a check-list for management of diabetic patients with preterminal renal failure.

- Reversible causes of renal failure present? (contrast media, urinary tract infection, angiotensin converting enzyme inhibitors, congestive heart failure)
- Hypovolaemia present?
- Coronary heart disease present (percutaneous transluminal angioplasty or coronary bypass surgery required?
- Cardiomyopathy or congestive heart failure present?
- Congestion due to hypervolaemia or heart failure?
- Early vascular access?
- Hypoglycemic episodes present? Adequate nutrient intake?
- Eye (examined and treated?)
- Foot (neuropathic? ischaemic? foot ulcers? infection?)
- Residual urine present, urinary tract infection?
- Normotension or antihypertensive treatment achieved?
- Orthostatic blood pressure drop?
- Gastroparesis or diarrhoeal episodes?

Table 1. Check-list for management of diabetic patients with preterminal renal failure

3. Option in uremia therapy

Determination of which treatment option is "best" for a particular diabetic ESRD patient, however, is an **individualized judgment** (table 2) depending on the patient's age, education, geographic location, family and social support systems, and the extent of co-morbid conditions, most importantly, of cardiovascular integrity. Major subjects which must be apprised when devising a longterm plan for ESRD management include anticipated patient compliance and potential to participate in self-treatment. Each ESRD treatment option must be explained in understandable terms covering the probable survival rate, the degree of rehabilitation and the expected stabilisation of extrarenal diabetics complications. Ideally, what has been termed a "life plan" should be constructed for every ESRD patient after consultation between the health care team, the patient, and the members of the patient's social support system.

While the best rehabilitation of diabetic ESRD patients is achieved in recipients of living related donor renal transplants, this superior outcome may reflect a selection bias in which younger, healthier patients are chosen for a transplant leaving a residual pool of more morbid dialysis patients. Morbidity from blindness and neuropathy (but not coronary artery or peripheral vascular disease) is decreased in diabetic kidney transplant recipients (9). Lacking randomized prospective trials of diabetics treated with dialytic therapy versus a kidney transplant, controlled for age, race, gender, and severity of extrarenal complication, caution must be exercised when assessing one ESRD therapy against another. A reasonable policy can be based on the premise that while the best rehabilitation is effected by renal transplantation, there is no distinctly superior treatment for the uraemic diabetic, and therefore, **assessment and treatment of diabetic with ESRD must be highly individualized** (10).

1. **Passive suicide which is the consequence of declining dialysis or kidney transplantation**
2. **Haemodialysis**
   - Facility haemodialysis
   - Home haemodialysis
3. **Peritoneal dialysis**
   - Intermittent peritoneal dialysis (IPD)
   - Continuous ambulatory peritoneal dialysis (CAPD)
   - Continuous cyclic peritoneal dialysis (CCPD)
4. **Renal transplantation**
   - Cadaver donor kidney
   - Living donor kidney
5. **Pancreas, plus kidney transplantation**
   - IDDM
   - ? NIDDM
   - islet-cell transplantation (type 1)

Table 2. Options in uremia therapy for diabetic ESRD patients

4. Timing the start of dialytic therapy

As residual creatinine clearance falls to about 20–30 ml/min, available ESRD options should be discussed and a selection made. In practice, bias by the patient's most trusted physician usually is the major factor determining which renal replacement therapy is chosen.

Diabetic complications which persist and/or progress during ESRD and on dialysis are: retinopathy, glaucoma, cataracts; coronary artery disease, cardiomyopathy; cerebrovascular disease; hypertension; peripheral vascular disease: limb amputation; motor neuropathy, sensory neuropathy; autonomic dysfunction: diarrhoea, constipation, hypotension; myopathy; depression; infections; bladder neuropathy; sexual disorders; impotence; eating disorders; gastroparesis with vomiting and food retention; alteration in the metabolic control and dyslipidaemias; ion imbalance and metabolic acidosis.

For the 80% of uraemic diabetic selecting haemodialysis (HD), the construction of a vascular access is of great importance. Once it is clear that uraemia is a near term probability (less than one year), an arteriovenous access should be constructed.

The first choice in HD access in diabetics is an autologous a-v fistula of the Cimino-Brescia type.

When peritoneal dialysis (PD) is selected advance planning should ensure that a suitable peritoneal catheter is *in situ* 2–4 weeks before starting dialysis.

Option for a kidney or a kidney plus pancreas transplant obviously demands referral to and evaluation by a transplant team. In the case of an intended living related donor transplant, interim dialysis can be avoided by proper planning, performing the transplant at an early stage of uraemic symptoms. A long wait is usual for a cadaver kidney.

Accordingly, patients should be entered on waiting lists when the creatinin clearance is about 10–15 ml/min.

5. Haemodialysis in diabetics

Haemodialysis has emerged as the most common treatment for all forms of renal failure including diabetic nephropathy. It is generally accepted that renal replacement therapy should be considered as a creatinine clearance of approximately 9–14 ml/min in non-diabetic uraemia patients (11).

In diabetic patients with ESRD, dialysis is started at creatinine clearance as high as 15–20 ml/min, at serum creatinine levels as low as 3–5 mg/dl.

In any case, HD should be started before the clinical status deteriorates, secondary to fluid overload, malnutrition, hyperkalaemia and infection. This is usually the case when the GFR declines below 20 ml/min.

Vascular access surgery (usually autologous arteriovenous fistula of the Cimino-Brescia type) some month before the initiation of the dialysis treatment helps to avoid central venous lines and their concomitant complications. Blood drawing for regular serum chemistry is restricted to the dorsal hand veins only.

5.1 Prognosis in patients with diabetic nephropathy on haemodialysis and in assessing the adequacy of haemodialysis

In the past, the prognosis for DN was discouraging, with 77% of patients dying within 10 years after the onset of persistent proteinuria. The survival of dialysed diabetics has improved over the past decade. No single factor is credited with reducing the death rate of haemodialysed diabetics, though better control of hypertension, a reduction in intravascular volume overload, better nutrition, and better vascular access surgery have contributed.

Table 3 compares actuarial 5-year survival of non-diabetic and diabetic patients on maintenance haemodialysis in different countries. It is obvious that in countries with a low prevalence of cardiovascular deaths in the general population, e.g. East Asian countries and, to a lesser extent, the Mediterranean countries, survival of diabetic patients on RRT is significantly better than that in countries with notoriously high cardiovascular death rates, e.g. USA and Germany.

	No diabetes	Diabetes
Australia	60	42/27 a
Japan b	64/73	50/40
Taiwan	65	37
Hong Kong	70	20
Italy (Lombardy)	61	28
Spain (Catalonia) c	65	30
Germany	–	38/5
USA d	35	21

Values are expressed as percentage of surviving patients.
[a] Reported as type 1 / type 2 diabetes.
[b] Reported as haemodialysis / continuous ambulatory peritoneal dialysis.
[c] Includes renal transplantation.
[d] Censored at first transplantation.

Table 3. Comparison of actuarial 5 year survival of non-diabetic and diabetic patients on dialysis treatment in different countries (1).

In table 4 are the causes of death in diabetic patients on HD.

	Type 1 diabetes (n = 67)	**Type 2 diabetes (n = 129)**
Myocardial infarction	8	12
Sudden death	7	13
Cardiac other	3	17
Stroke	0	6
Septicaemia	7	11
Interruption of treatment	2	8
Other	2	13
Total	29 (40%)	80 (43%)

Total cardiovascular mortality was 62% in type 1 and 60% in type 2 diabetes.

Table 4. Causes of death in diabetic patients 57 months after start of haemodialysis (12).

Cardiovascular disease and serious infections are the major causes of death in haemodialysed and transplanted diabetics. Despite recent improvement, rehabilitation of haemodialysed diabetics continues to be inferior to that of nondiabetics. Improvement of survival is a matter of reduction of cardiovascular death and infection.

5.2 Cardiovascular death and adequacy of dialysis

Cardiac death is strongly predicted by a *history of vascular disease* (peripheral vascular and/or carotid), *myocardial infarction* and *angina pectoris*. *Proliferative retinopathy* and *polyneuropathy* were associated with an increased cardiac risk, in the latter possibly due to an imbalance of autonomic cardiac innervation. *Hypotensive cardiac episodes* during dialysis are also predictive of cardiac death.

Haemodialysis procedures should be with low ultrafiltration rates and prolonged duration of dialysis sessions (13). In practice, ultrafiltration in diabetics should not exceed more than 500-600 ml/h on haemodialysis. This means dialysis sessions of more than 4h and, in larger patients, of more than 5h haemodialysis three times per week.

Guidelines have been created to assure adequate dialysis - "dose of dialysis".

According to DOQI (Dialysis Outcomes Quality Initiative), a *Kt/V* (indicator for adequacy of dialysis, where *K* is the dialyser clearance rate, *t* the net duration of dialysis and *V* the corrected body volume) of above 1.2 (e.g. a 70-kg patient dialysed for 5h) is adequate (14). Lower *Kt/V*, especially below 1, is associated with a higher mortality rate and this is particularly true of the patient with diabetic nephropathy.

Optimal dialysis in diabetic patients:

Need for a dialysis technique which will provide

- - absence of acetate
- - good cardiovascular stability
- - good acid-base correction
- - good solute removal
- - good biocompatibility

5.3 Special problems of diabetic patients on haemodialysis

5.3.1 Vascular access

In a diabetic patient it is often more difficult to establish vascular access because of a poor arterial inflow (atherosclerosis, media calcification of the artery) and venous run-off (hypoplasia or thrombosed veins) in chronically ill patients, with numerous stays in hospital. Arterio-venous anastomosis should be placed in the upper forearm to maintain adequate shunt blood flow. It is therefore advisable to **establish vascular access early, when creatinine clearance is above 20-25 ml/min (14, 15). In malnourished, older individuals, this level of GFR impairment can be reached even at a serum-creatinine of 2 mg/dl**.

One should patiently wait for maturing of the fistula: early puncture tends to be associated with haematoma formation, scarring, stenosis and thrombosis, and should be avoided, even if dialysis has to be performed by a central venous catheter. Some authors have reported poor functioning of the vascular access in diabetics, with only 64% of fistula functioning after 1 year compared to 83% in non-diabetic.

Radial steal syndrome, venous hypertension, infection/thrombosis (15, 16), and ischaemic monomelic neuropathy could be problems related to vascular access.

5.3.2 Metabolic control

In clinical practice, the need for insulin decreases upon the institution of maintenance HD. The fall in insulin requirements in no way signifies any improvement in the underlying disease. Also, good glucose control should remain a goal even after initiation of dialysis. It remains important to protect further injury to other organs such as the eyes. Glycaemic control may also be important for preserving residual renal function for as long as possible (17).

Most nephrologists prefer to dialyse against glucose (200 mg/dl) to achieve better stabilization of plasma glucose concentrations. One must consider, however, that glucose-containing dialysate does not guarantee normoglycaemia if the prescribed insulin dose is too high (18,19). "Tight" metabolic control - a key component in diabetic management - risks potentially fatal hypoglycaemic episodes in haemodialysed patients (14). Oral sulphonylurea must be avoided, in fact is strictly forbidden, because of prolonged hypoglycaemia in endstage renal failure (20).

If glucose-free dialysate is used, glucose loss (amounting to 80-100 g per dialysis session) may occur. It has been argued that the glucose loss into the dialysate contributes to catabolism but no convincing evidence for this was produced in a control trial (20).

Diabetic control is occasionally rendered difficult by diabetic gastroparesis and the tendency of gastric motility to deteriorate acutely during dialysis sessions.

Adequate control of glycaemia is important: hyperglycaemia causes intense thirst and subsequent increased fluid intake, as well as osmotic water shift and shift of potassium from the intracellular to the extracellular space, with the attendant risk of circulatory and pulmonary congestion and hyperkalaemia.

Poorly controlled diabetics are also more susceptible to infection.

The HbA1c should be < 8.0% (18, 19, 22).

5.3.3 Intradialytic and interdialytic blood pressure

Blood pressure in the diabetic is primarily volume-dependent. Consequently, *hypertension* tends to be more common in dialysed diabetics, who have higher predialytic blood pressures, require multidrug therapy more often than non-diabetic uraemic patients. About one-half of haemodialysed diabetics require antihypertensive medications, compared to 27.7% of non-diabetics (23). Betablockers should not be used in diabetics as they exacerbate hypertriglyceridemia, worsen glucose control and mask symptoms of severe hypoglycaemia. Improvement is typical in volumen-dependent hypertension after intradialytic fluid extraction. The problem is compounded by the fact that *intradialytic hypotension is more frequent in diabetics*; as a consequence it is often difficult to reach the target dry weight.

Hypotension is more prevalent in diabetic than in non-diabetic haemodialysis patients. Episodic hypotension is at least 20% greater in incidence while nausea and vomiting are three times more prevalent (23). Episodes of hypotension are highly predictive of cardiac death (24). Severe or sustained hypotension may precipitate *angina pectoris* culminating in acute myocardial infarction.

Intradialytic hypotension is a multi-factorial problem; inadequate circulatory adjustment to volume subtraction (as a consequence of autonomous polyneuropathy) and left ventricular diastolic malfunction (necessitating higher left ventricular filling pressures) have both been implicated in its genesis.

Hypotensive episodes have been associated with an increased risk of sudden cardiac death, acute myocardial ischaemia, deterioration of maculopathy and non-thrombotic mesenteric ischaemia.

The following suggestions could be useful for minimizing haemodialysis-induced hypotension in diabetics (9):

- bicarbonate rather than acetate dialysate,
- acetate free biofiltration,
- high sodium concentration (140–145 mmol/l) in dialysate,
- slow rate of ultrafiltration,
- schedule sequential ultrafiltration and dialysis in patients who are grossly
- oedematous,
- prime dialysis circuit with hypertonic albumin solution,
- maintain hematocrit at or above 30 vol% with erythropoietin,
- omit antihypertensive medications on morning of dialysis,
- leg toning exercises to improve venous return, and
- decrease dialysate temperature (particularly near conclusion of treatment).

High interdialytic weight gain. Diabetics gain near 30% more weight between haemodialysis than non-diabetics.

Intensified metabolic control facilitated by dietary counselling plus sodium modeling of dialysis, and sequential ultrafiltration curtails weight swings and their deleterious consequences.

5.3.4 Lipid abnormalities in diabetic patients with renal failure

Hypercholesterolaemia and hypertriglyceridaemia are strong predictors of coronary heart disease (25). Major dyslipidaemia is seen only in untreated type-1 diabetic patients. A strong correlation exists between HbA1c and plasma cholesterol, triglyceride and high-density lipoproteins (26). In type-2 diabetes, dyslipidaemia persists even when glycosaemia is well controlled, presumably due to an underlying genetic defect which predisposes to both diabetes and disturbed lipid metabolism (27, 28).

In a prospective study (29), a relationship between coronary risk and cholesterol concentrations in diabetics admitted for haemodialysis has been established.

Non-accumulating fibrates or HMG Co-reductase inhibitors are indicated for the treatment of dyslipidaemia which does not respond to dietary manipulation. Regular control of creatinin kinase (rhabdomyolysis) is recommended.

5.3.5 Erythropoietin and iron substitution in uraemic diabetic patients

Len venticular hypertrophy (LVH) is more prevalent in diabetics compared to non-diabetics with end-stage renal disease, and it is possible that the beneficial effects of erythropoietin on LVH could be particularly relevant for diabetic patients (30, 31).

Currently, there is no reason to recommend a different target haemoglobin for diabetic and non-diabetic patients; a haemoglobin of 11–12 g/dl is therefore also appropriate for diabetic patients.

Increases in blood pressure, vascular access clotting and even seizures have been observed more frequently in diabetic dialysis patients when haemoglobin was increased too rapidly.

A suggested mode of correction of anaemia in diabetic patients is as follows: a cautious dosage of erythropoietin (initial dose of 2000 three times weekly s.c., followed by increments of 2000 at monthly intervals) and careful adjustment of heparinisation during dialysis. If haemoglobin increases by > 1.3 g/dl over two weeks, the erythropoietin dose should be reduced. Once the target haemoglobin has been reached, the weekly dosage should be reduced and haemoglobin monitored at regular intervals.

It is important to establish adequate iron substitution in erythropoietin treated dialysed diabetic patients. In clinical practice intravenous iron substitution, at the end of the dialysis procedure, is safe and effective. A target ferritin level of above 250 mg/dl is advisable. During infection episodes, however, iron substitution should be temporarily stopped.

5.4 Malnutrition in dialysis – dependent diabetics

It is important that diabetic patients on dialysis maintain adequate energy (35–40 kcal/kg/day). In addition, protein intake should not be below 1.3 g/kg a day because of the known higher protein requirements of dialysis patients. Anorexia and prolonged habituation to dietary restrictions are important reasons for malnutrition of the diabetic patient on dialysis. Malnutrition is a common concern in dialysed diabetic patients.

5.5 Infections in uraemic diabetic patients

Bacterial infections are common complications in uraemic diabetic patients (32), in whom the polymorphnuclear leukocyte function is depressed, particularly when acidosis is present. Leukocyte adherence, chemotaxis and phagocytosis may be affected.

Uraemic diabetics have several particular sites where infections can occur: arteriovenous fistula and central venous catheters, CAPD catheter, the urinary tract, the sinus and diabetic foot ulcer. Infections of the dialysis access, either HD or CAPD, are mostly caused by *Staphylococcus* as a result of increased skin and mucosal colonization with these organisms and need specific therapy. Diabetic patients with prolonged hospital stay should be screened for methicillinresistant *Staphylococcus*. Diabetics are more prone to urinary tract infections due to diminishing residual diuresis, incomplete bladder emptying because of autonomic neuropathy and following diagnostic or therapeutical instrumentation of the urethra or bladder. Foot ulcer infections often progress to septic gangrene and amputation.

6. Microvascular complications

6.1 Diabetic retinopathy

Diabetic retinopathy occurs in 97% of uraemic diabetic patients and 25–30% are blind (33).

Visual loss results from proliferative retinopathy, cataracts, glaucoma,or vitreous haemorrhage.

Diabetic uraemic patients need regular ophthalmologic controls at a frequency of 3–6 months. Laser photocoagulation and other intervention are very frequent in all diabetics either prior to or during treatment for ESRD.

Anticoagulation (heparin) during the haemodialysis procedure and the application of platelet aggregation inhibitors (e.g. aspirin) can cause severe retinal bleeding and blindness.

6.2 Diabetic neuropathy

Many patients suffer from the consequences of a peripheral sensorimotor neuropathy, or from gastroparesis or other bowel disturbances caused by autonomic neuropathy.

These are very difficult to treat and respond poorly to conventional treatments. Neuropathy is less likely to progress in a renal transplant recipient. It also tends to be less severe in patients treated with PD, theoretically because of improved clearance of medium-sized molecules (33).

Many patients may also suffer from impotence caused by neuropathy, vascular disease, or medication. These patients may require specialist investigation and treatment.

7. Macrovascular complication

7.1 Peripheral vascular disease

Problems related to the diabetic foot are a major cause of hospital admission, and 50–70% of all nontraumatic amputations occur in diabetics. One UK study reported that 6.8% of diabetics receiving renal replacement therapy had a major amputation (34, 35).

There is no reported difference between CAPD and HD (34). The major contributory etiologic factors in diabetic foot problems are peripheral vascular disease, diabetic neuropathy and stress caused by inappropriate footwear.

To prevent diabetic foot complications, patients at risk, should be identified should perform education about foot care, have regular examination of the feet at clinic, provision of appropriate footwear and of podiatry services.

Some studies have reported a symptomatic deterioration in the lower limbs that correlates with falls in blood pressure. Therefore, care should be taken to avoid excessive ultrafiltration in diabetic patients undergoing dialysis. In type 2 diabetics, better glycaemic control is associated with fewer amputations.

The treatment of this condition requires a multidisciplinary approach, ideally in a combined clinic with a nephrologist, diabetologist, and a podiatrist. At the first sign of lower limb ischaemia, patients should be assessed by a vascular surgeon.

7.2 Hyperparathyroidism

Diabetics undergoing dialysis developed secondary hyperparathyroidism at a slower rate than nondiabetics and this may predispose to adynamic bone disease in which there is a reduced rate of bone turnover without an excess of unmineralized osteoid. The reduced bone formation may lead to enhanced deposition of aluminium at the ossification front. Diabetics appear to accumulate aluminium more readily and are more susceptible to bone pain and fractures related to aluminium bone disease, which may also be unmasked by parathyroidectomy.

The diabetic uraemic should be treated with calcium-containing phosphate binders, which are ingested with every meal (500–1000 mg according to the amount of food). Aluminium-containing phosphate binders should be avoided because of possible aluminium intoxication. Vitamin D supplementation (e.g. 10000 U 25-(OH) vitamin D3 once weekly) is recommended.

Serumphosphate control is important not only to prevent renal bone disease, but to prevent stiffness of the large arterial vessels. Increased stiffness of the aorta (36) is associated with reduced survival in end-stage renal disease and vascular stiffness is correlated with the increase in serumphosphate.

8. Peritoneal dialysis (PD)

8.1 Continuous ambulatory peritoneal dialysis (CAPD), continuous cycling peritoneal dialysis (CCPD), in diabetic patients

CAPD has both medical and social benefits and most patients with diabetes are eligible for it. This technique enable patients to stay at home, where they can rapidly be taught the home dialysis regime and allows flexibility in treatment. The medical benefits of CAPD include slow and sustained ultrafiltration and a relative absence of rapid fluid and electrolyte changes and preservation of residual renal function.

Parameters	**Peritoneal dialysis**		**Haemodialysis**	
	Advantages	**Disadvantages**	**Advantages**	**Disadvantages**
Technique	Peritoneal access is easy	Low technique survival rate, high hospitalization rate, higher rate of infection	Better technique survival rate, lower hospitalization rate, lower infection rate	Difficulty with vascular access
Blood pressure	Good blood pressure control, slow ultrafiltration and fewer episodes of cardiovascular instability	–	–	Difficult blood pressure control, frequent hypotensive episodes
Biochemical parameters	Steady-state biochemical parameters, preservation of residual renal function for longer	–	Efficient solute and water extraction	–
Social factors	Maintains independence	–	Can be performed at home	–
Nutritional factors	Fewer dietary restrictions	Excessive weight gain, poor nutrition, hyperlipidemia	–	Difficulty with fluid and dietary restrictions

Table 5. Comparison of dialysis options for the diabetic patient (37, 38)

In CAPD the major osmotic agent for water removal is glucose. It is therefore of note to consider an extra amount of glucose (approximately 600–800 kcal) per treatment-day in the uraemic diabetic. Insulin dosage has to be adjusted.

Some authors propose that insulin be administred via the CAPD fluid. This route of application is not without difficulties, because adsorption of insulin into the CAPD bag and possible infection by installation of insulin into the bag are possible.

In table 6 are given a comparison of dialysis options for the diabetic patient.

8.2 Assessing the quality of dialysis in CAPD

Adequacy of dialysis is an important issue in CAPD as well as in HD. According to the DOQI guidelines, which are based on numerous studies (37), a weekly Kt/V of 2 or even more (weekly peritoneal creatinine clearance of more than 70 l) is nowadays considered an adequate dose of dialysis. In most patients this is only achievable when a certain amount of peritoneal fluid (more than 50 l/week) and a considerable residual renal function are combined. This has two implications: a) CAPD in diabetic patients should be started early (as in haemodialysis, at a creatinine clearance of approximately 20 ml/min); and b) residual renal function has to be monitored vigorously. If there is substantial fall in residual renal function (below 5 ml/min), in many cases adequate peritoneal dialysis is impossible. Inadequate PD, has a high mortality rate and patients must be taken off PD and either transferred to HD or, if possible, transplanted.

8.3 Outcome of patients on PD (CAPD / CCPD)

CAPD / CCPD appears to be associated in different evaluations with different outcomes in diabetics. The data from the United States Renal Data System (USRDS) registry indicate that, within the first 2 years of therapy, outcomes were superior to those for patients on HD. The risk of all-cause death for female diabetics aged >55 years in contrast, was 1.21 (confidence interval 1.17–1.24) for CAPD / CCPD, and in cause-specific analyses, these patients had a significantly higher risk of infectious death (39). This was confirmed by data from the Lombardy Registry but interpreted as a result of a hidden negative selection of patients (40). In a single-centre evaluation, HD and PD patients had similar survival, whereas the elderly (> 75 years) had a better survival on CAPD (41). Data from a Canadian Registry did not show any difference between the modalities, but a better survival for patients on PD (42). These discrepancies relate most probably to differences in clinical and demographic setting, patient populations, study design, statistical methods, and interactions between the dialytic modality effect and various other covariables.

8.4 Renal and pancreas transplantation

Renal transplantation is a safe and effective treatment modality for diabetic subjects with ESRD. Studies have shown that besides the improvement in quality of life, there is also posttransplantation better survival in uraemic patients (43, 44, 45). Simultaneous pancreas and kidney transplantation can be recommended as it prolongs survival in patients with diabetes and end-stage renal failure (46, 47) compared with kidney transplantation alone. In another series, patient or graft survival in diabetic patients receiving living-related donor kidney transplants or simultaneous pancreas and kidney transplants were not different, whereas unadjusted graft and patient survival rates in diabetic recipients (older and longer on dialysis) of cadaveric renal transplant were significantly lower than in the other group (48).

Despite these encouraging data, acturarial patient survival post-transplant is less favourable in diabetes compared to other primary renal diseases. It is indispensable to examine a diabetic uraemic thoroughly for vascular complications and infectious foci before the patient qualifies for the transplant waiting list (49).

Living related donor graft survival is superior to cadaveric donor grafts in diabetics (80 versus 64%, 5-year survival) as in nondiabetics. The higher mortality rate seen in cadaveric graft recipients is probably a consequence of a higher cumulative burden of immunosuppression and co-morbidities (50, 51). The introduction of improved immunosuppressive agents should further improve patient and graft survival both in the diabetic and nondiabetic population.

Survival of the diabetic patient ranges from 45 to 75% at 5 years. This is significantly lower than in nondiabetic renal transplant recipients and is a consequence of cardiovascular disease: 36% of diabetic transplant recipients die from cardiovascular disease (51, 52). There is also an increased risk of death from infection, cerebrovascular disease, and peripheral vascular disease compared with nondiabetic graft recipients. The pretransplant presence of any vascular disease is reported to have a significant effect on mortality in diabetis transplant recipients, especially preexisting cardiac or peripheral vascular disease. Although patient survival is still suboptimal compared with nondiabetic subjects, it is better than that seen with dialysis. Transplantation is also associated with improved rehabilitation and a better quality of life than dialysis.

8.5 Pretransplant assessment

Most important is the vascular tree evaluation, the Achilles' heel of every successful transplantation procedure. Careful evaluation of pelvic and lower extremily arteries must be performed. Non-invasive methods (e.g. Doppler and Duplex techniques) as well as invasive procedures (e.g. angiography) may be applied. Plain radiography on the pelvis documents the magnitude of media calcification in the uraemic diabetic.

Coronary artery disease is an important issue in diabetic patients on dialysis. Non-invasive testing is often non substantial and coronary angiography is still the most helpful procedure to rule out severe coronary stenosis in this patient population.

Additional information on cardiac valves are no less important, since aortic stenosis is a common problem in dialysis patients.

Before transplantation, peripheral vascular surgery is mandatory, particularly on the ipsilateral side of the graft, to avoid post-transplant circulatory complications of the lower extremities.

Cardiac surgery (bypass or valve replacement) is nowadays a common procedure in non-diabetic and diabetic patients with an in-hospital mortality rate of 5.4%, which is roughly comparable to those of non-uraemic cardiac patients.

Chronic infections are common in diabetic patients and several sites of infections in diabetic patients have to be considered. Infection of the native kidneys may be due to renal calculi or papillary necrosis and secondary obstruction, and infection of the bladder is often due to multiresistant bacteria.

Cholecystolithiasis is common in diabetics and recurrent cholecystitis should be an indication for cholecystectomy. Uraemic patients often suffer from chronic constipation and colonic diverticula are common in female diabetic patients, gynaecological infections or tumours must be excluded by bacteriological work-up and cytology.

9. Post-transplantation in diabetics

9.1 Hypertension

Approximately 80–90% of adult renal transplant recipients develop hypertension post-transplantation (52, 53). This incidence is no different in diabetics. Hypertension is a major risk factor for post-transplant cardiovascular disease and should be very well controlled in the diabetic.

9.2 Hyperlipidemia

Hypercholesterolaemia and hypertriglyceridaemia following renal transplantation have been reported. Increased total serum cholesterol is usually from increases in low-density lipoprotein (LDL) cholesterol (74% of patients) (53.) Many patients also have elevated levels of triglyceride (29%) and very low-density lipoprotein (VLDL) cholesterol, especially in the presence of proteinuria and graft dysfunction. High density lipoprotein (HDL) cholesterol levels are normal or may be reduced in up to 10% of transplant recipients and the composition of HDL may be abnormal, leading to a reduced cardioprotective effect. The use of diet and pharmacologic approaches to treat hyperlipidemia is reasonable.

9.3 Infection

Diabetics are at increased risk of infection following transplantation. As well as the effects of immunosuppression, which are similar to those in nondiabetic patients, factors specific to diabetics include impaired chemotaxis, increased colonization, and the effects of hyperglycaemia on host defences. Cell-mediated immunity is essentially normal in diabetics. Diabetics are at increased risk of foot infections and fungal infections, especially candidiasis and mucormycosis. Urinary tract infections are more common in diabetic transplant recipients and often associated with glycosuria and urinary stasis as a result of poor bladder emptying. In this situation, antibiotic prophylaxis is often required.

9.4 Diabetic control and continuing complication of diabetes

Glycaemic control remains an important post-transplantation factor affecting the development of macrovascular disease and the development of recurrent disease. A number of factors result in altered blood glucose homeostasis. Corticosteroid therapy and cyclosporin (cyclosporin A) alter blood glucose control and insulin requirements. Cyclosporine and, particularly, tacrolimus may lead to *de novo* diabetes. Improved renal clearances may also change post-transplantation insulin requirements.

9.5 Recurrent diabetic nephropathy

Lesions consistent with diabetic nephropathy develop in almost all grafts, with basement membrane thickening and mesangial expansion reported after 2 years and hyalinization of arterioles after 4 years. The development of nodular glomerulosclerosis is, however, rare in the transplant.

Factor	Peritoneal Dialysis	Haemodialysis	Kidney Transplant
Extensive Extrarenal disease	No limitation	No limitation except for hypertension	Excluded in cardiovascular Insufficiency
Geriatric patients	No limitation	No limitation	Arbitrary exclusion as determined by programme
Complete Rehabilitation	Rare, if ever	Very few individuals	Common so long as graft functions
Death rate	Much higher than for nondiabetics	Much higher than for nondiabetics	About the same as nondiabetics
First year survival	About 75%	About 75%	> 90%
Survival to second decade	Almost never	Fewer than 5%	About 1 in 5
Progression of complications	Usual and unremitting. Hyperglycaemia and hyperlipidemia accentuated	Usual and unremitting. May benefit from metabolic control.	Interdicted by functioning pancreas + kidney. Partially ameliorated by correction of azotemia.
Special advantage	Can be self-performed. Avoids swings in solute and intravascular volume level.	Can be self-performed. Efficient extraction of solute and water in hours.	Cures uraemia. Freedom to travel.
Disadvantage	Peritonitis. Hyperinsulenemia. Long hours of treatment. More days hospitalized than either hemodialysis or transplant.	Blood access a hazard for clotting, haemorrhage and infection. Cyclical hypotension, weakness. Aluminium toxicity, amyloidosis.	Cosmetic disfigurement, hypertension, personal expense for cytotoxic malignancy. HIV transmission.
Patient acceptance	Variable, usual compliance with passive tolerance for regimen.	Variable, often noncompliant with dietary, metabolic, or antihypertensive	Enthusiastic during periods of good renal allograft function. Exalted when

		component of regimen.	pancreas proffers euglycaemia.
Bias in comparison	Delivered as first choice by enthusiasts though emerging evidence indicates substantially higher mortality than for haemodialysis	Treatment by default. Often complicated by in attention to progressive cardiac and peripheral vascular disease.	All kidney transplant programme preselect those patients with fewest complications. Exclusion of those older than 45 for pancreas + kidney simultaneous grafting obviously favoruably prejudices outcome.
Relative cost	Most expensive over long run	Less expensive than kidney transplant in first year, subsequent years more expensive.	Pancreas + kidney engraftment most expensive uraemia therapy for diabetic. After first year, kidney transplant C alone C lowest cost option.

Table 6. Comparison of ESRD options for diabetic patients

10. The future

In the future, new techniques such as insulin gene manipulation in autologous cells (e.g. myoblasts, hepatocytes or fibroblasts) or islet cell transplantation will be the procedure of choice. Such a graft is currently technically feasible in patients who are recipients of other, usually renal, grafts. Another possibility is to graft encapsulated xeno-islets, protected against immune attack by encapsulation in a biocompatible membrane.

Comparison of ESRD options for diabetics patients are given in table 6 (54).

11. Diabetics on dialysis in the Republic of Macedonia

Today the nephrologists are challenged both to control the underlying diabetic disease and also to provide an adequate renal replacement therapy. On the other hand, it has to be stressed that treatment of these patients and DM complications is very expensive. For example, in USA the cost of treatment of these patients per year was estimated to about 100 billion dollars, which is more than the whole health budget of a country like Italy (health budget estimated for 2001). Moreover, in USA around 2 billion dollars are being spent on dialysis treatments [55]. Recently performed, large epidemiological studies have demonstrated that CV morbidity and all cause mortality can be reduced with strict glycaemic and blood pressure control and with the use of anti-angiotensine agents and also lipid lowering agents [56-60]. Certain factors like age, time on dialysis, vascular access complications, co morbidities, type of dialysis membrane, time of dialysis and others have been identified to correlate with the survival of the patients on dialysis [61, 62]. These factors assume even greater importance in diabetics. Biocompatible membranes, ultrapure dialysis fluid and diffuse - convective techniques have also been promoted to reduce cardiovascular instability [63, 64] and to minimize the injuries of the excessive oxidative stress inherent in uremia and the dialysis treatment.

In Republic of Macedonia (RM) in last two decades there was an increase of number of diabetic patients. The number of patients with diabetic nephropathy progressing to the point of need for renal replacement therapy and renal transplantation is also increasing [65-67]. Given the fact of lack of data and valuable epidemiological studies in these patients, we performed a nation wide study with the aim of defining prevalence of these patients in RM, determining the standards of care in diabetics in term of methodological approach, dialysis and drug treatment and analysis of these patients on dialysis. The aim of the study was to make a closer observation in all dialysis centers in 2002 in the country and to compare data with those obtained 2006.

11.1 Patients and methods

Data were collected from medical histories of diabetic patients on dialysis in all dialysis centers in Republic of Macedonia by using a specially developed questionnaire for this purpose. Date of 31 December for 2002 and 2006 year was selected as a "critical day" for data collection. Besides demographic data (name, surname, sex, date of birth and profession), data for cigarette smoking and alcohol consuming were collected as well as type of diabetes (family history for diabetes, therapy, dose and type of the insulin intake, duration of diabetes and kidney disease), hypertension (family history, duration, therapy), other renal diseases including diabetic nephropathy, as well as laboratory findings (residual diuresis, blood glucose level, HbA1C, microalbuminuria, proteinuria, urea, creatinin blood level, creatinin clearance, thryglycerides (TG) blood level, cholesterol, HDL and LDL cholesterol, hepatitis B virus serological markers (HBs Ag, anti HBc-Ig G) , hepatitis C virus serological markers (anti HCV) and human imunodeficiency virus antibodies (anti-HIV); type of dialysis (bicarbonate or acetate); duration and frequency of dialysis sessions, medications used, hypoglycemic events, number of hospitalizations, complications: cardiovascular events (pectoral angina, heart attack, cerebrovascular insult), hypertension, peripherial vascular artheriopathy (diabetic foot), diabetic retinopathy, infection of the urinary system); cause of death - if patient died. The progression of other diabetic complications was obtained by roentgenograms, ECG, echocardiography and examination of eye fundus. Special attention was paid to data on vascular access (type of central venous catheter, A-V fistula, graft, complications on vascular accesses infection/thrombosis, other complications, as well as number of created vascular accesses).

Patients were treated according to the recommendations introduced by University Nephrology Clinic - Skopje, Faculty of Medicine, "Ss. Cyril and Methodius" University in Skopje, as a reference center for dialysis patients in Republic of Macedonia [68]. Duration of dialysis sessions was approximately three times four hours per week divided into three day sessions in same week. Low flux polysulphonic membranes, were used. Water was prepared by a reverse osmosis and blood flow in most of the cases was 250-280ml/min, whereas dialysis flow was usually 500 ml/min. Dialysis machines used were GAMBRO types AK 10, AK 100 and AK 95. There was no reuse of the dialysis filters. A low salt intake diet and malnutrition protective protein intake of 1gr/kg diet were recommended to all patients.

11.2 Results

Total number of dialysis patients in RM was 1114 and 1074 in 2002 and 2006 year, respectively (Figure 1, Table 7). There were 109 (9.78%) diabetic patients on dialysis, 60 (55%) male and 49 (45%) female in 2002. A slight increase of diabetics was determined in 2006, namely there were 115 (10.7%) diabetic patients on dialysis, 74 (64.35 %) male and 41 (35.65%) female in 2006 year, as to compare with 2000 when total number of dialysis patients was 1010 and number of diabetics on dialysis was 103 (10.19%) [65, 66] (Figure 2). There was a difference in distribution of diabetics on dialysis trough different dialysis centers in RM for 2002 and 2006 year (Table 8 and Table 9), respectively. Diabetics on dialysis were from 3% in Veles, to 21 % in Kavadarci for 2002. Similar diversity was obtained in 2006: from 2.43% in Skopje Military Hospital Dialysis Center to 22.07% in University Nephrology Clinic - Skopje. In 2002 most of the diabetics on dialysis (31 patients) were registered in University Nephrology Clinic - Skopje and in the Nephrology Institute - Struga (15 patients) similarly like 2006 when most of diabetics on dialysis (34 patients) were in University Nephrology Clinic - Skopje and in Nephrology Institute - Struga (16 patients). The mean age of all diabetics on dialysis in 2002 was 58±10.29 years (56±10.49 for males and 60±9.56 for females), and in all diabetics on dialysis in 2006 it was 56.5±10.71 years (55.06±8.82 for males and 57.92±12.56 for females) (Table 1). In 2002, 19 (17.43%) patients had DM1, while 90 (82.57%) patients had DM2. 28 (25.68%) patients were treated with oral anti-diabetic drugs and 62 (57.21%) patients were on insulin. In 2006, 15 (13.04%) patients had DM1 while 100 (86.96%) patients had DM2. 31 (26,96 %) of diabetics were treated with oral anti-diabetic drugs and 69 (60%) were on insulin. The mean age of DM1 patients in 2002 was 47±11.6 years, with a diabetic history of 16.2±9.7 years, while the mean age of DM1 patients in 2006 was 45±7.32 years, with a diabetic history of 24.07±11.07 years. The mean age of DM2 patients in 2002 was 60.37±8.33 with a diabetic history of 13.4±8.1 years and the mean age of DM2 patients in 2006 was 61.14±10.23 years with a diabetic history of 14.18±8.42 (Table 1). The mean dose of insulin intake was 9.5±6.63IU and 10.85±9.29IU, for 2002 and 2006 respectively. In 2002, 21% of diabetics on dialysis were smokers, 13% consumed alcohol, while 15% were engaged in sport, as compared to 2006 when 17.39% of diabetics on dialysis were smokers, 5.22% consumed alcohol and 3.48% were doing sport.

The mean duration of dialysis therapy in 2002 for DM type 1 patients was 54.3±44.4 months, whereas in DM type 2 was 34.3±36.3 months. The mean duration of dialysis therapy in 2006 for DM 1 patients was 76.29±74.96 months, whereas in DM 2 was 33.68±43.24. The mean body mass index (BMI) in 2002 was 26.4±3.28 kg/m^2 and 25.5±2.92 kg/m^2 in DM1 and DM2 patients, respectively. In 2006 BMI was 23.49±4.74 kg/m^2 and 24.77±3.70 kg/m^2 in DM1 and

DM2 patients, respectively. There was a need for urgent dialysis treatment and a first dialysis session a trough femoral venous catheter in 90.1% and 94.4% of diabetics on dialysis in 2002 and 2006, respectively. After a period of patient adaptation to dialysis procedure and in order to eliminate possible bacterial infection trough the femoral venous catheter, an arterio venous fistula (AVF) was created as a permanent vascular access for dialysis. Preventive AVF was created in 9.9% and in 5.6% of diabetics on dialysis in 2002 and 2006 respectively. Thrombosis of the newly created AVF was detected in 41% and 24.35% in 2002 and 2006 respectively, whereas AVF infection was detected in 58.6% of the patients in 2002. In 2002 there were 19.26% of patients on acetate dialysis and 80.74% on bicarbonate dialysis while in 2006 there were no patients on acetate dialysis, and all 110 diabetic patients (95.65%) were on bicarbonate dialysis modality (Figure 3).

It has to be stressed that a high rate of HCV infection was noticed in diabetics on dialysis, 57% and 37.39% of these patients were anti HCV positive in 2002 and in 2006, respectively. 81% and 86.09% of the patients were treated with erytropoethin in 2002 and 2006, respectively. In both years hypertension (HTA) was the most frequent co-morbid state: in 2002, 91% diabetics on dialysis had a HTA before dialysis program and following the start of dialysis sessions 40.54% (Table 10). Furthermore, in 2006 HTA was registered in 47.74% of diabetics before dialysis, and in 60% of patients during dialysis. Finally, family history for HTA was noticed in 43% and 29.57% patients, in 2002 and 2006, respectively. The most frequent cardiovascular co-morbidity in these patients for the year 2002 and 2006 are shown in Table 10.

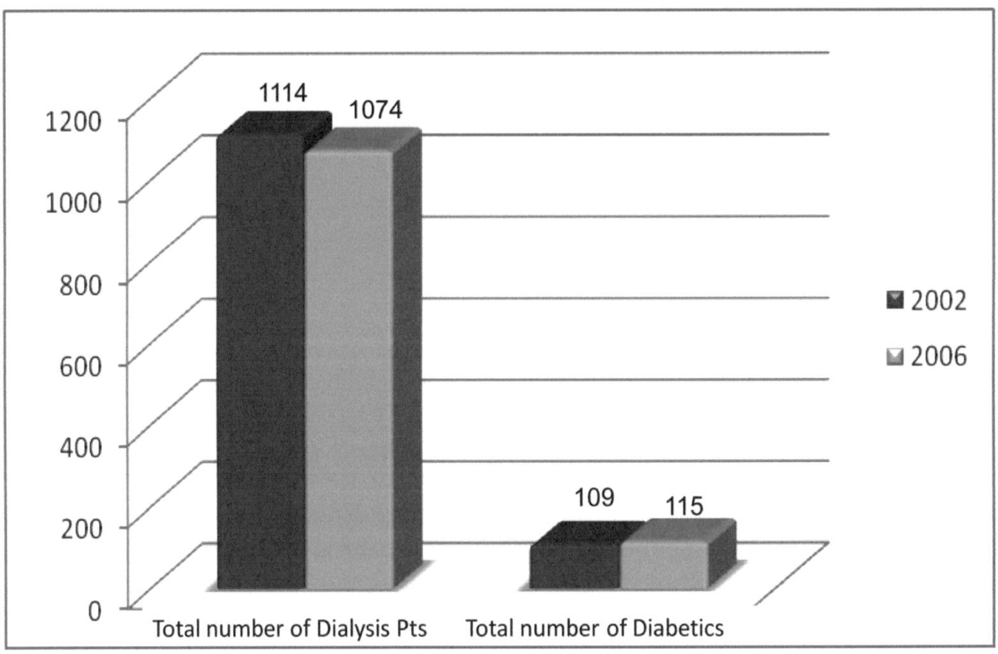

Fig. 1. Total number of patients on dialysis and diabetics on dialysis.

	2002 year	2006 year
N° dialysis patients	1114	1074
N° of diabetics	109 (9.78%)	115 (10.7%)
Male Pts	60 (55%)	74 (64.35%)
Female Pts	49 (45%)	41 (35.65%)
Mean age	58±10.29	56.5±10.71
Mean age male	56±10.49	55.06±8.82
Mean age female	60±9.56	57.92±12.56
Patients with DM1	19 (17.43%)	15 (13.04%)
Mean age DM1	47±11.6	45±7.32
DM history DM1 (years)	16.2±9.7	24.07±11.7
DM1 dialysis history (months)	54.3±44.4	76.29±74.96
Patients with DM2	90 (82.57%)	100 (86.96%)
Mean age DM2	60.4±8.33	61.14±10.23
DM history DM2 (years)	13.4±8.1	14.18±8.42
DM2 dialysis history (months)	34.3±36.3	33.68±43.24
On OADD	28 (25.68%)	31 (26.96%)
On insulin	62 (57.21%)	69 (60%)
Dose of insulin (IU)	9.5±6.63	10.85±9.29
BMI in DM1 kg/m^2	26.4	25.5
BMI in DM2 kg/m^2	23.49±4.74	24.77±3.70
First dialysis on FVC (%)	90.1	94.4
Preventive AVF (%)	9.9	5.6
Thrombosis of first AVF (%)	41	24.35
Anti HCV positive (%)	57	37.39

DM1 - Diabetes mellitus type 1, DM2 - Diabetes mellitus type 2 ; OADD – Oral antidiabetic drugs ; BMI – Body mass index; FVC – femoral vascular cathether ; AVF – Arterio venouse fistula

Table 7. Characteristics of diabetics on dialysis in Republic of Macedonia

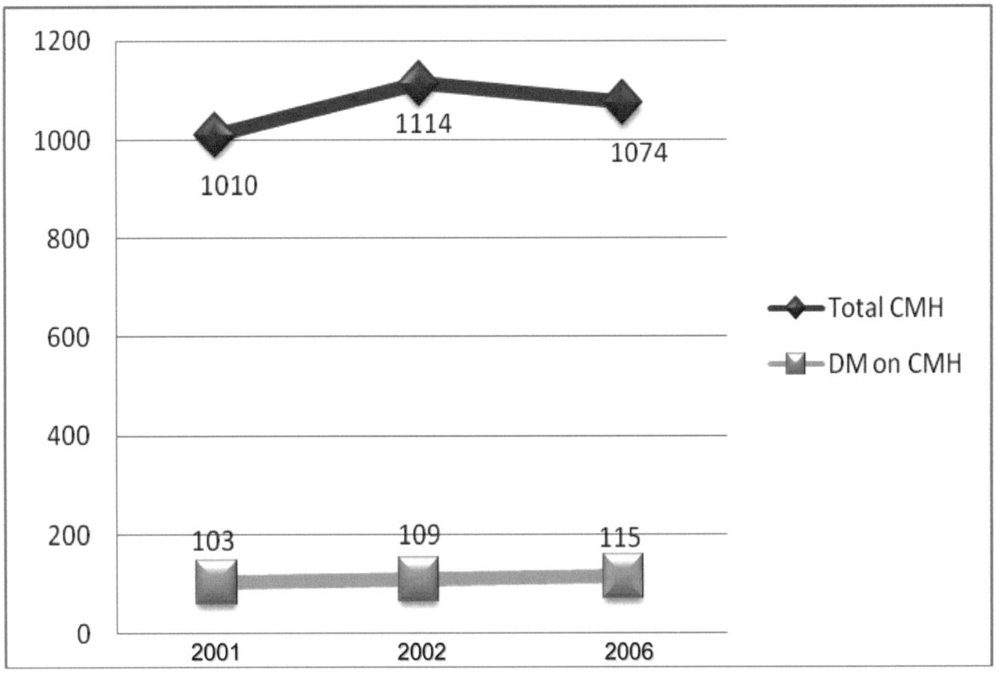

Fig. 2. Oscillations in the total number of dialysis patients and diabetics on dialysis period 2001 - 2006 in RM

Dialysis center	N° of Dialysis pts	N° of Diabetics	% DM
University Clinic of Nephrology, Skopje	201	31	15.42
Institute of Nephrology, Struga	204	15	7.35
Tetovo	63	9	14.28
Gevgelija	28	1	3.57
Debar	15	2	13.30
Gostivar	53	4	7.54
Kočani	24	3	12.50
Kumanovo	60	6	10.00
Delčevo	31	4	12.90
Strumica	46	4	8.69
Prilep	60	6	10.00

Bitola	38	4	10.52
Štip	49	3	12.50
Železara	125	5	4.00
Military hospital, Skopje	40	3	7.5
Veles	39	1	2.56
Kavadarci	38	8	21.50
Total	**1114**	**109**	**9.78**

Table 8. Distribution of dialysis patients by dialysis centers in RM, year 2002

Dialysis center	**N° of Dialysis pts**	**N° of Diabetics**	**% DM**
University Nephrology Clinic, Skopje	171	32	19.88
Nephrology Institute, Struga	171	16	9,36
Tetovo	69	11	15,94
Gevgelija	30	2	6,67
Kriva Palanka	26	3	11,54
Gostivar	46	4	8,70
Kočani	31	1	3,23
Kumanovo	49	7	14,29
Delčevo	32	7	21,88
Strumica	47	3	6,38
Prilep	56	6	10,71
Bitola	43	2	4,65
Štip	60	4	6,67
Železara	162	12	7,41
Military hospital	40	2	5
Veles	41	1	2,44
Total	**1074**	**115**	**10,71**

Table 9. Distribution of dialysis patients by dialysis centers in RM, year 2006

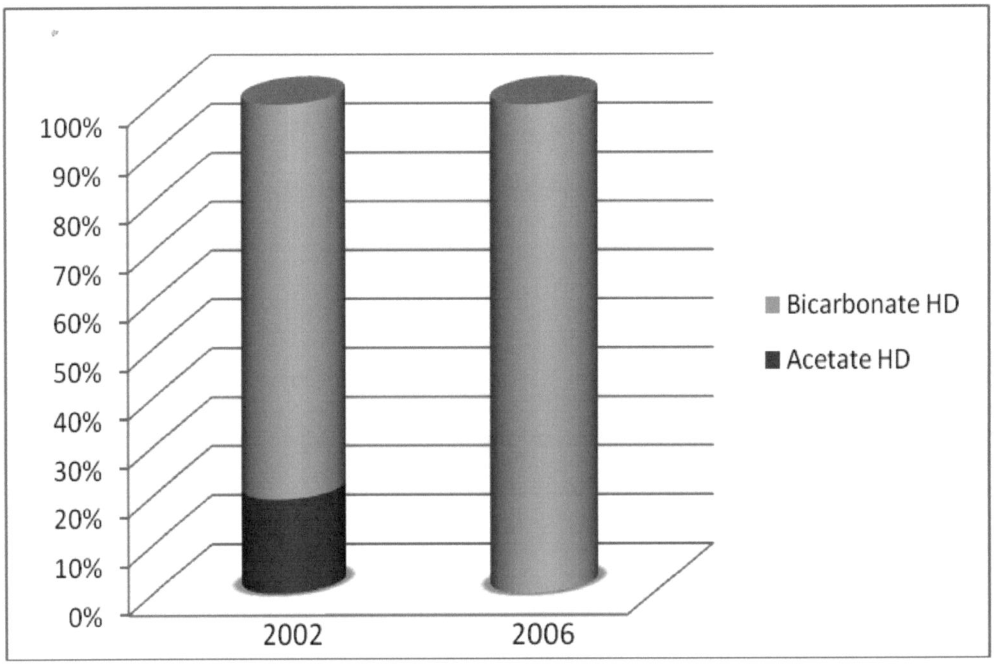

Fig. 3. Use of acetate and bicarbonate haemodialysis (HD) in 2002 and 2006

Condition	Before Dialysis (2002)	During Dialysis (2002)	Before Dialysis (2006)	During Dialysis (2006)
Pectoral angina	7.2%	19%	1.12%	3.4%
Heart attack	5.4%	5.4%	1.12%	4.43%
Intermitent claudication	10%	10%	2.25%	11.3%
Cerebrovascular attack	7%	8%	8.7%	9.57%
Hypertension (HTA)	91%	40.54%	47.74%	60%

Table 10. Distribution of the most frequent cardiovascular co-morbidity in diabetics on dialysis in 2002 and 2006.

11.3 Discussion

In the present analysis we have demonstrated an increase in the prevalence on diabetic dialysis patients in certain dialysis centers of RM. It has been reported before that the annual incidence of patients who initiate dialysis is constantly increasing in all industrialized countries and a significant part of this increase is explained by the influx of diabetic patients on dialysis [68, 69]. This study shows the importance of the need to increase the number of specialists nephrologists in RM who will take an important role in healthcare of these patients in collaboration with endocrinologists and other specialists practitioners.

We have previously shown that the number of diabetics on dialysis in RM enlarges slowly but progresively [65-68]. In current analysis, beside the fact that mean total prevalence of DM was just slightly increased as compared to our previous studies [66], we show that there is an important difference in prevalence of diabetics on dialysis between different dialysis centres. In certain dialysis in RM the prevalence of diabetics reached a level similar with that of Northern European countries [69] while in others it was lower than expected. This diversity in the number of diabetics on dialysis could be explained by the fact that RM is a developing country, geographically European with predominance of Mediterranean diet, and this difference could be due to a numerous economical, sociological, genetic, environmental and nutritional factors in different parts of the country.

We included in the study all diabetic patients on dialysis in RM, without differentiating diabetics who started dialysis because of diabetic nephropathy from those who started dialysis with other renal pathology. We show that diabetics with CKD in most of the cases were diagnosed at the University Nephrology Clinic - Skopje, and diagnosis most often was in developed phase of CKD. It has been shown that these patients present an extraordinary acceleration of all clinical complications and it is a well known fact that accelerated development of terminal uraemia constitutes a devastating clinical event [1, 55, 69, 70, 71]. Phase of the disease when diabetes is installed is accompanied usually with a certain variety of cardiovascular complications, predominatelly as a result of a long-term hypertension, nephrotic syndrome and infections. Metabolic and blood vessels modifications induce constant overweight and problems with vascular access leading to quality of life decrease in these patents. Consequently, as it has been showen by the others and us, the survival rate of diabetics on dialysis is significantly reduced, Figure 4 [72, 73]. When compared with other dialisys patients it has been shown that the best survival rate was observed in those with balkan endemic nephropathy and adult polycystic kidney disease. This observation goes in line with other studies confirming that in diabetics on dialysis the quality of life is impaired and survival is significantly curtailed [1, 74, 26]. It has been shown also that the clinical results depend on both the severity of complications present at the initiation of dialysis and on capacity to slow its evolution during dialysis [74]. In current analysis we did not evaluate the effect of patient therapies on the incidence of complications and on patient mortality.

Besides the fact that most of the nephrologists and internal medicine specialists in RM are aware of the importance of the timely initiation of dialysis for diabetic patients, this analysis underlines the fact that dialysis initiation often starts in emergency conditions and most of the patients start dialysis program at University Nephrology Clinic – Skopje trough urgently and temporary placed femoral venous catheter. We found that almost 90% of first dialysis sessions in 2002 as well as in 2006 were started in emergency conditions, confirming that diabetics are reffered to the nephrologists late in the course of CKD. Analysing why this happens, we think that a part of responsibility for the delay of dialysis initiation could be explained by patient mentality but it is also important to stress the important role of medical personnel in preparing the patient for dialysis. We have to underline insufficient coordination between physicians such as general practitioners, internists, endocrinologists and nephrologists, and lack of their influence on patient dialysis reality acceptance. It is also important to notice that in two dialysis centres where the prevalence in diabetics on dialysis is much higher, dialysis patients are followed by educated and well trained nephrologists. In these centres accessibility of other specialties practitioners is higher as compared to dialysis centres where patients are followed by internal medicine specialists and other specialized doctors are also accessible. This might explain the high difference in number of diabetic's among different dialysis centers and it also underlines the need for more trained nephrologists in the country and their more important implication in follow up of diabetics on dialysis.

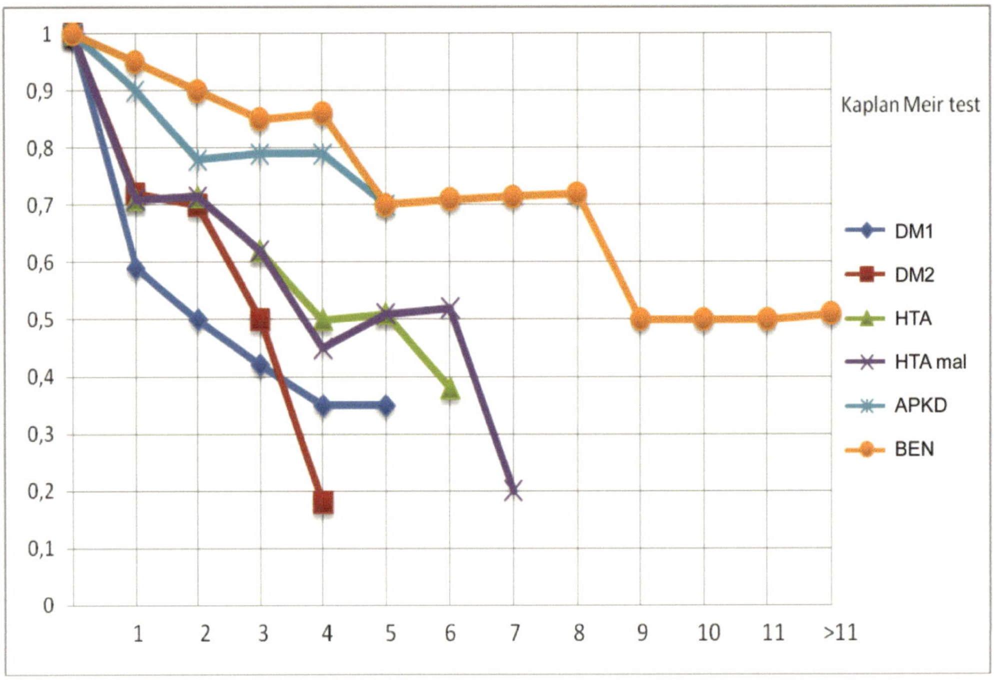

Fig. 4. Distribution of survival (Kaplan Meier test) of dialysis patients, distribution by basic renal disease (University Clinic of Nephrology - Skopje); abbrevations: Diabetes Mellitus Insulin Independent - DM1, Diabetes Mellitus Insulin Dependent DM2, Arterial Hypertension - HTA, Malignant HTA - HTA mal., Adult Polycystic Renal Diseases-APKD, Balkan Endemic Nephropathy - BEN).

It has been shown previously that a very large difference exists in the ratio of DM2 to DM1 on dialyisis in different European countries and among different regions in a same country [1]. A recent study of Italian population showed that most diabetics on dialysis were DM2 patients, probably because of high prevalence of this disease among the general population [75]. In our study we found that the ratio of DM2 to DM1 patients was approximately 4,3 : 1. As expected, patients with DM2 were older, with higher body weight and body mass index.

Epidemiological studies has also shown that cardiovascular morbidity and mortality can be reduced with pharmacological therapy that normalizes blood pressure values and controls hyperglicemia, hyperlipidemia, platelet agreggation and hypercoagulability [56-58]. Proportion of diabetics od dialysis treated with ACE inhibitors and / or angiotensin receptor blockers (ARB), beta blockers and antiplatelat drugs was still quite low as compared to propositions of the guidelines. There was a negligible number of patients treated with lipid lowering agents.

In conclusion, the present study underline the importance of an interdisciplinary approach in early diagnosis and treatment of diabetes, diabetic nephropathy and treatment of diabetics on dialysis, as well as importance of introducting preventive measures for progression of CKD in these patients. In most dialysis centres in the Republic of Macedonia prevalence of diabetics on dialysis did not increase in the period from 2002 to 2006 where these patients were followed mostly by internal medicine specialists. Frequency of complications was increased in DM2 compared to DM1 dialysis patients. Blood glucose level control is important as well as a strict control of the blood preasure. Bicarbonate dialysis is a dialysis of choice with an optimal duration of minimun 12 hours per week. More nephrologists need to be involved in the dialysis centres and together with an improvement of colaboration between general practitioners, internternal medicine doctors, endocrinologists, nephrologists, cardiologists, ophtalmologists, neurologists in order to improve health care for these patients. This kind of studies should be carried out on a regular basis in Republic of Macedonia.

12. Could we prevent or postpone diabetic kidney disease and development of chronic renal failure?

The World Kidney Day, 11 March 2010 was devoted to diabetic kidney disease, under the auspices of the International Society of Nephrology (ISN) and the International Federation of Kidney Foundations (IFKF), together with the International Diabetic Federation (IDF).

R.C. Atkins and P. Zimmet in their paper: *Diabetic kidney disease: act now or pay later* [76] point out the importance of a better understanding of the global pandemic of type 2 diabetes and diabetic kidney disease. They suggest that it is necessary to alert governments, health organizations, providers, doctors and patients to the increasing health and socioeconomic problems due to diabetic kidney disease and its sequels: end-stage kidney disease requiring dialysis, and cardiovascular death. It should be emphasized that its management involves prevention, recognition and treatment of its complications.

The most important measure is primary prevention of type 2 diabetes. It will require massive lifestyle changes in the developing world, supported by strong governmental commitment to promote lifestyle and societal change.

In the Republic of Macedonia there are about 100,000 patients with diabetes mellitus type 1 and 2; 85-95% have diabetes mellitus type 2. Around 28,000-30,000 patients are on therapy with insulin.

Some of them are candidates for development of diabetic kidney disease.

We should develop a strategy to detect early diabetic kidney disease by screening for albuminuria as well as reduced glomerular filtration rate. It is very important to introduce public education about the relationship between diabetes and kidney disease. There is a remarkable lack of awareness among patients about their condition.

In our papers: *Chronic Kidney Disease: a Hidden Epidemic* [77] and *Public Health Aspects of Renal Disease in the Republic of Macedonia* 1983–2007 [78] we have shown a continuous increase in end-stage renal disease and renal replacement therapy (RRT) in the Republic of Macedonia. In 2002, we had 1,056 patients on RRT compared to 1,216 in 2005. In some dialysis centres 20% of the patients on haemodialysis are diabetics. Our message was that there is an urgent need for a screening programme for the detection of Chronic Kidney Disease (CKD) in the Republic of Macedonia. Health authorities, nephrologists and general physicians should collaborate on the detection of CKD.

"There is evidence that early therapeutic intervention in patients with chronic kidney disease or diabetes can delay the onset of complications and improve outcomes. For example, the UKPDS [79, 80], STENO-2 [81] and ADVANCE studies [82, 83, 84] all demonstrated that tight control of blood glucose level and blood pressure (and lipids in STENO-2) significantly reduced the incidence and progression of diabetic kidney disease. In people with type 2 diabetes, inhibition of the renin-angiotensin-aldosterone system using an angiotensin-converting enzyme (ACE) inhibitor or an angiotensin II receptor blocker (ARB) decreased the progression from normoalbuminuria to microalbuminuria [85] and slowed the development of ESRD [86]. Thus the use of an ACE inhibitor or ARB is now standard therapy for patients with diabetic nephropathy, as well as glucose, lipid and blood pressure control." [76]

12.1 How should we act now?

We are going to repeat our message from 2008 [77]: "there is an urgent need for a screening programme for the detection of CKD" and we will add as well as of diabetic kidney disease in the Republic of Macedonia.

We can follow the steps suggested by Atkins and Zimmet (76):

"i. prevention of type 2 diabetes;
ii. screening for early diabetic kidney disease;
iii. increasing patient awareness of kidney disease;
iv. using medications of proven strategy"

"The ultimate challenge is to get action from primary health care to all higher levels, from the individual patient, to those at risk, in various health jurisdictions, in all countries despite varying economic circumstances and priorities. The problem is a global one and yet requires action at a local level; prevention screening and treatment strategies; education, including increasing awareness both in diabetic patients and those at risk of developing diabetes; and health priorities and governments. Basic research and clinical trials searching for a new understanding and therapies must be supported." [76]

In our country we should work harder on the prevention of diabetic kidney diseases, to stop or postpone the development of CKD and chronic renal failure with modern therapy and the need for RRT.

13. References

[1] Ritz E., Rychlik I., Locatelli F., Halimi S. (1999): End-stage renal failure in type 2 diabetes: a medical catastrophe of worldwide dimensions. Am J Kidney Dis. 34: 795-808.

[2] Ritz E., Orth S. R. (1999): Nephropathy in patients with type 2 diabetes mellitus. New Engl J Med. 341: 1127-1133.

[3] Stengel B., Billon S., Van Dijk C. W. Paul et al. (2003): Trends in the incidence of renal replacement therapy for end-stage renal disease in Europe, 1990-99. Nephrol Dial Transplant. 18: 1824-1833.

[4] Polenakovic M. (2002): Dialysis in adults in year 2000 in the Republic of Macedonia. Int J Artif Organs. 25(5): 386-390.

[4a] Polenakovic M. Sikole A., Nikolov IG. et al.: Diabetics on dialysis in the Republic of Macedonia: a nationwide epidemiological study. Prilozi, XXXI (1) 2010, 261-277

[5] Perez-Garcia R., Rodriquez Benitez P., Verde E., Valderrabano F. (1999):Increasing of renal replacement therapy (RRT) in diabetic patients in Madrid. Nephrol Dial Transplant. 14: 2525-2527.

[6] Marcelli D., Spotti D., Conte F. et al. (1995): Prognosis of diabetic patients on dialysis: analysis of Lombardy Registry data. Nephrol Dial Transplant. 10: 1895-1900.

[7] Friedman E. A., Beyer M. M. (1980): Uraemia in diabetics: the prognosis improves. Klin Wochenschr. 58: 1023-1028.

[8] Sawicki P.T., Kaiser S., Heinemann L., Frenzel H., Berger M. (1991): Prevalence of renal artery stenosis in diabetes mellitus - an autopsy study. J Intern Med. 229: 489-492.

[9] Legrain M., Rottemburg J., de Groc F. et al. (1986): Selecting the best uraemia therapy. In Diabetic Renal Retinal Syndrome, ed. by Friedman E.A., L`Esperance F.A., New York, Grune and Stratton, p. 453.

[10] Friedman E. A., Miles A. M. V. (1996): Dialytic management of diabetic uraemic patients. In Replacement of renal function by dialysis, eds. Jacobs C., Kjellstrand C. M., Koch K. M., Winchester J. F., Dordrecht/Boston/London, Kluwer Academic Pub., pp. 935-953.

[11] Hakim R. M., Lazarus J. M. (1995): Initiation of dialysis. J Am Soc Nephrol. 6: 1319-28.

[12] Koch M., Thomas B., Tschöpe W., Ritz E. (1993): Survival and predictors of death in dialysed diabetic patients. Diabetologia. 36: 1113-1117.

[13] Laureut G., Calemard E., Charra B. (1999): Haemodialysis for French diabetic patients. Nephrol Dialysis Transpl. 14: 2044-5.

[14] National Kidney Foundation. Dialysis outcomes quality initiative, DOQI. National Kidney Foundation, Inc., New York, 1997.

[15] Oncevski A., Dejanov P., Gerasimovska V., Polenakovic M. (2002): Approach to vascular access for haemodialysis: experiences from the Republic of Macedonia. Int J Artif Organs. 25(5): 354-365

[16] Gerasimovska V., Oncevski A., Dejanov P., Polenakovic M. (2002): Are ambulatory femoral catheters for haemodialysis a safe vascular access? The Journal of Vascular Access. 3: 14-20.

[17] Tzamaloukas A. H., Murata G. H., Eisenberg B., Murphy G., Avasthi P. S. (1992): Hypoglycaemia in diabetics on dialysis with poor glycemic control: haemodialysis versus continuous ambulatory peritoneal dialysis. Int J Artif Organs. 15: 390.

[18] Yu C. C., Wu M. S., Wu C. H. et al. (1997): Predialysis glycemic control is an independent predictor of clinical outcome in type II diabetes on continuous ambulatory peritoneal dialysis. Perit Dial Int. 17: 262–268.
[19] Wu M. S., Yu C. C., Yang C. W. et al. (1997): Poor pre-dialysis glycaemic control is a predictor of mortality in type II diabetic patients on maintenance haemodialysis. Nephrol Dial Transplant. 12: 2015–2110.
[20] Krepinsky J., Ingram A. J., Clase C. M. (2000): Prolonged sulfonylurea - induced hypoglycaemia in diabetic patients with endstage renal disease. Am J Kidney Dis. 35: 500–505.
[21] Farrel P. C., Hone P. W. (1988): Dialysis induced catabolism. Am J Clinic Nutr. 33: 1417–22.
[22] Levey A. S., Beto J. A., Coronado B. E. et al. (1998): Controlling the epidemic of cardiovascular disease in chronic renal disease. National Kidney Foundation on Task Force on Cardiovascular Disease. Am J Kidney Dis. 32: 853–906.
[23] Ritz E., Strumpf C., Katz F. et al. (1985): Hypertension and cardiovascular risk factors in haemodialyzed diabetic patients. Hypertension. 7 (Suppl. II): 118.
[24] Shideman J. R., Buselmeier T. J., Kjellstrand C. M. (1976): Hemodialysis in diabetics. Arch Intern Med. 136: 1126.
[25] Schömig S., Ritz E. (2000): Cardiovascular problems in diabetic patients on renal replacement therapy. Nephrol Dial Transplant. 15 (Suppl. 5): 111–116.
[26] Fontbonne A. (1989): Hypertriglyceridaemia as a risk factor of coronary artery disease mortality in subjects with impaired glucose tolerance. Diabetologia. 32:300–304.
[27] Semenkovic C. F., Ostlund R. E., Schechtman K. B. (1989): Plasma lipids in patients with type I diabetes mellitus: influence of race, gender and plasma glucose control. Arch Intern Med. 149: 51–56.
[28] Kostner G. M., Karadi I. (1988): Lipoprotein alterations in diabetes mellitus. Diabetologia. 36: 1113–17.
[29] Tschöpe W., Koch M., Thomas B., Ritz E. (1993): Serum lipids predict cardiac death in diabetic patients on maintenance haemodialysis. Nephron. 64: 354–8.
[30] Ismail N. (1997): Use of erythropoietin, active vitamin D3 metabolites and alkali agents in predialysis patients. Semin Nephrol. 17: 270–284.
[31] Sikole A., Polenakovic M., Spiroska V., Polenakovic B., Klinkmann H., Scigalla P. (2002): Recurrence of left venticular hypertrophy following cessation of erythropoietin therapy. Artif Organs. 26(2): 98–102
[32] Joshi N., Caputo G. M., Weitekamp M. R., Karchmer A. W. (1999): Infections in patients with diabetes mellitus. N Engl J Med. 341: 1906–1911.
[33] Miles A. M. V., Friedman E. A. (1993): Dialytic therapy for diabetic patients with terminal renal failure. Curr Opin Nephrol Hypertens. 2: 868–75.
[34] Tzamaloukas A. H., Yuan Z. Y., Balaskas E., Oreopoulos D. G. (1992): CAPD in end stage patients with renal disease due to diabetes mellitus - an update. Adv Perit Dial. 8: 185–91.
[35] Khanna R. (1994): Peritoneal dialysis in diabetic end-stage renal disease. In Gokal R., Nolph K. D. eds. Textbook of peritoneal dialysis. Dordrecht, Netherlands: Kluwer Academic; 639–59.
[36] Blacher J., Guerin A. P., Pannier B. et al. (1999): Impact of aortic stiffness on survival in endstage renal disease. Circulation. 99: 2434–9.

[37] Churchill D. N. (1998): Implication of the Canada-USA (CANUSA) study of the adequacy of dialysis on peritoneal dialysis schedule. Nephrol Dialysis Transpl. 13(6): 158–63.

[38] Car S. (2000): RRT for Diabetic Nephropathy. In Johnson R.J., Freehally J. eds. Comprehensive Clinical Nephrology. Mosby, London. 361–370.

[39] Collins A. J., Hao W., Xia H. et al. (1999): Mortality risks of peritoneal dialysis and haemodialysis. Am J Kid Dis. 34: 1065–1074.

[40] Malberti F., Conte F., Limido A. et al. (1997): Ten years experience of renal replacement treatment in the elderly. Geriatr Nephrol Urol. 7: 1–10.

[41] Maiorca R., Cancarini G. C., Brunori G. et al. (1996): Comparison of longterm survival between haemodialysis and peritoneal dialysis. Adv Perit Dial. 12: 79–88.

[42] Schaubel D. E., Morison H. I., Fenton S. S. (1998): Comparing mortality rates on CAPD/CCPD and haemodialysis. The Canadian experience: fact or fiction? Perit Dial Int. 18: 478–484.

[43] Bonal J., Cleries M., Vela E. (1997): Transplantation versus haemodialysis in elderly patients. Renal Registry Committee. Nephrol Dialysis Transpl. 12: 261.

[44] Luft V., Kliem V., Tusch G., Danneuberg B., Brunkhorst R. (2000): Renal transplantation in older patients: is graft survival affected by age? A case control study. Transplantation. 790–94.

[45] Schnuelle P., Lorenz D., Trede M, van der Woulde F. J. (1998): Impact of renal cadaveric transplantation on survival in endstage renal failure: evidence for reduced mortality risk compared with haemodialysis during long-term follow-up. J Am Soc Nephrol. 9: 2135–41.

[46] Becker B. N., Brazy P. C., Becker Y. T. et al. (2000): Simultaneous pancreas-kidney transplantation reduces excess mortality in type 1 diabetic patients with end-stage renal disease. Kidney Int. 57: 2129–2135.

[47] Smets Y. F., Westendorp R. G, van der Pijl et al. (1999): Effect of simultaneous pancreas-kidney transplantation on mortality of patients with type-1 diabetes mellitus and end-stage renal failure. Lancet. 353: 1915–1919.

[48] Rayhill S. C., D'Alessandro A. M., Odorico J. S. et al. (2000): Simultaneous pancreas kidney transplantation and living related donor renal transplantation in patients with diabetes: is there a difference in survival? Ann Surg. 231: 417–423.

[49] Zeier M. (2003): End-stage renal failure in diabetes mellitus: special problems of treatment and monitoring. In Diabetic nephropathy ed. by Hasslacher, Wiley and Sons, 299–313.

[50] Friedman E. A. (1995): Management choices in diabetic end-stage renal disease. Nephrol Dial Transplant. 10 (Suppl. 7): 61–69.

[51] USRDS (United States Renal Data System). Annual Data Report 1997. Bethesda, M.D.: The National Institutes of Health, National Institute of Diabetes and Digestive disease; April 1997.

[52] Raine A. E. G. (1992): Management of renal failure in Europe XXII, 1991. Cardiovascular mortality in patients on renal replacement therapy. Nephrol Dial Transplant. 7 (Suppl. 2): 7–35.

[53] Kasiske B. L. (1993): Risk factors for cardiovascular disease after renal transplantation. Miner Elektrolyte Metab. 19: 186–195.

[54] Friedman E. A. (2002): Diabetic Nephropathy: Improving Prognosis. Saudi J Kidney Dis Transplant. 13(3): 281–310.

[55] Locatelli F, Canaud B, Eckardt KU, Stenvinkel P, Wanner C, Zoccali C. (2003) The importance of diabetic nephropathy in current nephrological practice Nephrol Dial Transplant;18 9:1716-25.

[56] Gaede P, Vedel P, Larsen N, Jensen GV, Parving HH, Pedersen O. (2003) Multifactorial intervention and cardiovascular disease in patients with type 2 diabetes The New England journal of medicine;348 5:383-93.

[57] Gaede P, Vedel P, Parving HH, Pedersen O. (1999) Intensified multifactorial intervention in patients with type 2 diabetes mellitus and microalbuminuria: the Steno type 2 randomised study Lancet;353 9153:617-22.

[58] Hansson L, Zanchetti A, Carruthers SG, Dahlof B, et al. (1998) Effects of intensive blood-pressure lowering and low-dose aspirin in patients with hypertension: principal results of the Hypertension Optimal Treatment (HOT) randomised trial. HOT Study Group Lancet;351 9118:1755-62.

[59] Hayashino Y, Fukuhara S, Akiba T, Akizawa T, et al. (2007) Diabetes, glycaemic control and mortality risk in patients on haemodialysis: the Japan Dialysis Outcomes and Practice Pattern Study Diabetologia;50 6:1170-7.

[60] Nissen SE, Tuzcu EM, Schoenhagen P, Brown BG, et al. (2004) Effect of intensive compared with moderate lipid-lowering therapy on progression of coronary atherosclerosis: a randomized controlled trial Jama;291 9:1071-80.

[61] European Best Practice Guidelines for Haemodialysis. Available at http://ndt.oxfordjournals.org/content vol17_7 index.dtl.

[62] NKF-K/DOQI. (2006) Clinical practice guidelines for hemodialysis adequacy. Am J Kidney Dis;48:S2-S90.

[63] Panichi V, Migliori M, De Pietro S, Taccola D, et al. (2000) The link of biocompatibility to cytokine production Kidney Int Suppl;76:S96-103.

[64] Verzetti G, Navino C, Bolzani R, Galli G, Panzetta G. (1998) Acetate-free biofiltration versus bicarbonate haemodialysis in the treatment of patients with diabetic nephropathy: a cross-over multicentric study Nephrol Dial Transplant;13 4:955-61.

[65] Polenakovic MH. (2002) Dialysis in adults in year 2000 in the Republic of Macedonia The International journal of artificial organs;25 5:386-90.

[66] Polenakovic MH, Stojceva-Taneva O, Grcevska L. (2000) Diabetic nephropathy - a challenge for the new millennium. Mac J of Med;45:5-13.

[67] Polenakovic M., Dimitrovski Ch. (2010): How to prevent and manage diabetic kidney disease in the Republic of Macedonia. Prilozi, XXXI (1) 2010, 235-239

[68] Polenakovic M, Sikole A, Grozdanovski R, Amitov V, et al. (2003) Лекување на возрасни пациенти со дијабетес мелитус и терминална бубрежна инсуфициенција со дијализа во 2000 година во Р.Македонија Македонски Медицински Преглед:137-41.

[69] Van Dijk PC, Jager KJ, Stengel B, Gronhagen-Riska C, Feest TG, Briggs JD. (2005) Renal replacement therapy for diabetic end-stage renal disease: data from 10 registries in Europe (1991-2000) Kidney international;67 4:1489-99.

[70] Sorensen VR, Mathiesen ER, Heaf J, Feldt-Rasmussen B. (2007) Improved survival rate in patients with diabetes and end-stage renal disease in Denmark Diabetologia;50 5:922-9.

[71] Sorensen VR, Mathiesen ER, Watt T, Bjorner JB, Andersen MV, Feldt-Rasmussen B. (2007) Diabetic patients treated with dialysis: complications and quality of life Diabetologia;50 11:2254-62.

[72] Polenakovik M, Sikole A, Stojcev N, Spasovski G, et al. (1999) Survival of patients on chronic hemodialysis: single center experience Artificial organs;23 1:61-4.

[73] Sikole A, Nikolov V, Dzekova P, Stojcev N, et al. (2007) Survival of patients on maintenance haemodialysis over a twenty-year period Prilozi / Makedonska akademija na naukite i umetnostite, Oddelenie za bioloski i medicinski nauki = Contributions / Macedonian Academy of Sciences and Arts, Section of Biological and Medical Sciences;28 2:99-110.

[74] Schrier RW. (2000) Treating high-risk diabetic hypertensive patients with comorbid conditions Am J Kidney Dis;36 3 Suppl 1:S10-7.

[75] Stack AG, Bloembergen WE. (2001) Prevalence and clinical correlates of coronary artery disease among new dialysis patients in the United States: a cross-sectional study J Am Soc Nephrol;12 7:1516-23.

[76] Panzetta G, Basile C, Santoro A, Ancarani E, et al. (2008) Diabetics on dialysis in Italy: a nationwide epidemiological study Nephrol Dial Transplant;23 12:3988-95.

[77] Atkins R.C., Zimmet P. (2010): Diabetic kidney disease: act now or pay later. J Nephrol; 23(01): 1–4.

[78] Polenakovic M., Sikole A. (2008): Chronic Kidney Disease: a hidden epidemic: Prilozi; 29(1): 5–9.

[79] Kosevska E., Kasapinov B., Pollozhani A. et al. (2009): Public health aspects of renal diseases in the Republic of Macedonia 1983–2007; Prilozi; 30(2): 139–157.

[80] Holman RR., Paul SK., Bethel MA. et al. (2008): 10-year follow-up of intensive glucose control in type 2 diabetes. N Engl J Med.; 359: 1577–1589.

[81] Bilous R. (2008): Microvascular disease: what does the UKPDS tell us about diabetic nephropathy? Diabet Med.; 25(Suppl2): 25–29.

[82] Gaede P., Lund-Andersen H., Parving HH., Pedersen O. (2008): Effect of a multifactorial intervention on mortality in type 2 diabetes. N Engl J Med.; 358: 580–591.

[83] Patel A; ADVANCE Collaborative Group, MacMahon S. et al. (2007): Effects of a fixed combination of perindopril and indapamide on macrovascular and microvascular outcomes in patients with type 2 diabetes mellitus (the ADVANCE trial): a randomized controlled trial. Lancet.; 370: 829–840.

[84] ADVANCE Collaborative Group, Patel A., MacMahon S. et al. (2008): Intensive blood glucose control and vascular outcomes in patients with type 2 diabetes. N Engl J Med.; 358: 2560–2572.

[85] Zoungas S., de Galan BE., Ninomiya T. et al.; on behalf of the ADVANCE Collaborative Group (2009): Combined effects of routine blood pressure lowering and intensive glucose control on macrovascular and microvascular outcomes in patients with type 2 diabetes; new results from the ADVANCE trial. Diabetes Care; 32: 2068–2074.

[86] Ruggenenti P., Fassi A., Ilieva AP. et al. (2004): Preventing microalbuminuria in type 2 diabetes. N Engl J Med. 351: 1941–1951.
[87] Parving HH., Lehnert H., Bröchner-Mortensen J. et al. (2001): The effect of irbesartan on the development of diabetic nephropathy in patients with type 2 diabetes. N Engl J Med.; 345: 870–878.